Allergic Contact Dermatitis

Acknowledgement

This independent review was commissioned and sponsored by the European Cosmetic, Toiletry and Perfumery Association (COLIPA) as the major part of a three-year research project undertaken by the authors within the Section of Molecular Toxicology, Division of Biomedical Sciences, Imperial College School of Medicine, London, UK. The authors would like to thank members of the COLIPA Skin Sensitisation and Skin Tolerance Task Forces for their support and advice during the preparation of the manuscript.

Allergic Contact Dermatitis

Chemical and Metabolic Mechanisms

Camilla K. Smith (D.Phil)*
and
Sharon A.M. Hotchkiss (PhD)
Section of Molecular Toxicology
Imperial College
School of Medicine
Sir Alexander Fleming Building
South Kensington
London, UK

Commissioned by the European Cosmetic Toiletry and Perfumery Association (COLIPA)

*Present address:
SEAC Toxicology
Unilever Research Colworth
Colworth House
Sharnbrook
Bedford, UK

TAYLOR & FRANCIS
ALERE FLAMMAM
Founded 1798

London and New York

First published 2001 by Taylor & Francis
11 New Fetter Lane, London EC4P 4EE

Simultaneously published in the USA and Canada
by Taylor & Francis Inc,
29 West 35th Street, New York, NY 10001

Taylor & Francis is an imprint of the Taylor & Francis Group

Typeset in Stone Serif by Wearset, Boldon, Tyne and Wear
Printed and bound in Great Britain by TJ International Ltd,
Padstow, Cornwall

British Library Cataloguing in Publication Data
A catalogue record for this book is available from the British Library

Library of Congress Cataloging in Publication Data
Smith, Camilla K., 1971–
Allergic contact dermatitis : chemical and metabolic mechanisms / Camilla K. Smith, Sharon A.M. Hotchkiss.
p. ; cm.
Includes bibliographical references and index.
1. Contact dermatitis. I. Hotchkiss, Sharon A.M. II. Title.
[DNLM: 1. Dermatitis, Allergic Contact–etiology. 2. Allergens–adverse effects. 3. Skin–drug effects. 4. Skin Absorption–physiology. 5. Xenobiotics–metabolism. WR 175 S644a 2001]

RL244 .S65 2001
616.97'3–dc21 00-064911

ISBN 0-415-25047-1

Contents

Figures

Colour section between pp. 110–111

Schemes

Tables

Acknowledgements

We would like to thank the following people for their contributions to the manuscript. In particular, we acknowledge the significant contribution of Dr David Roberts (Unilever, Port Sunlight, Wirral, UK) in discussions relating to the hypotheses presented in Chapter 5. Also, we thank Dr David Basketter (Unilever, Bedford, UK) for providing us with information for many of the compounds discussed in Chapter 5. For the production of original figures, we thank the Audio Visual Archives Department at St Mary's Hospital, Imperial College School of Medicine (Figure 1.1), Dr Connie Cheung (Imperial College School of Medicine, London, UK) (Figures 4.1 and 4.2), Dr Thomas Hurley, Indiana University Purdue University Indianapolis (IUPUI, USA) (Figures 3.2 and 3.3), Prof. Bi-Cheng Wang (University of Georgia, USA) (Figure 3.4) and Dr Johan Wouters (Facultes Universitaires Notre-Dame de la Paix, Namur, Belgium) (Figure 3.5). Also, many thanks for the support and comments from members of the COLIPA skin sensitisation task force, all of whom have been involved during preparation of the manuscript.

The authors would like to pay special tribute to Gilles Dupuis and Claude Benezra, who pioneered this field of research.

Acknowledgements

Preface

Allergic contact dermatitis (ACD) is a skin condition that has been estimated to affect a significant proportion (1–4%) of the general world-wide population. ACD may arise following skin contact with a variety of exogenous small molecule (xenobiotic) sensitisers. Such xenobiotics may be commonly encountered in the workplace, in the natural environment and at home, and as a result the risk of skin exposure to xenobiotics continues to present a serious problem to both industry and the consumer. However, it is only in recent decades that the classes of sensitising chemicals and the molecular mechanisms in skin, which can contribute to the generation of ACD, have begun to be appreciated (Chapter 1). In light of the recent move by industry, towards increasing the use of *in vitro* alternative methods, for identifying and classifying potential sensitisation hazards, it is vital to establish a thorough understanding of the molecular principles underlying ACD. This book aims to provide an overview of recent research in the field of ACD. In addition, we aim to highlight some of the major questions that remain unanswered with respect to the biochemical mechanisms of ACD, provide some mechanistic hypotheses, and lend some appreciation to the overall immunological context within which these mechanisms may apply.

Since the pioneering work of Landsteiner and Jacobs in the 1930s, the idea that a 'carrier protein' is required to elicit an immune response, has been propagated, i.e. the small molecule xenobiotic covalently conjugates to skin protein (thus acting as a hapten) to form a macromolecular immunogen. This 'hapten hypothesis' was extensively discussed in the review by Dupuis and Benezra (1982) and will be expanded upon to provide a new working hypothesis for ACD. It is hypothesised that in the early stages, within the first 24 hours after skin exposure to a chemical, cutaneous metabolism may play a role in detoxifying potentially toxic chemicals that are absorbed. Of particular concern, however, is that cutaneous metabolism may also activate seemingly innocuous chemicals (prohaptens) into protein-reactive haptens.

A small molecule cannot act as a hapten, however, until it has been absorbed into the skin and a discussion of the factors affecting percutaneous absorption of xenobiotics is presented in Chapter 2. As metabolism is hypothesised to play a role in ACD, a general discussion of xenobiotic metabolism performed by liver enzymes (presented in Chapter 3) provides the basis from which many skin metabolic pathways may be supposed. Many enzymes analogous to those found in the liver have been detected in skin (either at the protein or mRNA level), and a review of these enzymes is presented in Chapter 4. In Chapter 5, we postulate mechanisms for the protein-binding capacity and metabolism of ~200 chemicals that exhibit varying levels of contact sensitisation *in vivo*. In Chapter 6, we focus on how the protein/peptide binding of haptens may result in specific antigen formation and subsequent recognition by the major histocompatibility molecules (MHCs) and T cells of the immune system. Finally, in Chapter 7, we extend the original hapten hypothesis to include the likely roles of MHCs and peptide-hapten recognition in the generation of ACD. This book reveals many gaps in our current knowledge of ACD and will hopefully stimulate further research in this area.

CHAPTER

1

Allergic Contact Dermatitis to Small Molecule Xenobiotics

'Allergic and irritant dermatitis (contact dermatitis) is overwhelmingly the most important cause of occupational skin diseases, which account for 15% to 20% of all reported occupational diseases. There is virtually no occupation or industry without potential exposure to the many diverse agents that cause allergic and irritant dermatitis. Research is needed to better identify the prevalence, causes, exposure assessment methods, and early biologic markers of this ubiquitous condition.'

(Statement from the National Occupational Research Agenda, NIOSH, USA)

Contents

Human skin abnormalities can result following a variety of chemical or physical insults to the tissue. One area of particular concern, to both individuals and industry, is the occurrence of skin allergies following skin contact with small chemicals (xenobiotics typically of molecular weight <600 g/mol). Such exposure to xenobiotics may occur either in the workplace, in the natural environment or at home. The concern arises from the present difficulties in predicting which chemicals will cause skin allergies upon exposure (from chemical knowledge alone) and also that some individuals appear to be more susceptible to suffering from contact allergies (to specific chemicals) than others. The causes and mechanisms of contact allergy have only begun to be understood within the last few decades. It is apparent that the physico-chemical properties of the molecule, as well as genetic and metabolic factors in an individual, may all play roles in the manifestation of skin allergies to xenobiotics, and that the allergic response is induced and elicited by complex T-cell mediated immune mechanisms. Recent research and hypotheses relating to all of these mechanistic factors will be discussed in subsequent chapters. This introductory chapter provides a definition of xenobiotic-derived allergic contact dermatitis, and the basic immune mechanisms, clinical diagnosis, treatment and epidemiology of the condition are discussed.

1.1 DEFINITION OF ALLERGIC CONTACT DERMATITIS

Allergic contact dermatitis (ACD) is the clinical definition of an eczematous skin reaction that results from (specifically) delayed type IV hypersensitivity (DTH) (as defined by Coombs and Gell (1975)), which occurs at the site of secondary skin contact with a small molecule allergen.[1] Some examples of the clinical appearance of ACD (in particular to para-phenylenediamine in hair dye, sesquiterpene lactones in chrysanthemums and epoxy resins in a synthetic watch strap), are shown in Figure 1.1 (see colour plate section). The elicited skin reaction (i.e. the generation of erythema and oedema in the epidermis) is maximal typically at 48–72 hours subsequent to allergen challenge, and only occurs in individuals that have become sensitised previously with the same (or cross-reactive) allergen (see section 1.2 below).

In contrast to other forms of hypersensitivity, DTH cannot be transferred from one animal to another via serum but it can be transferred via T-helper (T_H1) cells. Therefore, this condition is believed to occur as a result of undesired hyper-responsiveness to an exogenous agent by the T-cell mediated immune system (see section 1.2).

1.2 SENSITISATION AND ELICITATION PHASES OF ACD

There are two phases that contribute to the manifestation of ACD, namely sensitisation and elicitation.

1.2.1 Sensitisation

In humans, sensitisation to a chemical takes between 10–14 days to occur, after skin exposure to a sensitising dose. The mechanisms thought to be involved during the sensitisation phase of ACD are illustrated schematically in Figure 1.2.

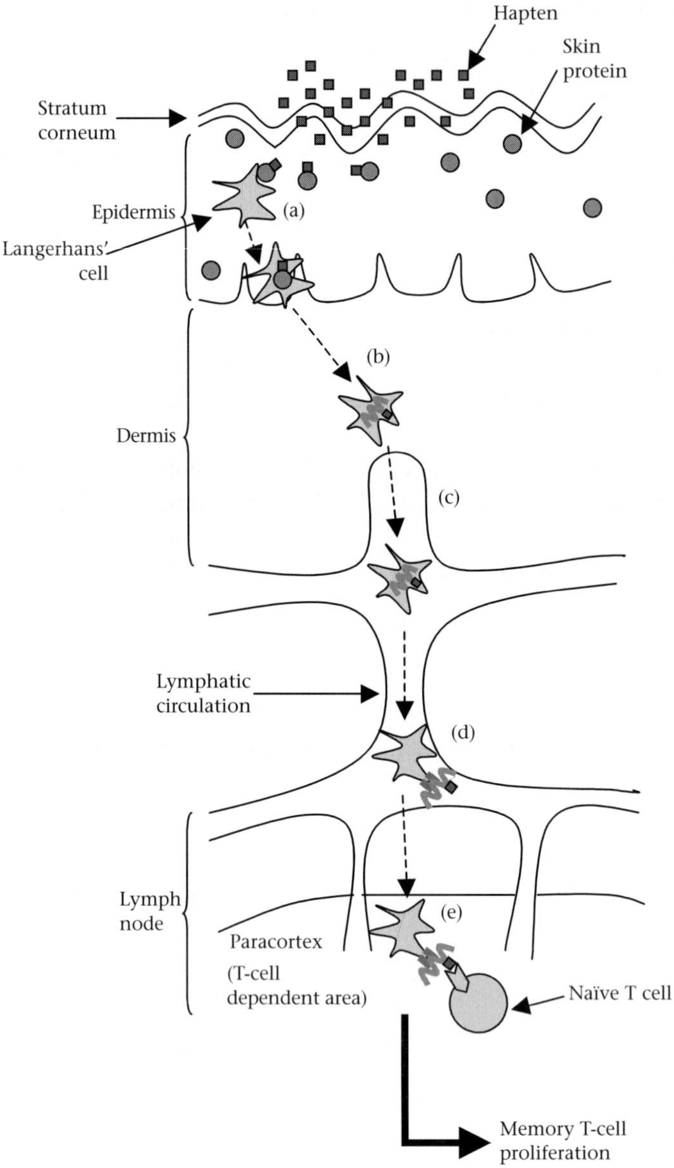

Figure 1.2: Mechanisms of sensitisation in delayed-type IV hypersensitivity. This schematic represents the current theory of the processes involved during the sensitisation phase of ACD. A hapten (square) must first penetrate the stratum corneum and be absorbed into the epidermis, where it can bind to skin protein, thus forming an immunogen. These modified-proteins may then be recognised and internalised by a Langerhans' cell (LC) (a). The LC then migrates from the epidermis into the dermis (b) and finally to the draining lymph node (c), whilst maturing into a dendritic cell. The LC processes the immunogen into peptides (c) that 'carry' the hapten, which is bound covalently, and display them on their surface (d). The peptide-hapten complexes are then recognised by the TCR of a naïve $CD4^+$ T cell residing in the paracortex of the lymph node (e). This recognition, then stimulates the generation and proliferation of a population of memory T cells.

1.2.1.1 Concepts of carrier-protein/peptide and the hapten hypothesis

A small molecule xenobiotic does not occupy a sufficient molecular volume to stimulate an immune response by cellular/antibody recognition mechanisms. Hence, it has long been hypothesised that once a small molecule allergen has penetrated the outer barrier of the skin (stratum corneum) and been absorbed into the epidermis (Figure 1.2), it binds covalently to skin protein/peptide (see Chapters 5 and 6) to form a macromolecular immunogen. The self-protein/peptide acts effectively as a 'carrier-protein' for the small molecule, which acts as the antigenic 'hapten'.[2] This is the classical 'hapten hypothesis' that was originally proposed by Landsteiner and Jacobs (1936) and subsequently revisited by Dupuis and Benezra (1982), and has become widely accepted in the field of ACD (Figure 1.3). The exact nature of hapten-carrier complex formation is unproved. However, the carrier is believed to be an epidermal protein/peptide (see Chapter 6).

It was originally thought that the macromolecular (haptenated) immunogen would react with antibodies (secreted by B cells) but it is now considered that ACD is a purely T-cell mediated disease. It is also known that some molecules that do not have the capacity to bind to protein can act as skin sensitisers. It was hypothesised by Dupuis and

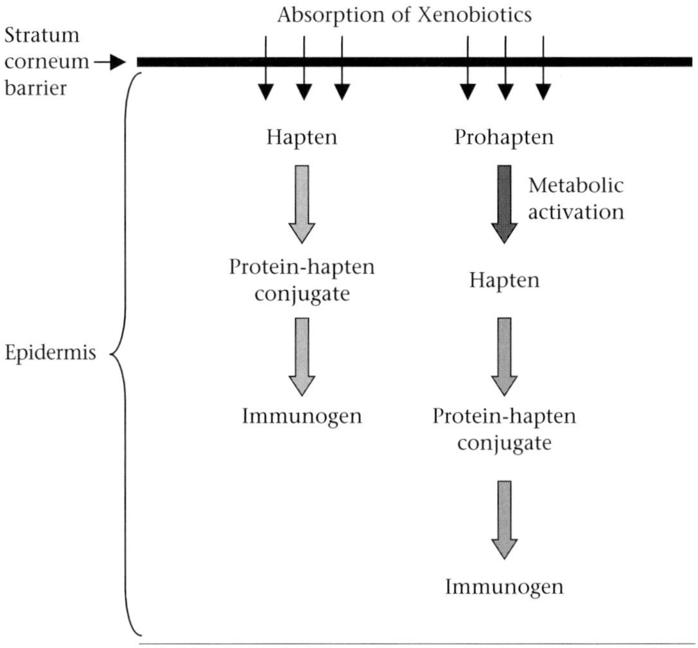

Figure 1.3: The original prohapten/hapten hypothesis. Proposed by Dupuis and Benezra (1982). Once a sensitising xenobiotic has been absorbed into the skin it can act as a hapten by binding covalently to skin protein to form an immunogen. Alternatively, the xenobiotic can be a prohapten that requires metabolic activation by cutaneous enzymes to become a hapten.

Benezra (1982) that such molecules (called 'prohaptens') are actively metabolised to protein-reactive haptens by cutaneous enzymes (Figure 1.3; see Chapters 4 and 5). The existence of cutaneous xenobiotic-metabolising enzymes has only been shown within the last 10–15 years (see Chapter 4). Also, recent evidence suggests that small molecule allergens may non-covalently associate with molecules of the immune system (Zanni *et al.*, 1998). Hence, the basic hapten hypothesis now requires some modification and expansion (see Chapter 7) to account for recent findings in the field of ACD, which will be discussed throughout this review.

1.2.1.2 The roles of Langerhans' cells

The skin possesses a unique type of antigen-presenting cell (APC) called the Langerhans' cell (LC). LCs are immature dendritic cells that are derived from the bone-marrow and are present in the epidermis (Figure 1.2), constituting a population of ~3% of all epidermal cells. LCs possess a range of cell surface markers, including the CD1 molecule and major histocompatibility complex II antigen (MHC class II; in humans, human leukocyte antigen DR (HLA-DR)). It is hypothesised that LCs recognise the hapten-carrier complex and internalise it, though the mechanisms by which LCs perform this recognition and process the complex into a specific hapten-peptide antigen are unknown. Internalisation and antigen recognition signals the LC to mature into a dendritic cell (DC), whilst migrating from the epidermis via the dermis into the efferent lymphatic system. LC migration has been shown to be crucial to the generation of sensitisation and dependent upon the expression of the cytokines, tumour necrosis factor-α (TNF-α) and interleukin 1β (IL-1β), and other cytokines/chemokines (Enk and Katz, 1992; Kimber *et al.*, 1998a; Kimber *et al.*, 2000). Upon arrival of the mature LC-derived DC in the paracortical (T-cell dependent) areas of the regional lymph node, the antigen (hapten-peptide complex) is presented by MHC class II to a $CD4^+$ naïve T cell (lymphocyte) (Figure 1.2).

1.2.1.3 Proliferation of antigen-specific memory T cells

On presentation of the antigen to $CD4^+$ naïve T cells in the lymph node, a population of antigen-specific memory T cells proliferates. This T-cell proliferation is the result of the sensitisation phase and the individual becomes primed with a population of circulating T cells that can recognise specifically the same (or cross-reactive) hapten upon subsequent challenge.

1.2.2 Elicitation

The elicitation phase of ACD (Figure 1.4) occurs locally in the skin, upon subsequent exposure to a hapten in an individual that has been sensitised previously with that hapten. The hapten binds to a carrier protein (as yet unidentified), as described previously for sensitisation. However, during elicitation, antigen presentation performed by APCs (LC/macrophages) to memory T cells occurs both in the skin (memory T cells migrate from the blood circulation into the dermis) and in the lymph nodes (Figure 1.4).

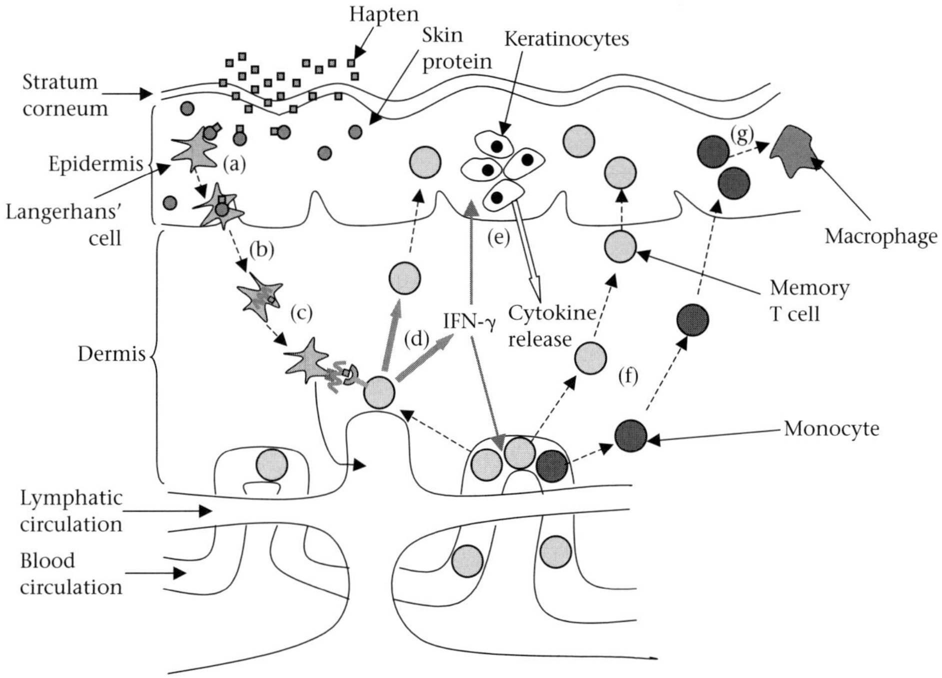

Figure 1.4: Mechanisms of elicitation in delayed-type IV hypersensitivity. This schematic represents the current theory of the processes involved during the elicitation phase of ACD. During elicitation, which occurs on subsequent exposure to the same compound, the hapten is absorbed and binds to protein (as described for sensitisation) (a). The immunogen is recognised and internalised by an LC or an antigen-presenting cell (APC) and processed into peptides (b). This peptide is then recognised by a memory T cell that is present in the dermis (c). The recognition of the antigen stimulates the migration of the T cell into the epidermis and also stimulates the release of cytokines and chemokines (d). The action of interferon-γ release from the activated T cell stimulates keratinocytes to secrete cytokines (e), which in turn stimulates monocyte, macrophage and T cell (both $CD4^+$ and $CD8^+$) infiltration into the epidermis (f and g).

Antigen recognition by memory T cells in the skin signals the release of the cytokine interferon-γ (IFN-γ) from the activated T cell. This cytokine has multiple stimulatory influences, including inducing the expression of cellular adhesion molecules (such as ICAM-1), MHC class II molecules and proinflammatory cytokines such as interleukin (IL)-1β, IL-6 and granulocyte macrophage colony stimulating factor (GM-CSF) from epidermal keratinocytes. The local release of these proinflammatory cytokines signals the recruitment of monocytes and lymphocytes (predominantly non-antigen specific T lymphocytes) from the blood and lymphatic circulations via the dermis and into the epidermis at the site of contact (Figure 1.4). The infiltration of cells into the epidermis, which causes the clinical symptoms of erythema and oedema, is maximal between 48–72 hours. Macrophages are also present in the skin and become recruited and activated locally. After 72 hours, down-regulation of the immune response starts to occur, which may be effected by eicosenoids (such as prostaglandins that are produced by keratinocytes and macrophages, and inhibit IL-1 and IL-2 production) or inhibitory cytokines, such as TGF-β or IL-10. Alternatively, T cells may bind to keratinocytes, thus initiating the enzymatic and cellular degradation of the hapten-carrier complex.

Although the T cells that infiltrate the epidermis are predominantly antigen-independent cells (i.e. they are not T cells that specifically recognise antigen), elicitation is a very specific end response to a particular compound. Recent studies have suggested that both $CD4^+$ (MHC class II-restricted) and $CD8^+$ (MHC class I-restricted) memory T cells are important in the development of the elicitation phase of ACD (Abe *et al.*, 1996; Kalish and Askenase, 1999). If this is the case, then the APC could either be a Langerhans' cell, keratinocyte or macrophage and may possibly involve hapten-peptide antigen-recognition by both MHC class I and MHC class II molecules (see Chapter 6). However, the exact mechanisms of antigen specificity in both sensitisation and elicitation remain unknown.

1.2.3 The roles of keratinocytes in the immune system

The major epidermal cell type, which forms the structural integrity of the epidermis, is the keratinocyte. As well as possessing metabolic capacities, keratinocytes also have the potential to play a role in the immune responses within the skin, as they possess MHC class II molecules and intercellular adhesion molecules (such as ICAM-1) on their surface. They also release cytokines including interleukin (IL)-1β, IL-3, IL-6, IL-8, IL-12, GM-CSF, macrophage colony stimulating factor (M-CSF), tumour necrosis factor (TNF)-α, tumour growth factor (TGF)-α, TGF-β, macrophage inflammatory protein (MIP)-2, interferon-induced protein (IP)-10 (Kimber *et al.*, 1995) and the recently identified chemokine CTACK (also named CCL27, ESkine) (Morales *et al.*, 1999; Homey *et al.*, 2000). The complex mechanisms of action of such cytokines on the immune response, as a result of contact allergen stimulation, are beginning to be elucidated. However, extensive discussion on the action of cytokines and chemokines in ACD is outside the scope of this review.

1.3 ACD VS IRRITANT CONTACT DERMATITIS (ICD)

The generation of ACD may be dependent upon the exposure frequency and concentration of specific types of chemical that are absorbed by the skin. It is often the case that allergenic chemicals only sensitise the immune system between minimum and maximum threshold doses. Above the maximum dose (a specific dose of hapten per unit area of skin for each chemical), the chemical can act as an irritant. Repeated exposure to very low concentrations of hapten (per unit area) of chemical can lead to ACD in an individual following long-term exposure without ICD (i.e. immediate reddening and inflammation at the site of contact) occurring. However, most allergens can act as irritants at a high enough dose.

In contrast, the majority of exogenous chemicals encountered can, at a specific and often relatively high concentration, cause irritant contact dermatitis (ICD). However, not all chemical irritants can act as allergens i.e. induce systemic sensitisation of the immune system and locally elicit delayed reactions.

It has been postulated that differential cytokine expression may discriminate between irritant and allergic reactions (Muller *et al.*, 1996). Although, the mechanisms of irritancy appear to be distinct from those of hypersensitivity reactions in the initial stages of xenobiotic contact, there are some similarities between ACD and ICD in the events that occur in the skin later, following exposure to both irritants and allergens. For example, the skin becomes infiltrated with monocytes, lymphocytes and macrophages following exposure to an irritant, in a similar way to that seen in the elicitation stage of ACD following secondary contact with allergen (Figure 1.4). Hence, there is the potential for some overlap to occur between allergenic and irritant mechanisms in the skin upon contact with a chemical.

1.4 DIAGNOSIS AND TREATMENT OF ACD

At first sight the eczematous conditions of ACD and ICD (often occurring on the hands or face) appear to be rather similar (both clinically and histologically) on presentation to the clinician. For this reason, it is difficult to diagnose clinically whether an individual is suffering from ACD or ICD. It is often only by discussion of an individual's history of encounters with chemicals, that true cases of ACD can be discerned from ICD. However, occupationally and environmentally relevant series of chemicals have been developed, to which an individual can be patch tested, to aid in the diagnosis of whether the eczema/dermatitis is specifically a result of contact allergy to a chemical.

1.4.1 Patch testing

It is important to diagnose the specific chemical cause of ACD correctly, in order that the affected individual can avoid the allergen. On presentation of dermatitis derived from an unknown cause, the dermatologist will perform 'patch testing' using a battery of suspected common standard allergens. Patch test chemicals can be obtained commercially at standardised sensitising doses in pre-prepared syringes (and, most importantly, not at irritant concentrations). Different standard series of chemicals are used in different countries (e.g. the European Standard Patch Test Allergen series) and some series have been designed to particularly test individuals working in different occupations depending upon the chemicals they are likely to encounter (see Table 1.1). Up to 20 chemicals are applied to the back, either in defined volumes in aluminium cups or as thin layers of chemicals painted onto water-impermeable patches. The latter method, called the thin-layer rapid use epicutaneous test (TRUE-test) (Fischer and Maibach, 1985) has become the most popular choice in the US for ready-to-use patch testing due to the increased accuracy in reproducing the dose per unit area required (Prue *et al.*, 1998). Cups or patches are taped in place for 48 hours. Occlusion of the chemicals encourages the skin penetration of the allergen. The positions of the patches are marked and removed, then the skin is inspected both immediately and after 96 hours following application. The reactions are graded as either no reaction (o) doubtful reaction (±), weak (non-vesicular) reaction (+), strong (oedematous) reaction (++), extreme reaction (+++) of irritant (IR). It is important that the results are interpreted carefully in light of the patient's history to make an accurate diagnosis, as a positive reaction may not necessarily be relevant to the appearance of the presented dermatitis.

1.4.2 Treatment of ACD

Once the condition of ACD has been successfully diagnosed, avoidance of the offending chemical(s) can be an effective cure. However, in the short-term, the condition may require treatment and even when avoidance of known allergens is put into practice, on occasions a cross-reactive allergenic chemical may be encountered unwittingly, thus causing a recurrence of ACD.

Topical corticosteroids may be prescribed as anti-inflammatories. However, such corticosteroids themselves may act as sensitisers (see Figure 5.23) and topical corticosteroid preparations may contain other small molecule sensitisers in their formulations (e.g. propylene glycol, cetostearyl alcohol and hydroxybenzoates) (British National Formulary, 2000). Hence, care must be taken when using topical corticosteroids to treat ACD as the condition may worsen rather than improve, depending on the corticosteroid allergy susceptibility or cross-reactivity of the individual. Whilst the symptoms of ACD are present, avoidance of physical trauma to the skin, such as excessive exposure to sunlight, wind, or rapid temperature changes is recommended by dermatologists.

1.5 EPIDEMIOLOGY OF ACD

The epidemiology of ACD is poorly understood, for a number of possible reasons. The difficulties in diagnosing ACD from ICD, as outlined in sections 1.3 and 1.4, may contribute to an uncertainty in the number of cases of ACD. Also, ACD is an uncomfortable and debilitating condition but is not a life-threatening disease, and often improves with no treatment (upon avoidance of the allergen) over a period of days to weeks. Hence, individuals may not report their symptoms to general practitioners or dermatologists. There may also be a risk of response bias in population based surveys as they depend upon voluntary participation. Although the purpose of such surveys is to randomly sample the whole population, it is often seen that certain individuals (e.g. extremes of age, retired, unemployed individuals) may be more or less likely to respond to questionnaires than others (Gill *et al.*, 2000). Hence, the incidence and prevalence statistics for ACD that have been reported may be much lower than the true number of sufferers in the general population.

1.5.1 Incidence and prevalence statistics for ACD in the general population

It was estimated from studies performed in Sweden, Gothenburg and the Netherlands, that the prevalence of ACD in the general population is ~1% (Burr, 1993). Meding and

Swanbeck (1982) have provided estimates (derived from 16 584 individuals in Gothenburg) for the prevalence of ACD according to age and gender; for men the prevalence statistics were 0.25% (20–29 yrs), 0.35% (30–39 yrs), 0.49% (40–49 yrs), 0.38% (50–59 yrs) and 0.40% (60–69 yrs); and for women 2.3% (20–29 yrs), 1.6% (30–39 yrs), 1.7% (40–49 yrs), 1.5% (50–59 yrs) and 1.8% (60–69 yrs). This data indicates that ACD is typically 3–6 times more prevalent in women than in men.

Data for the incidence and prevalence of ACD in the general population is scarce. More commonly, statistics are reported for the frequency of sensitisation to particular chemicals, within groups of patients known to be suffering from ACD and attending dermatology clinics (see section 1.5.4 below).

1.5.2 Individuals at risk from chemical allergens in the home

Almost everyone comes into contact with potential allergens in the home environment. Consumer products such as perfumes, soaps, cosmetics, hair dyes, paints, polishes, rubber, dyes in clothing and shoes, spectacle frames, sun tan lotion, toothpaste, mouthwash, scented tissues and fabric softeners etc. can all contain low levels of potentially sensitising chemicals. The majority of people use such products with no problems at all as these products undergo rigorous toxicological testing procedures prior to approval for public use. However, some individuals, who may be unusually sensitive to a particular chemical or who use a product in extreme excess of the recommended usage may be at risk from developing ACD.

Naturally occurring allergens are also present in and around the home; for example poison ivy and other plants (such as chrysanthemums and tulips), barks, fruit (citrus peel), kitchen spices (e.g. cinnamon, vanilla, clove and cardamom) and burned incense oils (such as patchouli and myrrh). Natural flavours are found in soft drinks, liqueurs, cakes, pastries, chewing gum, sauces, soups and tobacco etc. and these ingredients may be the cause of allergic reactions on the hands and mouths of some individuals when they contact these products.

Some prescribed drugs, most notably antibiotics (such as neomycin, bacitracin, chloramphenicol, gentamycin, nitrofurazone), 'caine ester' anaesthetics (e.g. benzocaine and tetracaine), topical corticosteroids and the anti-alcoholism drug, antabuse (disulfiram) have been seen to cause ACD in some individuals. In addition to these organic substances, nickel and chromium in jewellery and studs on clothing are also common allergens (see Table 1.2).

1.5.3 Individuals at risk from chemical allergens at work

Occupational contact dermatitis presents a significant socio-economic problem, predominantly in the developed world. Over 13 million workers in the US are believed to be at risk from exposure to chemicals that can be absorbed by the skin (unpublished communication from the National Institute for Occupational Safety and Health, US).

Exposure to sensitising chemicals may result from direct skin contact with contaminated surfaces, deposition of aerosols, immersion or from splashes.

It has been estimated that of all occupationally related conditions, occupational skin disease accounts for ~40% (US Bureau of Labor Statistics 1973–1984; Mathias and Morrison, 1988; Lodi *et al.*, 2000). Of all occupational skin disease, contact dermatitis (both ACD and ICD) has been reported to constitute ~90% of cases (Occupational Disease Statistics Unit, San Francisco, 1982; Lushniak, 1995). Recently, contact dermatitis has been estimated to account for an estimated 10–15% of all occupational illnesses (unpublished communication from NIOSH, US). A report from Italy has stated that more than 50% of occupational disease workers' compensation has been due to occupational contact dermatitis (Moroni *et al.*, 1985). This figure is in agreement with compensation statistics from a study in South Carolina (48%) (Keil and Shmunes, 1983). The US Bureau of Labor Statistics estimated in 1988 that annual costs for occupational contact dermatitis cases (due to lost work days, medical care and disability payments) were in the range $222 million–$1 billion (Mathias and Morrison, 1988). Recently, the level of compensations due to occupational contact dermatitis has been estimated at >$1 billion (unpublished communication from NIOSH, US). This cost is high, even though compensation is only given when the employee can prove that their dermatitis has resulted from contact to an allergen in the workplace, according to strict criteria (Mathias, 1985). Hence, contact dermatitis is a significant economic problem to industry. ACD has been estimated to account for ~25% of all occupational contact dermatitis (Marks and DeLeo, 1997).[3] Some of the occupations that show high incidences of ACD to particular chemicals are presented in Table 1.1.

It can be seen from Table 1.1, that those occupations affected represent a diverse population of individuals who present allergies to many different types of chemical allergen. However, some chemicals are known to cause allergies more frequently than others.

1.5.4 Frequency of sensitisation to common allergens

Of those people who are diagnosed as suffering from ACD, the most frequent allergens, as determined from patch test positive reactions, are those listed in Table 1.2 (showing data from selected world-wide studies). In all studies, nickel is the most common allergen world-wide. However, nickel (and cobalt) may cause allergy by mechanisms other than the hapten hypothesis (Figure 1.3) for small organic molecules and hence will not be discussed in mechanistic detail in this review (see review on nickel contact allergy by Maibach and Menne, 1989).

The components of the most common organic allergen, fragrance mix, are listed in Table 1.3: of these chemicals cinnamic alcohol, cinnamaldehyde, eugenol, α-amyl cinnamaldehyde, hydroxycitronellal and isoeugenol are all sensitising (with different potencies) when tested individually *in vivo*. Studies relating to the potential metabolism and protein-binding capacity of these compounds are discussed in Chapter 5.

TABLE 1.1

Occupations where increased risk of exposure to contact allergens leads to increased incidences of occupationally-related ACD

Occupations	Potential allergens encountered
Aircraft and automobile assemblers	Epoxy resins, formaldehyde resins, rubber, dimethacrylate resins, chromates, nickel, cobalt
Artists	Pigments, dyes, colophony, epoxy resins, oxidised turpentine
Bakers and confectioners	Flavours and spices (e.g. cinnamon, citrus fruits, vanilla) essential oils, dyes, benzoyl peroxide, ammonium persulphate
Bookbinders	Glues, resins, leathers
Butchers	Nickel, sawdust
Carpenters	Pine dust, tar
Cashiers and bank tellers	Nickel, cobalt
Construction workers	Chromates, cobalt, cement, epoxy resins, rubber, woods, leathers
Chemical industry workers	Miscellaneous sensitising chemicals
Cleaners	Polishes, rubber gloves, fragranced cleaning materials
Coal miners	Rubber boots and masks
Cooks and caterers	Foods, e.g. onions, garlic, spices, flavours, sodium metabisulphate, lauryl and octyl gallate, formaldehyde
Dental workers	Local anaesthetics, mercury, methacrylates, eugenol, disinfectants, rubber, epoxy resins, acrylate resins, glutaraldehyde, formaldehyde resins
Electricians	Epoxy resins, colophony, rubber
Electronics workers	Nickel, chromium, cobalt, epoxy resins, acrylate resins, colophony
Embalmers	Formaldehyde, glutaraldehyde, rubber
Farm workers	Carbamates, fungicides, pesticides, poison ivy, rubber, oats, barley, plants, wood preservatives, cement, veterinary medicaments
Florists and gardeners	Sesquiterpine lactones, tuliposides, pesticides, rubber gloves
Foundry workers	Colophony, phenol-and-urea-formaldehyde resins
Hairdressers	Para-phenylenediamine (PPD) in hair dyes, Kathon CG, persulphates, nickel, fragrances, formaldehyde, resorcinol, pyrogallol, glycerol thioglycolate
Housekeepers and home-makers	Nickel, rubber, formaldehyde, glutaraldehyde, foods, spices, flavours, polishes, chromates, Kathon CG
Jewellers	Nickel, chromium, leather
Machinists	Nickel, formaldehyde, colophony, Kathon CG
Mechanics	Nickel, chromium, epoxy resins, rubber, colophony, PPD
Medical workers	Rubber, acrylate resins, formaldehyde, glutaraldehyde, anaesthetics, antibiotics, antiseptics, phenothiazines, hand creams
Office workers	Epoxy resins, rubber, nickel
Painters and decorators	Paints, dyes, oxidised turpentine, thinners, cobalt, chromates, polyester resins, formaldehyde, epoxy resins, adhesives, colophony
Photo processors	Metol, thiourea, formaldehyde, phenidone, para-aminophenol, rubber, colour developers, hydroquinone, chromates, sodium metabisulphate
Plastics industry workers	Hardeners, phenolic resins, polyurethanes, acrylics, plasticisers
Printers	Chomium, epoxy resins, acrylate resins, formaldehyde resins, PPD
Roofers	Tar, colophony
Rubber workers	Rubber, dyes, colophony
Shoemakers	Epoxy resins, leather, rubber, turpentine
Tannery workers	Leather, chromates, formaldehyde, tanning agents, fungicides, dyes
Textile workers	PPD, dyes, formaldehyde resins, chromates, nickel, rubber, epoxy resins
Veterinarians	Anaesthetics, rubber, medicaments
Welders	Colophony, chromium, nickel

TABLE 1.2

Selected studies (between 1989–1999) illustrating percentage frequencies of patch test positive reactions to standard chemicals, in patients with ACD

	GIRDCA	Zurich	China	NACDG	India	Leeds, UK
No. individuals	42839	5565	107	3120	200	100
Time period	(1989–1993)	(1990–1994)	(1990–1991)	(1994–1996)	(1997)	(1999)
Nickel	31.1	18.5	14	14.3	16.5	21
Fragrance mix	6.2	9.6	15	14.0	7.5	22
Balsam of Peru	4.4	6.9	3	10.4	1.5	–
Cobalt	8.3	6.8	4	8.0	8.0	8
Thiomersal	4.2	4.7	–	10.4	–	–
Potassium dichromate	8.7	4.4	2	2.0	20.5	6
Neomycin	2.0	4.0	0	11.6	5.0	–
Para-phenylenediamine	3.7	3.7	16	6.8	11.5	1
Kathon CG	3.0	3.2	–	3.0	1.0	–
Colophony	1.8	2.5	4	2.6	5.5	3
Wool alcohol	1.4	1.7	2	3.3	4.0	5
Epoxy resin	0.7	1.1	0	2.2	1.5	3
Quaternium 15	0.3	–	1	9.2	2.5	–
Formaldehyde	1.4	–	8	9.2	6.5	3
Ethylenediamine	3.3	–	1	2.9	–	3
Formaldehyde resin	1.8	–	2	2.7	1.0	–
Benzocaine	1.4	–	6	2.6	2.5	1
Cinnamaldehyde	–	–	–	2.4	–	–
Tixocortol pivolate	–	–	–	2.3	–	1
Black rubber mix	–	–	1	2.3	1.5	–
Mercapto mix	–	–	0	2.2	5.0	–
Glutaraldehyde	–	–	–	2.2	–	–
Mercaptobenzothiazole	0.9	–	–	2.1	–	–
Ethyl acrylate	–	–	–	1.8	–	–
Methyl methacrylate	–	–	–	1.2	–	–
Propylene glycol	–	–	–	1.1	–	–
Sesquiterpene lactone mix	–	–	–	0.9	14.0	–

Italian Group of Research on Contact Dermatitis (GIRDCA) (Sertoli *et al.*, 1999); Zurich (Bangha & Elsner, 1996); China (Bian & Weixin, 1991); North American Contact Dermatitis Group (NACDG) (Marks *et al.*, 1998); India (Sharma & Chakrabarti, 1998); Leeds, UK (Goulden & Wilkinson, 2000).

TABLE 1.3

Components of the European Standard Patch Test Allergen, Fragrance Mix, from the highest to lowest constituent chemical

Chemical	Properties	Usage
Cinnamic alcohol (see Figure 5.4d)	Natural: cinnamon hyacinths balsam of Peru	Perfumed cosmetics Deodorants Laundry products Paper Flavours Toothpaste
Cinnamaldehyde (see Figure 5.6c)	Natural: cinnamon	Bath oils Hair cosmetics Lipsticks Toothpaste Mouthwashes Soaps/detergents Flavours Vermouth/bitter Chewing gum Soft drinks
Eugenol (see Figure 5.4b)	Natural: cloves cinnamon leaf	Perfumes/colognes Tonics Surgical dressings Hair cosmetics/creams Dental impression material Inhalants Antiseptic Toothpaste
α-amyl cinnamaldehyde (see Figure 5.6c)	Synthetic: jasmine oil	Perfumes/fragrances Cosmetics Soaps Industrial products Toothpaste
Hydroxycitronellal (see Figure 5.5)	Synthetic: floral fragrance	Perfumes/fragrances Cosmetics Eye cream Aftershave
Geraniol (see Figure 5.3a)	Natural: rose, geranium, lavender, jasmine and other essential oils	Perfumes/fragrances Lip salve Cosmetics Skin care products
Isoeugenol (see Figure 5.4b)	Natural: clove ylang ylang oil nutmeg	Perfumes/fragrances Aftershave Eye cosmetics
Oak moss absolute	Natural: oak and tree moss	Perfumes/colognes Aftershave
Sorbitol sequioleate		Used as an emulsifier

There are slight variations in the ranking order of the chemicals between studies, i.e. from the most frequent to the least frequent allergen. Also, some substances are much more frequent allergens in some studies than in others. For example, para-phenylenediamine (PPD) is a much more frequent allergen in China (16%) (Bian and Weixin, 1991) and India (11.5%) (Sharma and Chakrabarti, 1998) than in Europe (3–5%) (Bangha and Elsner, 1996; Sertoli *et al.*, 1999; Goulden and Wilkinson, 2000) and the USA (6.8%) (Marks *et al.*, 1998) (Table 1.2). Also, potassium dichromate and sesquiterpene lactone mix (plant extracts) are much more frequent allergens in the study from India (20.5% and 14.0%, respectively) than in the other studies (2–6% (all studies) and 0.9% (NACDG only; Marks *et al.*, 1998), respectively) (Table 1.2). These differences may reflect societal differences (i.e. the increased use of natural dyes in these countries) or may be a result of the lower test populations (107 (China) and 200 (India) in comparison to >3000 in the NACDG, Zurich and GIRDCA studies).

In all of these studies, it was seen that ACD occurs in women more frequently than in men, possibly due to a higher exposure to cosmetics, perfumes and toiletries, jewellery, hair dyes and dyes in clothing/shoes etc. in women. Alternatively, factors pertaining to the skin in women may be different to those in men e.g. absorptivity of the skin, metabolic activity, immunogenicity etc., but such sex-related differences require much further research.

1.6 FACTORS CONTRIBUTING TO XENOBIOTIC-DERIVED ACD

As shown in the sections above, many individuals may be exposed to a wide variety of different chemical allergens both at home and in the workplace. However, not all individuals who come into contact with potential allergens suffer from ACD and those who do, often react specifically to only a few types of chemically related allergens. Also, some chemicals are more potent than others i.e. a lower dose per unit area is required to cause sensitisation as determined by *in vivo* assay. Factors that may contribute to the occurrence of ACD in an individual include both the physico-chemical properties of the chemical and factors pertaining to the individual. Such factors will be discussed throughout this monograph within three different areas:

- i Skin Absorption of Xenobiotics — the generation of ACD may depend upon the concentration, lipophilicity and solubility of the chemical, and also on the anatomical site of exposure (discussed in Chapter 2).
- ii Skin Metabolism of Xenobiotics — the generation of ACD may depend upon the metabolic capability of the skin at the site of exposure and whether the chemical is a suitable substrate for xenobiotic-metabolising enzymes upon skin absorption (discussed in Chapters 3, 4 and 5). Haptens may be detoxified by metabolism; prohaptens may be activated to haptenic metabolites.
- iii Protein-reactivity and Immunogen Formation of Xenobiotics — the generation of ACD may depend on the chemical reactivity of the hapten with particular

protein/peptide residues and the recognition of specific antigens by immune system components (discussed in Chapter 6).

The first of these areas to be discussed is the nature of skin absorption.

NOTES

1 It is important to stress that not all types of contact allergy are defined as ACD. Only those delayed type IV reactions to small molecules are clinically diagnosed as ACD. Other contact allergies to macromolecular allergens (e.g. proteins, and also the common allergen latex in rubber gloves), which involve the production of IgE antibodies as well as T-helper cells, are classified as type I contact allergy, and will not be discussed in this review.

2 The protein-binding reactivity of a chemical is therefore considered to be important in the generation of sensitisation, and such reactivities are discussed for a range of sensitising and non-sensitising chemicals in Chapter 5.

3 Health and safety guidelines recommend that the worker wears protective clothing to prevent skin contact with allergens, which is often the most effective measure to control and prevent ACD. Such guidelines however, may not always be adhered to by an individual or the level of protection may not always be adequate.

CHAPTER

2

Skin Absorption of Chemical Allergens

Contents

In order for a chemical to cause allergic contact dermatitis following topical exposure, it must first enter the skin, from the skin surface, and diffuse across the various structures of the tissue to the site of action, the epidermis. This process of skin uptake, whereby the chemical becomes bioavailable at the site of toxicity, is a fundamental first step for the generation of an allergic response. Once in the epidermis, the chemical is then able to bind to proteins, forming a complete antigen, and interact locally with epidermal Langerhans' cells to initiate a chain of events in the immunological cascade that ultimately results in allergic contact dermatitis.

2.1 SIGNIFICANCE OF SKIN ABSORPTION IN ALLERGIC CONTACT DERMATITIS

During the passage of a chemical allergen from outside the skin into the body, a process known as percutaneous absorption, its topical fate or 'life cycle' can be subject to modulation at almost every step (Figure 2.1). Immediately following skin exposure to a chemical allergen, prior to uptake into the tissue, there is the potential for surface loss via the processes of evaporation, sweating, washing, abrasion and bacterial degradation. The chemical may then be taken up into the skin, the extent of which depends upon a number of factors such as the physicochemical properties of the compound in question (its lipophilicity, aqueous solubility, size, volatility etc.), the dose and concentration applied, the vehicle of application, the surface area of application, the time of skin contact, occlusion of the skin surface, the extent of skin hydration, skin temperature and the degree of skin barrier compromisation by disease or physical damage. The precise site of application is also a factor determining the rate and extent of skin uptake, as is its age and structural differences such as its thickness and the number of hair follicles. Once in the skin, the chemical allergen may be sequestered in the lipid-rich stratum corneum, forming a reservoir, or may diffuse deeper into the epidermis where it may be subjected to metabolism by enzymes present in this region. It is here, within the living tissue of the epidermis, that skin sensitisation may be initiated. Subsequently, the parent compound and/or its metabolites may diffuse into the upper dermis and thence be absorbed into the systemic circulation via the dermal microvasculature, and into the lymphatic system via the draining lymph nodes, to be distributed to distant sites of the body.

Percutaneous absorption studies have shown that human skin may absorb some chemicals very poorly (e.g. hippuric acid $<1\%$) whilst others are extensively taken up (e.g. coumarin $>70\%$) (Beckley-Kartey *et al.*, 1997; Feldmann and Maibach, 1967). Similarly some chemicals show 1000-fold differences in their rates of absorption. In an analogous fashion, it can be assumed that such variations in absorption will exist for potential chemical allergens. Essentially all low molecular weight chemical allergens (<1000 g/mol) have the potential to be absorbed into the skin. Some chemicals will be absorbed more effectively than others and, naturally, this will have an impact on whether they will become sensitisers or not. Those that are not absorbed will be unable to initiate toxicity, whilst those that are absorbed will be bioavailable within the skin

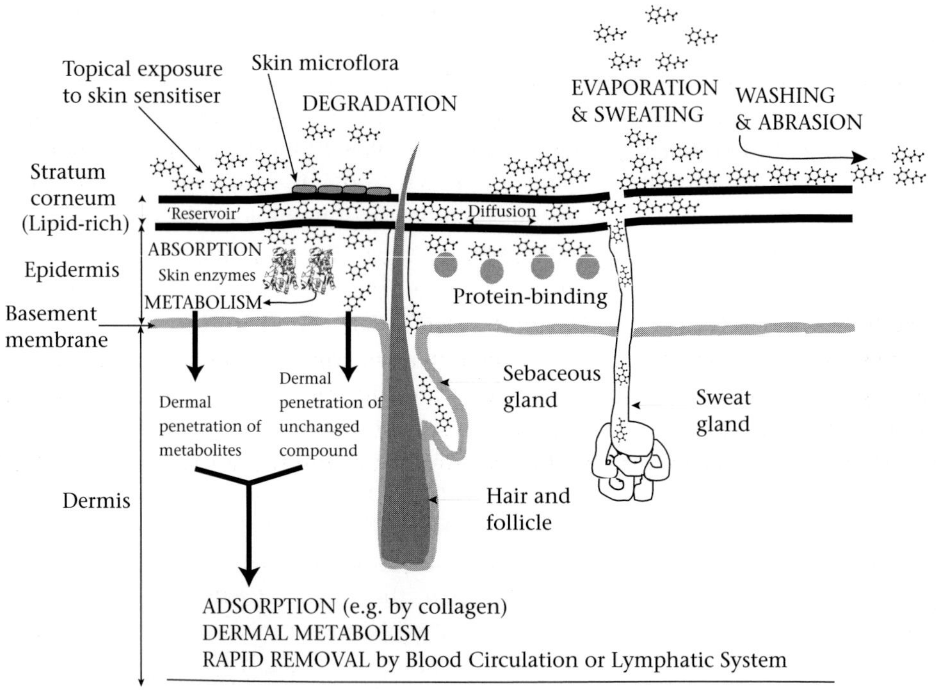

Figure 2.1: The life cycle of a xenobiotic following topical exposure. This schematic illustrates the possible fate of a xenobiotic once it has contacted the skin. It may be absorbed into the skin, degraded on the surface by skin microflora or removed from the surface. Xenobiotics may also travel down hair follicles and glands. Upon absorption, the xenobiotic may be metabolised, may bind to protein, or be excreted from the skin.

and may be in a position to induce an immune response. However, although skin absorption is essential for allergic contact dermatitis to develop, skin sensitisation potency does not necessarily correlate with the extent of percutaneous absorption: some well absorbed chemicals are only weak/intermediate sensitisers (e.g. eugenol, isoeugenol) whilst others are not sensitising at all (e.g. coumarin). This is because skin penetration is only one of a number of factors of importance in mediating sensitisation, including protein reactivity (Chapter 5), metabolic activation and clearance (Chapters 4 and 5), and immune competence (Chapter 6).

2.2 SKIN BARRIER FUNCTION AND THE STRATUM CORNEUM

Prior to a discussion of the role of percutaneous absorption in chemical induced cutaneous allergy, it is appropriate to describe, briefly, the structure of the skin, in order to establish how a chemical may penetrate the tissue, and the factors influencing this process, including where and how a chemical may be metabolised and the proteins that are likely to be available for covalent modification by the compound during its absorption.

The structure and function of the skin has been reviewed by many authors, including (Scheuplein and Blank, 1971; Barry, 1983; Holmann *et al.*, 1990; Payne, 1991; Rongone, 1987; Schaefer and Redelmeier, 1996; Roberts and Walters, 1998). The skin is the largest and heaviest single organ of the human body, accounting for approximately 10% of the total body weight. It has been estimated that the adult human male has a total skin surface area of 1.8–2.2 m^2, a thickness of about 3 mm, as well as receiving about 7% of the cardiac output, roughly 450 ml/min for an average 70 kg male (Emmett, 1991; Marzulli and Maibach, 1987; Patrick and Maibach, 1989).

The skin comprises two main layers: the outer epidermis and the inner dermis, separated by the basement membrane, with an underlying supportive hypodermis situated below the dermis (Figure 2.2). At the outermost region of the epidermis, in contact with the external environment, lies the stratum corneum or horny layer (about 20 μm thick

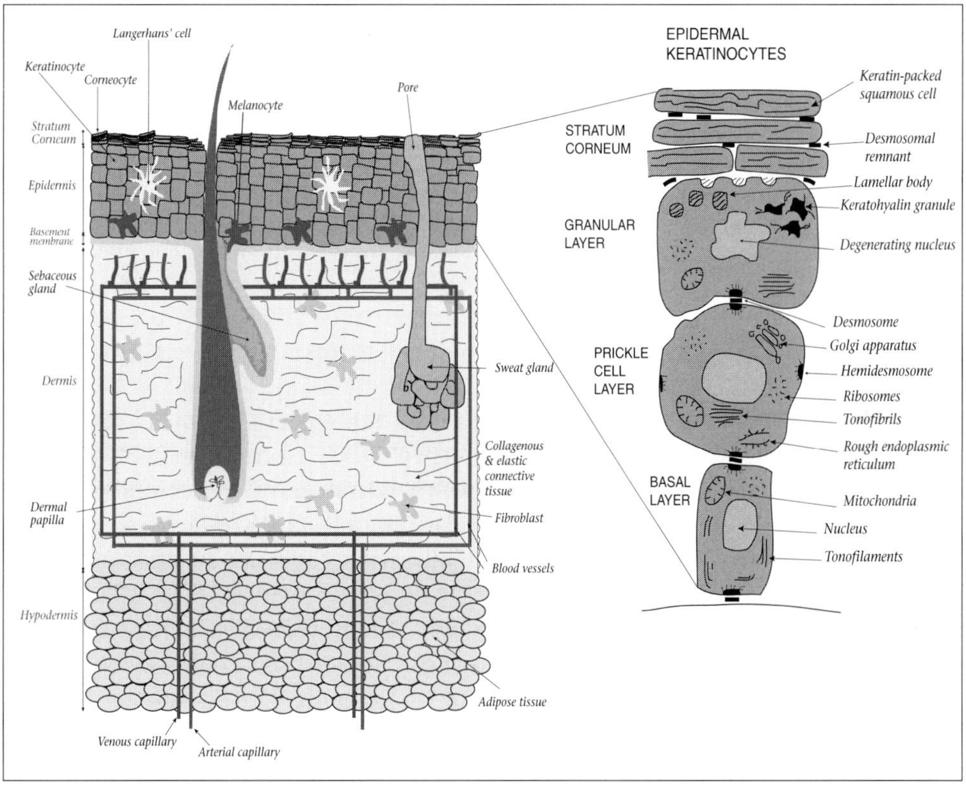

Figure 2.2: Structure of the skin. Schematic diagram showing the individual structural components of the skin as labelled. The epidermis has been expanded to illustrate the different types of keratinocytes (and their sub-structure) present in the basal layer through to the stratum corneum.

■ CHAPTER 2 ■

in humans but ranging from 10 μm (eyelids/scrotum) to 1 mm (palm and soles)), which is composed of densely packed, non-viable, flattened keratinocytes (corneocytes); and it is this structure that is considered to be the major barrier to percutaneous absorption of chemical allergens (Marzulli and Tregear, 1961; Scheuplein and Blank, 1971; Scheuplein and Bronaugh, 1983; Elias *et al.*, 1987; Potts and Francoeur, 1991; Potts *et al.*, 1992; Weigmann *et al.*, 1999). The corneocyte (approximately 1 μm thick) is packed with keratin, whilst the extracellular region contains various lipid lamellae structures (the so-called 'bricks and mortar'). Most biological membranes are comprised of phospholipid bilayers interspersed with proteins, of approximately 70Å (7 nm) thickness. The stratum corneum intercellular lipid lamellar membrane is unique, with its structure composed of three major fractions: ceramides, cholesterol and free fatty acids, in the lipid mass ratio 50:25:10. These lipids play an important role in epidermal barrier function (Elias, 1981; Wertz *et al.*, 1987). The high lipid content of the extracellular matrix and highly organised intracellular protein fibrils (keratin and keratohyalin) in the stratum corneum gives rise to an ideal environment for limiting the passage of exogenous compounds through the skin, as well as acting as a depot for topically applied compounds. The outermost layers of the stratum corneum are continuously shed at a rate of approximately one layer (1 g) of cells per day, in the process of desquamation or exfoliation, so that the stratum corneum is replaced every 14 days in the average adult (Barry, 1983).

Beneath the stratum corneum lies the viable epidermis which consists mainly of keratinocytes (95% cells) in various stages of development (Figure 2.2), together with antigen presenting Langerhans' cells (3–5% cells), melanocytes (which produce and distribute melanin for pigmentation and protection against u.v. irradiation), and Merkel cells (which may have a role in sensory function) (Lynch *et al.*, 1987). The epidermis is approximately 200 μm thick in humans, but varies with skin site from 60–800 μm, with skin on the eyelids being thinner than that on the palms and soles. The epidermis is avascular, and therefore relies on the diffusion of nutrients from the capillaries in the upper dermis for its viability. The epidermal keratinocytes arise as small (8–14 μm diameter) undifferentiated basal cells at the base of the epidermis which are actively involved in DNA synthesis and replication. They divide to form stem cells (which remain at the basal layer) and keratinocytes which migrate outwards, continuously differentiating, to form spinous cells, then granular cells and finally the cornified cells of the stratum corneum (Figure 2.2), a process that takes about 28–30 days in healthy human skin (Barry, 1983).

Below the epidermis, the dermal-epidermal junction provides mechanical support for epidermal growth and is a means of attachment of epidermal cells to the dermis, as well as acting as a semi-permeable filter excluding compounds with a molecular weight greater than 40 kDa. Deeper still, the dermis is a relatively thick structure (1 mm (scalp) to 4 mm (back)), and is comprised of a dense matrix of connective tissue (predominantly collagen (75%), with some elastin (4%) and reticulum (0.4%)), embedded in a matrix of polysaccharides (glycosaminoglycans e.g. chondroitin sulphate and heparin) and salt and water (20%), and various cells including fibroblasts (which synthesise fibrous proteins), macrophages, mast cells and lymphocytes (all involved in immune/inflammatory responses in the tissue), together with nerves, blood vessels and lymphatics (Singh and Singh, 1993; Wilkes *et al.*, 1973). The dermis also contains a variety of 'epidermal' appendages such as hair follicles, eccrine and apocrine sweat glands and sebaceous glands. An average human skin surface possesses between 10 and 70 hair follicles per cm^2, with these hair follicles occupying 0.1% of the total human skin surface (Katz and Poulsen, 1971). Underneath the dermis lies the hypodermis, which consists mainly of adipose tissue, with collagen linkage between the adipose cells. The arteries lying in the hypodermis give rise to the cutaneous plexus at the hypodermis-dermis junction and the papillary plexus in the upper dermis. The cutaneous circulation functions to supply nutrients and carry away waste products, and assists in thermoregulation.

Bearing in mind the structure of the skin (Figure 2.2), one can hypothesise the types of chemical allergen that may permeate its barrier. In essence, for a chemical to enter the lipid-rich stratum corneum it must be lipophilic in nature: hydrophilic substances are generally poorly absorbed. However some degree of aqueous solubility is also required since the chemical allergen must then be absorbed from the stratum corneum into the relatively aqueous regions of the epidermis, where allergic contact dermatitis may be initiated. The size of the molecule is also an important factor in skin uptake (although much less so than lipid solubility), with low molecular weight allergens best absorbed and increasing molecular size having an inverse affect on absorption.

2.3 PATHWAYS OF ALLERGEN ABSORPTION

In order for a chemical allergen to cause cutaneous toxicity — other than by directly damaging the stratum corneum — it must enter the tissue from the skin surface. Thus, for a chemical allergen encountering the skin surface to be absorbed into the skin, it must first negotiate the stratum corneum barrier, and three major pathways by which this may occur have been postulated (Figures 2.1 and 2.3) (Barry, 1983, 1987):

i transcellular route — the chemical passes alternately into the keratin-packed corneocytes and the lipid-rich extracellular region by partitioning into and out of the keratinocyte cell membranes;
ii intercellular route — the chemical passes around the corneocytes in the lipid rich extracellular lamellar regions;
iii appendageal route — the chemical by-passes the corneocytes and lipid lamellae by entering the shunts provided by the hair follicles, sweat glands and sebaceous glands. These routes of entry are also known as shunt pathways because they bypass the necessity to penetrate the stratum corneum.

It is generally accepted that all three routes are likely to play a role in percutaneous absorption, although consensus appears to favour the intercellular pathway as providing the most important molecular diffusion pathway for both lipophilic and hydrophilic

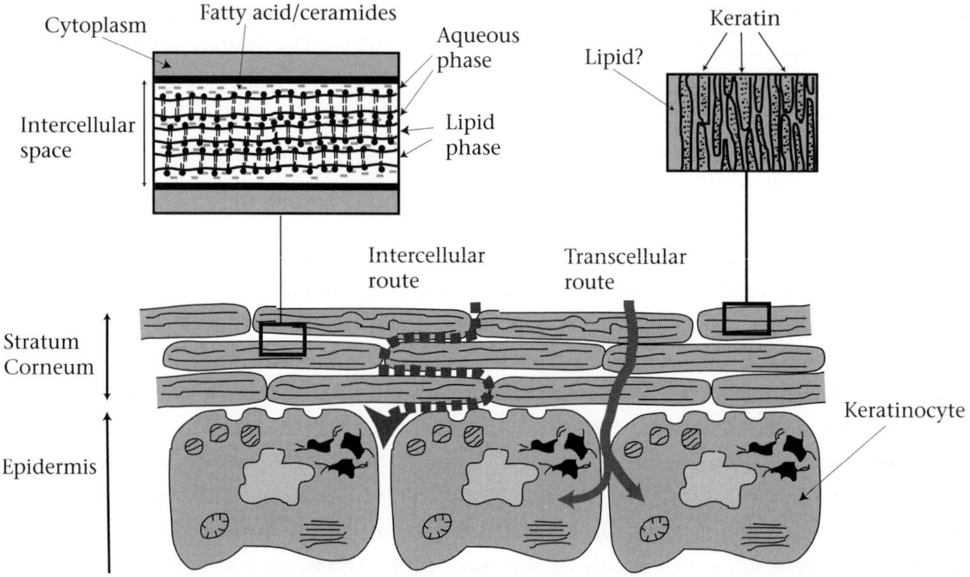

Figure 2.3: Routes of xenobiotic absorption. A xenobiotic may penetrate the stratum corneum by either transcellular or intracellular routes as shown. The insets illustrate the dual lipid and aqueous nature of the intercellular space and the densely packed keratin of the intracellular matter.

compounds, with lipophilic compounds traversing via the lipid lamellar acyl chain regions whilst the polar compounds traverse via the lipid polar head group regions (Elias, 1981).

The issue of which route predominates has been the subject of much debate. Theoretical considerations supporting the transcellular route arise from the observation that this route comprises 90–99% of the stratum corneum volume, whilst the intercellular region around the cells would appear to be too small (0.01–0.1% of the stratum corneum volume) to account for significant absorption. In addition, the transcellular diffusion path length is only 25 μm compared to 350 μm for the intercellular pathway and 200 μm for the transfollicular route (Zatz, 1984). Observations and theories supporting the predominance of the intercellular route includes the fact that the transcellular route requires multiple partitioning steps between corneocytes and lipid, so providing a tortuous route for any chemical (Guy and Hadgraft, 1989; Elias *et al.*, 1981). Furthermore, delipidisation of the stratum corneum has been observed to increase absorption, supporting the intercellular route (Anderson and Rayker, 1989). Hydrophilic compounds (e.g. water) have been postulated to pass through holes in the intercellular lipid matrix (Potts and Francoeur, 1991).

The transappendageal route has been postulated to be of significance for chemical absorption across the skin since early observations that compounds (e.g. tracer dyes, heavy metals) may accumulate around the hair follicles and further studies have confirmed the involvement of this route, particularly in haired species. Kao *et al.* (1988) reported that the absorption of benzo(a)pyrene was greater in haired than in hairless mice, concluding that the follicular route was important in skin penetration; similar conclusions were also drawn by Illel *et al.* (1991) and Hueber *et al.* (1992). Human volunteer studies have revealed the increased penetration of methyl nicotinate through skin with higher hair follicle densities (Tur *et al.*, 1991). It has been proposed that the absorption of coumarin, propranolol and griseofulvin in human skin involves movement via sebaceous ducts with sebum acting as a vehicle (Ritschel *et al.*, 1989). However, since the total surface area of the appendages is small in humans (<1% skin surface) this route is unlikely to provide a major quantitative means of skin absorption for most chemical allergens. It is thought that skin appendages are most likely to be of importance during the early stages of chemical absorption, before steady state diffusion is reached (Potts *et al.*, 1992).

Microautoradiographic studies have shown that the contact allergens, eugenol and isoeugenol, penetrate the stratum corneum into the epidermis and also accumulate in the hair follicles/sebaceous glands, suggesting that both the stratum corneum and hair follicle pathways play a role in the absorption of these chemicals, at least in the rat (Figure 2.4, see colour plate section). In theory, once an allergen has entered the hair follicle, lateral absorption in the hair shaft may allow access to the epidermis, and hence to epidermal Langerhans' cells, enabling the immune response to proceed, whereas absorption from deeper regions of the hair follicle/sebaceous gland may by-pass these epidermal mechanisms and allow direct entry into the dermis/microvasculature, possibly attenuating/obliterating the response.

Furthermore, particulate matter (<5 μm diameter) may accumulate down the hair follicles, and, where chemical allergens are adsorbed onto particle surfaces, the hair follicles may, in theory, provide a route of entry into the skin.

2.4 MECHANISMS OF ALLERGEN ABSORPTION

For a chemical allergen to be absorbed from the skin surface into the tissue, and across the tissue into the systemic circulation, the following partitioning and diffusional processes must occur (Barry, 1983):

- i partitioning of the chemical allergen from a vehicle/formulation into the stratum corneum;
- ii diffusion across the stratum corneum;
- iii partitioning into the viable epidermis (the site of allergy induction);
- iv diffusion across the viable epidermis;
- v partitioning into the upper dermis;
- vi diffusion across the upper dermis;
- vii partitioning into the capillaries of the papillary plexus and lymphatics in the upper dermis with subsequent distribution into the systemic circulation and clearance from the body.

It should be noted that the terms 'skin uptake' and 'percutaneous absorption' are not synonymous: strictly speaking the former refers to the first steps (i–vi) in the skin absorption process, namely the movement of the compound from the skin surface into the various regions of the skin. Technically, the latter refers to the whole transfer process, involving steps (i) to (vii), whereby a compound passes from the skin surface into the systemic circulation. In toxicological terms, both uptake and percutaneous absorption are important. However, for manifestation of allergic contact dermatitis, it is the uptake of the allergen into the skin, and consequent bioavailability at the site of toxicity, which is of major significance.

The absorption of a chemical allergen through the skin can be regarded as a passive diffusion process. Percutaneous absorption relies on transport across various biological membranes, including the lipid lamellae of stratum corneum, the plasma membrane of keratinocytes, the basement membrane separating the epidermis and dermis, the endothelial cell membrane of the dermal microvasculature and intracellular membranes such as those of the endoplasmic reticulum. In general, passive diffusion requires:

i a concentration gradient across the membrane;
ii that the compound is lipid soluble (lipophilic); and
iii that the compound is non-ionised.

The pH partition theory states that only non-ionised, lipophilic compounds may move by passive diffusion down a concentration gradient across a semi-permeable membrane. As the skin is a dynamic biological system, the concentration gradient across the stratum corneum will normally be maintained by removal of the compound (by metabolism and distribution into the blood, lymphatics, fat etc.) and thus an equilibrium will not be reached. The degree of ionisation of the molecule is also important since only non-ionised forms can cross lipid structures by passive diffusion. The Henderson-Hasselbach equation states:

$$pH = pKa + Log\frac{[A^-]}{[HA]}$$

where pKa is the dissociation constant for the acid HA,

and $HA \rightarrow H^+ + A^-$

$$pH = pKa + Log\frac{[A]}{[HA^+]}$$

for the base A, and where $A + H^+ \rightarrow HA^+$

The pKa of a chemical is the pH at which it is 50% ionised. The pH of the skin surface is usually between 4 and 5. The pH of the viable epidermis, dermis and blood is 7.4. Hence from the above equations, and a knowledge of the pH of the skin and pKa of the chemical allergen, the amount of chemical in its unionised form, and therefore available for absorption, can be calculated.

In regarding allergen uptake as a passive diffusion process, it is therefore governed by Fick's first law of diffusion at steady state, where the absorption rate (flux) is proportional to the concentration gradient across the membrane (skin) (Wepierre and Marty, 1979; Scheuplein and Blank, 1971). Immediately following skin exposure, there is a period of time, the lag-time, where diffusion increases to reach steady state. The duration of this is compound specific, ranging from minutes to days. Once the system reaches steady state, the rate of absorption is proportional to the applied concentration, i.e. a first-order rate process exists, and can be represented by the following equations:

$$Js \propto C$$

where Js is the rate of absorption or the steady state flux ($\mu g/cm^2/h$) and C is the concentration of the penetrant.

If the concentration gradient of the chemical across the skin is considered, and a proportionality constant is added, then the steady state flux per unit area and concentration can be derived:

$$Js = Kp \times \Delta C$$

where Kp is the permeability coefficient (cm/h) and ΔC is the concentration gradient across the membrane.

The permeability coefficient (Kp) can also be calculated using the following equation:

$$Kp = \frac{KD}{L}$$

where K is the stratum corneum/vehicle partition coefficient, D is the membrane diffusion coefficient and L is the diffusion path length (stratum corneum thickness) through the skin barrier (cm).

Thus the permeability coefficient increases with the solubility of the penetrant in the stratum corneum and decreases with increasing skin thickness.

If the latter two equations are combined, then at steady state, flux will be dependent on D and K, which are governed by solute size and lipophilicity, respectively. The calculation of D is often difficult, therefore lipophilicity is usually measured by log P (the partition coefficient, normally between octanol and water).

$$Js = \frac{K \times D \times \Delta C}{L}$$

The parameter Kp is of particular value since it is independent of the applied dose. Kp can also be calculated using the following equation:

$$Kp = \frac{A}{(SA \times C \times t)}$$

where A is the amount (μg) of penetrant absorbed through the skin, SA is the surface area to which the dose is applied (cm^2), C is the concentration of compound ($\mu g/cm^3$) and t is the elapsed time (h).

These equations may be applied to most skin absorption studies and, with certain exceptions, will give reasonable approximations.

The profiles of absorption, often displayed graphically, for most chemicals fall into two types:

- i infinite dose-approximate steady state absorption over the entire time course, where either the dose is high or the absorption through the skin is very slow and does not result in a significant depletion from the skin surface of the material remaining to be absorbed; and
- ii finite dose-decreasing rate of absorption, where either the dose is low or the rate of absorption is so rapid that there is depletion of the compound on the skin surface.

2.5 THE SKIN RESERVOIR

The skin is known to exhibit reservoir characteristics, whereby compounds may be rapidly absorbed from the surface into the tissue but only slowly released into the systemic circulation (Vickers, 1963). Thus, following topical exposure, a depot of the chemical may accumulate in the skin, resulting in continued local exposure even after skin contact has ceased. Such chemicals may pose a hazard to the skin itself, where high levels are sequestered, or to other organs which may be continually exposed to low levels of the compound for some considerable time afterwards. For the carcinogenic aromatic amines, 4′4-methylene-bis (2-chloroaniline) (MbOCA) and 4′4-methylenedianiline (MDA), a reservoir has been observed *in vitro* in human skin, 30 minutes following skin contact, although this human skin reservoir would appear to exhibit a lower capacity than that formed in rat skin (Hewitt *et al.*, 1993; 1995). Maximum reservoir formation was observed within 1 h and removal of these compounds from the skin surface after this time had no significant effect on reducing the subsequent percutaneous absorption across the skin over 72 h (Hewitt *et al.*, 1995). The precise location of the skin reservoir for most chemicals would appear to be the outer region of the skin, the stratum corneum (Rougier *et al.*, 1983; 1985). Following *in vitro* topical application of MbOCA and MDA to rat skin and removal of the stratum corneum by taking sequential tape-strips, a considerable amount of the total skin residue (ca. 65%) is recovered from the stratum corneum layers (Hewitt *et al.*, 1993; 1995). Hence, roughly two thirds of the total skin depot for these aromatic amines resides in the outermost stratum corneum, a structure which comprises less than 2% of the total skin thickness (35 mm thick compared with 2 mm for whole skin in the rat).

There is considerable debate over whether one should consider the material present within the skin reservoir as bioavailable, and hence of toxicological relevance. In theory, a chemical allergen within the stratum corneum is available for subsequent diffusion into the viable epidermis (and then into the systemic circulation), and will not be removed by conventional washing procedures. In support of this, a linear relationship has been shown to exist between the amount of a chemical present in rat stratum corneum at 30 minutes following application *in vivo*, and the total amount absorbed (excreted and in epidermis and dermis) in 4 days (Rougier *et al.*, 1983), indicating that measurement of the amount of chemical in the stratum corneum may allow the prediction of total systemic absorption. However, it is quite possible that in some cases, the kinetics of diffusion of the allergen from the stratum corneum into the viable epidermis (and then into the systemic circulation) may be so slow, that skin desquamation may remove the stratum corneum reservoir layers before further absorption may occur. The presence of a cutaneous reservoir for potentially hazardous allergenic compounds may mean that local (and systemic) exposure may continue to occur even after topical contact has ceased, or the skin surface has been washed, and as such, this has important toxicological implications.

2.6 FACTORS INFLUENCING ALLERGEN ABSORPTION

Any factor that enhances the absorption of an allergen into the skin and/or reduces its subsequent clearance from the skin into the systemic circulation may potentiate cutaneous toxicity by increasing the exposure of the target organ to the compound. Vice versa, any factor reducing absorption into the skin and/or enhancing clearance into the blood may reduce cutaneous toxicity. In relation to the latter, relatively recent studies have investigated the ability of topical skin protectants to protect against contact dermatitis to urushiol (Vidmar and Iwane, 1999). Many factors appear to be important in determining just how well a chemical penetrates into the skin (Hotchkiss, 1995; 1999). These factors can be broadly divided into (a) chemical (related to the allergen), and (b) physiological (related to the skin) (Table 2.1). In the following sections these factors,

TABLE 2.1
Factors influencing allergen absorption

Chemical (Allergen-related)	Physiological (Skin-related)
Aqueous solubility	Age
Binding	Anatomical site
Concentration	Blood flow
Contact time	Disease/damage
Dose	Gender
Ionisation (pKa/pKb)	Hair follicle density
Lipophilicity	Hydration
Melting point	pH
Molecular weight/volume	Metabolism
Protein reactivity	Occlusion
Vehicle	Species/strain
Volatility	Surface area
	Temperature
	Thickness

and their influence upon skin uptake/penetration, are described. Although much of the data has been derived for chemicals that are not allergens, the principles and mechanisms apply equally well to allergenic chemicals.

2.6.1 Chemical factors

2.6.1.1 Physicochemical properties

The physicochemical properties of a chemical allergen will determine its degree of skin uptake. Solubility of the chemical allergen in the stratum corneum is the major determinant of percutaneous absorption potential and therefore lipophilic compounds are generally well absorbed whilst hydrophilic substances are less well absorbed. For series of structurally related chemicals, there is often a relatively good correlation between lipid solubility and skin absorption. However, for structurally unrelated chemicals this is not necessarily the case. Human *in vitro* skin absorption experiments with a series of unrelated chemicals have determined that the optimum Log P for maximum absorption is 2, with rapid loss of absorption at Log P values either side. Some degree of aqueous solubility is also important, especially to enable the xenobiotic to move from the lipophilic stratum corneum to the aqueous epidermis, dermis and bloodstream. The lipid solubility of a compound is described in terms of its partition coefficient (P or Log P) usually between octanol and water, i.e. Log P o/w. The higher the Log P the more lipophilic the molecule. Owing to the fact that the skin is a considerably more complex membrane than most other biological membranes, the role of lipophilicity is not clear-cut. Certainly, not only lipophilic compounds penetrate the skin: small, polar, water soluble compounds can be absorbed in amounts sufficient to cause both local and systemic toxicity.

Although an optimal partition coefficient between lipid and aqueous phases has been determined for various homologous series, and a Log P o/w of 2 has been described, in contrast, for chlorinated organic solvents, a partition coefficient close to unity has been associated with highest skin absorption. For a series of phenols, a good correlation between Log P o/w and permeability has been reported, and the absorption of a series of alcohols through human skin *in vitro* has been observed to increase with increasing lipid solubility, with low absorption of ethanol and high absorption of octanol. Higher alcohols are less well absorbed, neat alcohols are absorbed slower than those in aqueous solution and esters are absorbed faster than the corresponding alcohol. As expected, in other studies, lipophilic chemicals have been observed to permeate the skin better than hydrophilic ones. However, unlike structurally related series of chemicals (e.g. phenols, alcohols, hydrocortisone esters), the permeability coefficients of 91 unrelated chemicals do not correlate well with lipophilicity (Log P o/w), indicating that factors other than lipophilicity e.g. molecular weight, molecular volume, melting point etc., are likely to be of importance (Flynn, 1990). A relationship between percutaneous absorption and ΔlogP has also been observed. This parameter (the difference between two permeability coefficients) is thought to provide a measure of the hydrogen-bond donor acidity of solutes, which may be important in membrane permeability.

The size of the molecule is also an important factor in percutaneous absorption, although much less so than solubility: increasing molecular weight or molecular volume will have an inverse affect on absorption. However, small hydrophilic molecules are absorbed (albeit to a lesser extent than lipophilic molecules): the small polar molecule, water, is absorbed through skin with a permeability coefficient (Kp) of 10×10^{-4} cm/h. Large molecules (molecular weight >500) will generally only be absorbed very slowly, if at all. Electrolytes in aqueous solution are not well absorbed probably because of the increased size of the hydration sphere. Absorption will decrease if the allergen possesses one or more polar groups or is charged or hydrated.

A compound that has a high Log P o/w value will partition well into the stratum corneum, but may not pass freely through the aqueous environment of the epidermis and dermis. Such compounds may have a high predicted penetration value, but in reality only diffuse from the stratum corneum through the skin very slowly. Increasing Log P for many compounds will not result in an increased absorption: typically a parabolic relationship is obtained between skin permeability and the water-ether partition coefficients of nicotinic acid esters. Other authors have reported that the dermis may present a degree of barrier function for some highly lipophilic chemicals.

Under certain conditions, the chemical may exist as a gas and exposure may therefore be to the vapour. Here the volatility (vapour pressure) of the compound will be important.

2.6.1.2 Binding

Certain chemicals, once absorbed into the skin, may become bound to skin proteins such as keratin in the epidermis or possibly even serum albumin, which may diffuse from damaged blood vessels in the dermis during inflammatory reactions. This may be of particular significance for protein reactive chemicals (as most allergens are), a factor that is dealt with in much greater detail in subsequent chapters.

Diethylphosphite binds keratin and the organophosphate insecticide, sarin is adsorbed onto callus. Binding will usually result in retarding penetration across the skin and a build up of the chemical within the tissue. Bound and unbound chemical will be in equilibrium and therefore bound material may act as a depot, so prolonging the toxicological effect of the chemical. Specific information on which proteins are bound is limited. Surfactants bind keratinous tissue, with the extent of binding dependent upon the structure of the detergent. Some detergents penetrate both the amorphous region of keratin and the crystalline microfibrils, hence changing their structure and tensile properties. Testosterone binds components in the dermis of human skin whilst diazepam, ketoconazole, popranolol, phenytoin and warfarin have been found to bind to constituents of both the epidermis and dermis (Menczal and Maibach, 1972; Walter and Kurz, 1988). A specific type of binding of xenobiotics with melanin can occur in skin: phenothiazines such as chlorpromazine and the antimalarial chloroquine concentrate in melanin-containing tissue, e.g. skin and eye, the latter resulting in retinopathy and blindness.

2.6.1.3 Contact time

The length of time for which the skin is exposed to a given xenobiotic with affect uptake into the tissue. The aromatic amines, 4′4-methylene-bis (2-chloroaniline) (MbOCA) and 4′4-methylenedianiline (MDA), are rapidly taken up into the skin within the first hour following exposure. Washing human skin at times between three and 30 minutes following application to these compounds results in the efficient removal of unabsorbed chemical from the skin surface and hence reduces skin absorption five- to six-fold (Hewitt *et al.*, 1993; 1995). However, removal of these compounds after this time has no significant effect on reducing the subsequent percutaneous absorption through the skin over the next 72 hours. Similarly, for the pesticides lindane and azodrin, washing the skin of human volunteers at early times (15 min to 4 h) following topical application, significantly reduced absorption compared to skin which remained exposed for 24 h (Wester and Maibach, 1985). However, this effect would appear to be compound-specific, since for malathion and parathion there was no difference in absorption between application times of 15 min, 4 h or 24 h.

2.6.1.4 Dose/concentration

In general, increasing the dose of a chemical will increase absorption, since from Fick's law, the rate of diffusion is proportional to the amount of diffusant. For example, the absorption of benzyl acetate through rat and human skin is observed to be directly related to the amount applied, over a dose range including levels of likely skin exposure (Hotchkiss *et al.*, 1990). However, at high doses where the rate of absorption reaches a maximum or where the chemical causes cutaneous toxicity, then this dose-response relationship will break down e.g. oestradiol (Chanez *et al.*, 1989) and ibuprofen (Akhtar and Barry, 1985).

2.6.1.5 Particle size

In addition to direct contact with chemicals, the skin is also exposed to particulate matter and aerosols in the environment and during certain occupational activities. Particles deposited on the skin surface may lodge in crevices or hair follicles, allowing any adsorbed chemical allergen to partition into the skin. Large particles ($>20\ \mu m$) are likely to remain on the skin surface and are thus unlikely to be of importance (unless the tissue is damaged), however smaller particles (submicron) may enter the hair follicles, and may pose a toxicological hazard.

2.6.1.6 Vehicle/formulation

Chemicals may come into contact with the skin either as the neat compound, or, more typically, in a mixture or formulation together with other compounds. The absorption of a chemical will most likely differ if applied in a vehicle or formulation than if applied as the neat compound, and a number of recent studies have investigated such effects (Dias *et al.*, 1999; El-Kattan *et al.*, 2000; Fishbein *et al.*, 2000; Hood *et al.*, 1999; Kim *et al.*, 1999; Martin *et al.*, 2000; Muller-Goymann, 1999; Obata *et al.*, 2000; Wong *et al.*, 1999; Yang *et al.*, 1999a; Zhao and Singh, 1999; 2000).

The test vehicle used in skin sensitisation studies is often acetone:olive oil (4:1) and this has been shown to affect the absorption (and sensitisation potential) of a number of chemicals. The absorption rate of the potent allergen DNCB (applied as a 10% solution) across human skin *in vitro* was approximately 30-fold lower in acetone:olive oil (4:1) than in dimethylformamide vehicle (Scott *et al.*, 1986).

Ethanol is also often employed in skin sensitisation studies. The vehicles, ethanol, 2-phenylethanol and DMSO have been shown to enhance the skin absorption of many xenobiotics, including benzyl acetate (Hotchkiss *et al.*, 1992). Ethanol/propylene glycol affects the *in vitro* percutaneous absorption of aspirin, and the biophysical properties of the skin (Levang *et al.*, 1999) and linolenic acid/ethanol or limonene/ethanol vehicles modulate absorption of LHRH (Bhatia and Singh, 1999). Various urea derivatives also act as penetration enhancers (Han *et al.*, 1999).

Vehicles may enhance skin absorption by various mechanisms including perturbing the skin barrier or altering the partition coefficient of the xenobiotic between the vehicle and the stratum corneum. Lipophilic compounds readily penetrate into the stratum corneum from aqueous solutions owing to the preferential partitioning into the relatively lipid skin. In contrast, a lipophilic chemical will partition less well into the skin from a lipophilic vehicle. The water soluble N-nitrosodiethanolamine has been observed to penetrate the skin 200 times faster from a lipophilic vehicle (olive oil) than from an aqueous vehicle (water).

Solvents such as ethanol probably increase the absorption of xenobiotics by directly extracting the lipids from the stratum corneum, thus damaging the barrier properties of the skin (Guy *et al.*, 1990). Other absorption enhancers, such as dimethylsulphoxide, propylene glycol, sodium lauryl sulphate and oleic acid, are thought to function by solvation of the polar head groups of the stratum corneum lipids, while azone acts through direct fluidisation of the stratum corneum lipids (Barry, 1983).

2.6.2 Physiological factors

2.6.2.1 Age

It is generally regarded that skin permeability to chemicals is higher in premature infants and lower in the elderly. For instance, the skin of infants is more permeable than adult and older children's skin to hydrocortisone, whilst absorption of steroids is lower in people over 65 years compared with those aged 18–40 years. The penetration of tri-n-propyl phosphate (TNPP) through human skin *in vitro* decreases with increasing age from three to 57 years (Marzulli, 1962). The *in vivo* percutaneous absorption of testosterone is higher in younger subjects (aged 19 to 30 years) than in older subjects (aged 71 to 82 years) (Christopher and Kligman, 1965). In two groups of subjects, the first aged 18–40 years and the second aged >65 years, absorption of a series of compounds with different physicochemical properties (testosterone, benzoic acid, estradiol, hydrocortisone, acetylsalicylic acid and caffeine) was observed to decrease in the older subjects for the steroids, but was unaffected by age for the other more hydrophilic compounds

(Roskos and Maibach, 1992). The skin of premature infants is particularly permeable, for instance premature infant skin is three times more permeable to ethanol than the skin of full-term infants and is almost 50 times more permeable to benzyl alcohol. The skin of pre-term infants has been shown to be up to 1000 times more permeable to some chemicals than that of full-term infants (Hammarlund and Sedin, 1979; Wilson and Maibach, 1982). This impaired barrier function is only temporary, with full-term infants exhibiting a fully functioning barrier (McCormack *et al.*, 1982). However, not all chemicals exhibit age-related differences in absorption: the absorption of benzoic acid and caffeine are independent of age (Roskos and Maibach, 1992).

In animals, limited age-related changes have been observed. There was no age-related effect for the percutaneous absorption, through rat skin, of 14 pesticides (Shah *et al.*, 1987), nor for water and mannitol (Dick and Scott, 1992), although decreased absorption of PCBs (Banks *et al.*, 1990) and 2,3,7,8-tetrachlorodibenzo-*p*-dioxin (Anderson *et al.*, 1993) in older rat skin, has been reported.

The mechanisms underpinning age-related changes in absorption are uncertain but are likely to be due to a combination of changes in stratum corneum hydration, skin structure, surface lipids and possibly skin blood flow. The morphology and thickness of human stratum corneum does not change with age but the lipid content and intercellular cohesion decreases. The observation of reduced absorption in the elderly is in line with studies showing the water content of skin from people over 40 years' old is lower than that in younger people, whilst older subjects demonstrate a decreased concentration of surface lipids. The dermal-epidermal junction alters with age, so that the blood circulation to the skin decreases, reducing clearance of the chemical from the epidermis.

2.6.2.2 Anatomical region

Regional variations in chemical absorption exist with inter-site differences that are apparently compound-specific. The *in vivo* absorption of hydrocortisone in human skin is greatest through the scrotum and decreases in the order: scrotum > jaw > forehead > scalp > forearm > foot arch, with scrotal skin 42 times more permeable than the forearm and plantar skin (from the foot arch) the least permeable (0.14 times that of the forearm) (Feldmann and Maibach, 1967). The absorption of methyl salicylate decreases in the order: abdomen > forearm > instep > heel. The penetration of the pesticides malathion and parathion decrease: scrotum > scalp = face > palms = soles > forearm. It would appear that in comparison with the palm of the hand, the abdomen and dorsum of the hand is twice as permeable, the scalp, jaw and forehead are four times as permeable and the scrotum almost 12 times as permeable. These data are in broad agreement with site-dependent differences in stratum corneum thickness: the stratum corneum thickness is thinnest on the eyelids and scrotum (10 μm) and thickest on the palms and soles (1 mm).

Interestingly, in contrast to that expected from stratum corneum thickness, the palms and soles have been observed to be as permeable to water and some other chemicals as other body regions with thinner stratum cornea, decreasing in the order: soles > scrotum > palms > back of the hand > forehead > arms = legs = trunk.

Site-dependent differences in animals have also been observed, e.g. the penetration of water, urea and hydrocortisone through rat skin is site-specific, with back skin more permeable than abdominal skin (Bronaugh *et al.*, 1983).

However, for some chemicals percutaneous absorption is independent of anatomical site: the *in vivo* absorption of paraquat is similar through human skin from the leg, hand and forearm (Wester *et al.*, 1984) and no differences were observed for fentamyl and sufentamyl (Roy and Flynn, 1990).

The mechanisms involved in these regional variations probably include a combination of differences in stratum corneum thickness, diffusivity, transepidermal water loss, hair follicle size and density.

2.6.2.3 Blood flow

Theoretically, alterations in the dermal blood flow will affect skin clearance and systemic uptake of chemicals from the skin into the bloodstream, potentially modulating skin toxicity. However, in practise this will only be a serious consideration for compounds that penetrate quickly, since it is the stratum corneum that usually provides the rate-limiting step to absorption. For example, the absorption of the high penetrant chemical, caffeine, through hairless rat skin is significantly impeded when blood flow is reduced, causing accumulation of caffeine in the upper dermis (Auclair *et al.*, 1991). In contrast, for the poorly absorbed compound, urea, and the intermediate compound, progesterone, this effect is not observed. Regional differences in blood flow have been postulated to account for inter-site variations in chemical absorption. Inflammatory reactions in the skin will also increase cutaneous blood flow and may therefore increase the percutaneous absorption of certain compounds.

2.6.2.4 Disease/damage

The barrier properties of the skin are diminished or even lost if its integrity is compromised by damage or disease. If the skin is damaged (for example, cut or abraded) then the absorption of many chemicals into the tissue is enhanced. Physical damage such as abrasion may result in almost complete loss of barrier properties towards certain chemicals such as water.

Chemical damage, such as that mediated by corrosive chemicals, (e.g. phenols and concentrated acids and alkalis), can dramatically increase permeability through the skin. For example, the percutaneous absorption of hydrocortisone through mouse skin pretreated with 10% acetic acid is increased (Soloman and Lowe, 1979). Mixtures of polar and non-polar solvents, such as methanol and chloroform, will remove the lipids from the stratum corneum, forming artificial shunts through the membrane (Blank and Scheuplein, 1969). Certain solvents, e.g. dimethylsulphoxide, dimethylacetamide and dimethylformamide, are used clinically to enhance the absorption of topically applied drugs. Skin that has been burned is also more permeable than normal healthy skin and this has been shown to be due to disruption of the keratin structures within the tissue (Baden *et al.*, 1973). For example, the penetration of butanol and octanol through heat-treated hairless mouse skin is increased, whereas the penetration of water, methanol and ethanol is unaffected (Behl *et al.*, 1980b). Scratching the skin enhanced the absorption of benzoic acid several fold through guinea pig skin (Moon *et al.*, 1990).

Ultraviolet radiation causes structural damage to the skin (and inflammation) enhances the absorption of nicotinic acid through rat skin (Bronaugh and Stewart, 1985) and the absorption of a range of chemicals is enhanced or unchanged through heat-treated mouse skin. Defatted skin, as a result of solvent treatment (e.g. with chloroform:methanol 2:1 or ether:ethanol 10:1), exhibits a severely damaged stratum corneum with the potential for consequently high absorption. Solvents may burn the skin and result in increased absorption. Soaps and detergents, anionic and cationic surfactants and aprotic solvents like DMSO may also damage the skin resulting in the potential for higher absorption.

A correlation exists in human and rat skin between the rate of percutaneous absorption of seven test chemicals (benzoic acid, caffeine, cortisone, nicotinic acid, phenol, propylene glycol, urea) and enhancement of penetration due to damage, with the greatest increase in penetration for the most poorly absorbed compounds. Perturbation of human skin also affects barrier properties towards salicylic acid (Benfeldt *et al.*, 1999) and a recent paper has reported the effects of industrial detergents on the barrier function of human skin (Nielsen *et al.*, 2000).

Skin barrier function may be modulated through disease. Psoriasis and eczema are characterised by hyperproliferation of keratinocytes, resulting in a rapidly produced stratum corneum which may be structurally flawed, with an impaired barrier function (Kligman, 1983a), demonstrating enhanced permeability to testosterone. The absorption of hydrocortisone and triamcinolone acetamide is enhanced through eczematous monkey skin (Bronaugh *et al.*, 1986b) whilst skin absorption of both hydrocortisone and benzoic acid is enhanced through diseased guinea-pig skin.

Occasional anecdotal evidence of enhanced absorption following occupational exposure in workers with diseased skin can be found in the literature. Higher organochlorine plasma levels are reported in a pesticide formulator with scleroderma than in other workers with non-diseased skin. Occupational skin diseases such as irritant and allergic contact dermatitis are known to be common, for instance in bricklayers and cement workers, and these may be postulated to affect the percutaneous absorption of chemicals. As well as having effects at the stratum corneum level to reduce barrier function, the inflammation of the skin present in these (and other) diseases may lead to enhanced blood flow to the tissue with a concomitant increase in skin absorption.

2.6.2.5 Hair follicle density

There is controversy as to the significance of hair follicles in xenobiotic absorption across the skin. Hair follicles may contribute to the increased absorption of some topically applied xenobiotics, for example the percutaneous absorption of benzo(a)pyrene is significantly greater through the skin of haired mice than hairless mice, suggesting that the follicular route is of importance for percutaneous absorption of this compound in rodents (Kao *et al.*, 1988). The absorption of benzo(a)pyrene in the mouse has been observed to correlate with hair follicle density, with extensive localisation of the compound in the hair follicles. Human volunteer studies have also shown an increased penetration of methyl nicotinate through skin with higher hair follicle densities, although this route is generally regarded as being of less significance in humans (Tur *et al.*, 1991). Several lipophilic compounds (coumarin, griseofulvin and propranolol hydrochloride) are reportedly absorbed across human skin with the involvement of ducts of the sebaceous gland, by using the sebum as a vehicle. However, the small skin surface area covered by these appendageal routes of entry does make it unlikely that these are important in absorption once steady state has been reached. Hair follicle density is low in human and pig skin (11 ± 1 per cm^2) compared with rat (289 ± 2), mouse (658 ± 38) or hairless mouse (75 ± 6), and species differences in absorption have been attributed in some cases to differences in hair follicle density.

2.6.2.6 Hydration

The degree of hydration of the stratum corneum may affect the percutaneous absorption of chemicals, with increasing stratum corneum hydration enhancing percutaneous absorption of some compounds up to ten-fold. Application of water to the skin will hydrate it and will enhance skin absorption. Increased water levels in the stratum corneum can be achieved when the skin is subjected to high levels of humidity or by covering the skin surface with an impermeable barrier (occlusion), such as clothing, bandages, plastic films or the vehicle of application itself, thus preventing the normal loss of water by evaporation. Increased hydration and occlusion have been shown to increase percutaneous absorption of nicotinic acid, salicylic acid, corticosteroids, acetone, various alcohols and benzyl acetate (Cronin and Stoughton, 1962; McKenzie and Stoughton, 1962; Scheuplein and Ross, 1974; Behl *et al.*, 1980a; Hotchkiss *et al.*, 1992a), although in other cases increased hydration does not enhance absorption (Bucks *et al.*, 1991; Treffel *et al.*, 1992). The degree of enhancement will be dependent upon the physicochemical properties of the penetrant.

The mechanisms underpinning permeability increases due to hydration are complex. Under normal conditions, the stratum corneum is hydrated as a result of water diffusing upwards from the underlying epidermal layers, resulting in the tissue softening, swelling and wrinkling. The basal level of stratum corneum water content is 5–15%, but this can be elevated to 50%, for example by occlusion of the skin surface (Bucks *et al.*, 1989). Hydration of the keratin and the regions of lipid polar head groups alters the structure of the skin, presumably allowing permeability to increase.

2.6.2.7 Inter-individual variation

As for most biological processes there is often considerable inter-individual variation between humans in the percutaneous absorption of xenobiotics, with variations up to ten-fold recorded for some compounds. The aromatic amines, MbOCA and MDA exhibit a three- to four-fold range in absorption between ten different human subjects. Similarly, a four-fold variation in diethyl phthalate absorption through eight subjects' skin has been observed.

2.6.2.8 Metabolism

There is now considerable evidence that the skin is a living tissue, containing many of the xenobiotic metabolising enzymes previously identified in the liver (Pannatier *et al.*, 1978; Hotchkiss, 1992, 1998) (see Chapter 4). Although specific activities of many cutaneous enzymes are lower than in liver, when the large surface area of the skin is considered, it is apparent that the tissue is an efficient xenobiotic metabolising organ, which is likely to make a significant contribution to the overall metabolic disposition of topically applied compounds.

It is not clear whether skin metabolism affects skin absorption or whether skin absorption affects skin metabolism. In theory both could occur. Skin absorption (and therefore skin toxicity) may be affected by skin metabolism since the metabolites of a compound may be absorbed at different rates from the parent chemical owing to their different physicochemical properties. Conversely, skin metabolism may be affected by skin absorption since the slower a chemical is absorbed, the greater the time it will be available at the cutaneous site of enzyme metabolism.

Metabolism is a major factor influencing the skin penetration of benzo(a)pyrene in six species including human: skin absorption of benzo(a)pyrene in non-viable skin *in vitro* is negligible whereas permeation in viable skin is significant. In addition, the *in vitro* absorption of benzo(a)pyrene is reduced by the metabolic inhibitor KCN.

The skin sensitiser, cinnamaldehyde, is metabolised following *in vitro* absorption into human skin, to cinnamic acid and cinnamyl alcohol metabolites (presumably by cutaneous aldehyde dehydrogenase (ALDH) and alcohol dehydrogenase (ADH) enzymes), and utilisation of the ADH inhibitor, pyrazole, affects not only the metabolism but also the absorption of cinnamaldehyde, suggesting that the absorption and metabolism are intrinsically linked (Smith *et al.*, 2000a).

Theoretically, skin absorption may affect skin metabolism, since the slower a chemical is absorbed, the longer it will be in contact with cutaneous drug metabolising enzymes and the greater the opportunity for it to be metabolised. The degree of cutaneous metabolism is an important factor since it will determine whether a chemical is absorbed across the skin barrier intact or as one or more metabolites, and hence affect the exact nature and extent of systemic absorption of potentially toxic chemicals. Skin metabolism, and its role in the manifestation of cutaneous allergy, is considered in more detail in later chapters of this book.

2.6.2.9 Occlusion

Occlusion of the skin surface following exposure to a xenobiotic may enhance the penetration of the compound across the skin. As described above, occlusion may be achieved by a number of means, including clothing, plastic and occlusive vehicles. The absorption of MDA through unoccluded human skin *in vitro* (13%) is increased by occlusion to 32% and increases for other chemicals of up to five-fold have been observed (Hotchkiss *et al.*, 1993). The major mechanism of permeation enhancement by occlusion is probably a reduction in transepidermal water loss, which results in an increase in skin hydration, although an increase in skin temperature may also be involved. Occlusion may increase skin temperature by preventing the cooling evaporation of water, with increases up to 5°C being observed, although occlusion does not always enhance skin temperature.

In addition to affecting the initial diffusion of a chemical from the skin surface into the tissue, occlusion may alter the disposition of any chemical that has already partitioned into the stratum corneum reservoir. Many lipophilic chemicals are rapidly absorbed into the skin forming a reservoir in the stratum corneum, and the increase in skin hydration and/or temperature that accompanies occlusion may act to increase the diffusion out from this reservoir into the systemic circulation, with its associated toxicological consequences.

2.6.2.10 Race

Limited, conflicting data are available concerning inter-racial differences in percutaneous absorption. The stratum corneum of black skin is the same thickness as that of Caucasian skin, however black skin has a much more compact barrier with a greater number of corneocyte layers than that from Caucasian skin (22 layers compared with 17 layers) (Weigand *et al.*, 1980) and black skin reacts less strongly to irritants than Caucasian skin. Percutaneous absorption of some chemicals, e.g. flucinolone acetate (Stoughton, 1969) may be reduced in black skin whereas in other cases e.g. benzoic acid, caffeine or acetyl salicylic acid (Lotte *et al.*, 1993) no inter-ethnic differences have been observed between Asians, Blacks or Caucasians.

2.6.2.11 Sex

Limited evidence is available of sex differences in absorption in animals (not humans) e.g. benzoic acid absorption is slower in male than in female rats (Bronaugh *et al.*, 1983), possibly due to effects of testosterone increasing stratum corneum and epidermal thickness in the male (McCormick and Abdel-Rahman, 1991).

2.6.2.12 Surface area

The surface area of skin exposed to the chemical will affect its percutaneous absorption. In general, the greater the surface area exposed, the greater the absorption. The 'rule of nines' has been applied to the estimation of the surface area of human body regions, with the head and neck accounting for 9%, each upper limb 9%, each lower limb 18%, and the front and back each 18%. The total body surface area of an average adult human is 18 000 cm^2 and that of a neonate is 1920 cm^2. For estimation of occupational and environmental exposure, the typical exposed surface area of skin is estimated to be 2940 cm^2 in a clothed adult (EPA, 1989).

2.6.2.13 Species

Species differences in the skin absorption of chemicals exist, and in general, although not always, human skin is less permeable to xenobiotics than the skin of most laboratory animals (Bartek *et al.*, 1972; Wester and Noonan, 1980; Garnett *et al.*, 1994; Mint *et al.*,

1994; Beckley-Kartey *et al.*, 1997; Hotchkiss *et al.*, 1992). Skin absorption would appear to be relatively high in the mouse, rat and rabbit and lower in the pig and monkey. The latter two species may provide a closer approximation than rodents to human skin, although there are still some significant variations (Wester and Noonan, 1980). However, on occasions, and particularly under occlusive conditions, the percutaneous absorption of some chemicals (e.g. phenol and MDA) is greater through human skin than through rat tissue (Hotchkiss *et al.*, 1993). The potent skin allergen DNCB exhibits species differences in absorption, with mouse and rat skin six and four times, respectively, more permeable than human skin (Scott *et al.*, 1986).

The absorption of six compounds in four species shows human skin is least permeable in comparison to rat, rabbit and pig; with pig skin providing the closest match to human and a rank order of rabbit > rat > pig = monkey > human.

The pesticide DDT, is poorly absorbed in human and squirrel monkey skin, with higher absorption in the rabbit and pig. The pesticides, lindane, parathion and malathion are all best absorbed in rabbit skin, with the squirrel monkey closest to human for lindane and the pig closest to human for parathion. Malathion shows similar absorption in human, monkey and pig skin. Some authors have reported that pig skin is anatomically and biochemically similar to human skin, and hence this species' skin is employed in numerous skin absorption studies e.g. of sunscreens in micro-yucatan pig skin. The Rhesus monkey appears to be very similar to humans in terms of the absorption of a group of ten selected compounds and a group of five nitroaromatic compounds. Species differences in absorption of a number of other chemicals has also been investigated (Mathews *et al.*, 1997; Moody *et al.*, 1995; Roper *et al.*, 1998).

Inter-species differences in absorption probably result from differences in skin anatomy, such as the thickness, organisation and lipid content of the stratum corneum, the number of hair follicles and sweat glands, the distribution of blood vessels, the ability to sweat and the general condition of the skin. The lower percutaneous absorption (increased barrier property) of human skin compared with rat tissue is possibly due to a combination of the increased skin thickness (3 mm compared to 2 mm) and decreased hair follicle density ($10/cm^2$ compared to $300/cm^2$) of human skin compared with rat tissue, notwithstanding the increased thickness of male rat stratum corneum (which is approximately 35 μm thick) compared with that of human stratum corneum (which is approximately 20 μm thick).

2.6.2.14 Temperature

Since the process of skin absorption is governed, in the main, by diffusion across the stratum corneum, temperature will inevitably affect the skin penetration of xenobiotics (Barry, 1983). Under normal conditions, skin surface temperature is approx. 32°C, although this varies with factors such as external air temperature, clothing, occlusion, rubbing and exercise. A number of authors have reported the enhanced absorption of chemicals such as levamisole, salicylate and phenols through animal skin as its temperature is increased, although absorption is not always enhanced by increasing skin temperature (Jetzer *et al.*, 1988; Arita *et al.*, 1970; Roberts *et al*, 1978; Cummings, 1969). An increase in skin temperature may also have an effect on the stratum corneum reservoir, releasing those chemicals sequestered there out into the systemic circulation. Reducing skin temperature from 30°C to 20°C decreases the percutaneous absorption of salicylic acid through guinea pig skin five-fold (Arita *et al.*, 1970).

In addition to its affect on diffusion across the stratum corneum, the mechanisms by which an increase in temperature may modulate percutaneous absorption may also include increased cutaneous blood flow. The homeostatic control of body temperature involves regulation of cutaneous blood vessels: increased skin temperature causes increased blood flow through the distal capillaries to facilitate heat loss. This enhanced perfusion of the tissue will have the effect of increasing the local clearance of any penetrant compound present in the upper dermis. The absorption of methyl salicylate is increased three-fold in humans who are exposed to high ambient temperatures or who undergo strenuous exercise, due to increased blood flow, with contributions from increases in skin hydration and sweating (Danon *et al.*, 1986).

2.7 SUMMARY

The skin is exposed to a considerable number of chemicals that induce allergic contact dermatitis. In order for a chemical to manifest such toxicity, it is essential that it is absorbed into the skin and the major barrier to skin uptake for most chemicals is the outermost stratum corneum. This structure must therefore be breached for the chemical allergen to reach the viable epidermis where cutaneous toxicity may develop. In addition, as outlined here and discussed in detail in later chapters, the skin is not an inert membrane, but possesses considerable metabolic activity, that may activate or detoxify chemical allergens during absorption (Figure 2.5).

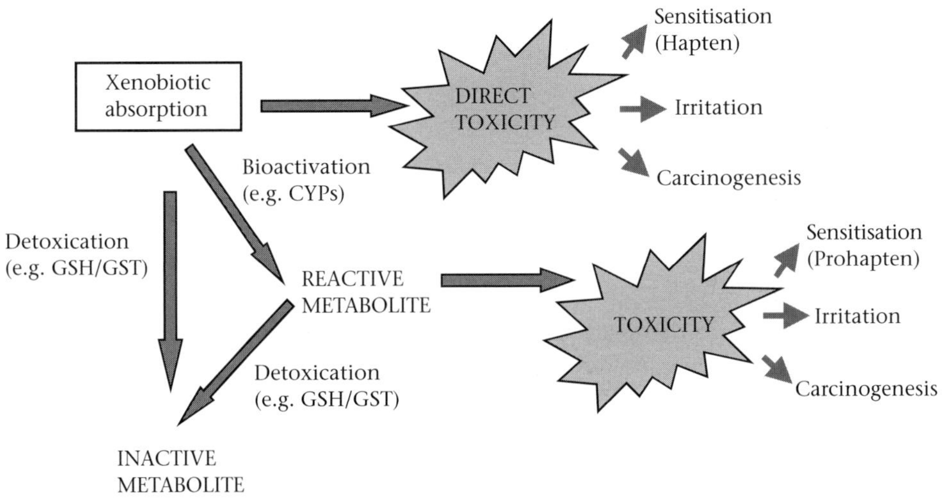

Figure 2.5: Balance of activating and detoxifying metabolism can contribute to skin toxicity derived from absorbed xenobiotics.

The balance between bioactivation and detoxication mechanisms within the skin will be of fundamental importance in the generation of allergic contact dermatitis. The parent compound and/or active metabolites, once bioavailable within the relevant region of the skin, may then be positioned to act at specific target sites within the tissue, to initiate the immune response.

The following chapters provide an overview of mammalian xenobiotic-metabolising enzymes and the reactions that these enzymes perform (Chapter 3), and the activity, expression and localisation of analogous enzymes within the skin (Chapter 4).

CHAPTER

3

Enzymes and Mechanisms of Xenobiotic Metabolism

'The essential design principle of these enzymes is non-selectivity: they recognise common, general, chemical features of organic molecules, not the molecules themselves. This system of xenobiotic metabolism, which is adapted to molecular invasion, is as vital to mammalian survival as the immunological apparatus, which has been adapted to deal with invasion by organisms. At the molecular level, they share the same design principles of non-selectivity. Built-in non-discriminatory activity has, however, got a down side: the immunological system sometimes sees self as foreign and becomes self-destructive: the xenobiotic metabolic system sometimes generates products more reactive and biologically destructive than the original substrate.'

(Sir James Black, Nobel Laureate in Medicine)

Contents

Metabolism is a complex phenomenon in mammals that is essential to survival. In general, it is hypothesised that metabolism has evolved to provide energy for cellular processes through metabolic turnover and to provide protective mechanisms against the generation of toxicity from exposure to xenobiotics. The metabolic system involves a wide variety of enzymes that are expressed in varying levels in all tissues. However, metabolism is regarded as being most dominant in the liver, which is the first organ to encounter ingested substances that have passed through the gastrointestinal tract, either intact or as transformed by gut bacteria/enzymes. As a result, most studies on metabolism have been conducted using liver derived enzymes from a variety of species but it is increasingly becoming apparent that extrahepatic organs also have major roles to play in metabolic processes, and such metabolism may influence both local and systemic toxicity.

As discussed in the previous chapter, an important route for exogenous material to enter the body is via skin absorption and penetration. It is known that skin contains metabolising enzymes (see Chapter 4) and it has been hypothesised that, as well as providing protection by acting as a physical barrier to exogenous substances (xenobiotics), it also possesses activating and detoxifying metabolism. In order to understand skin metabolism, however, it is first necessary to gain an appreciation and understanding of metabolism in general from the wealth of studies on hepatic enzymes, some of which may be extrapolated to analogous cutaneous mechanisms. Although, the levels of skin metabolising enzymes are often appreciably lower than their hepatic counterparts, the same considerations and general principles, with respect to basic reaction mechanisms, are expected to apply even though their kinetics may be somewhat different.

Metabolising enzymes in all tissues biotransform both endogenous and xenobiotic substrates which, when adequately controlled, may result in a number of positive effects. These include:

a the activation of substrate functional groups for subsequent specific mechanisms;
b the deactivation/detoxication of toxic species, which often aids excretion;
c the regulation of intracellular concentrations of small molecules;
d the generation of intracellular energy;
e the regeneration of essential cofactors and substrates etc.

In certain circumstances, however, it is conceivable that the first of these points, the activation of xenobiotic substrates, may lead to detrimental effects, especially when concentrations of an active xenobiotic become too high or too potent to be adequately controlled. Xenobiotic-metabolising enzymes are also, by the nature of their evolution, promiscuous in that each family of enzymes often metabolises a wide variety of related substrates. When sterically allowed, it is often the case that these enzymes utilise functional groups of a molecule rather than a specific substrate as a whole. In order to predict xenobiotic metabolism fully, it is essential to understand this multiplicitous nature of metabolising enzymes.

This chapter provides an overview of the major metabolising enzymes that have been identified to date (mainly in the liver), and illustrates the reactions they perform with selected substrates and discusses some of the factors that may influence the balance of these reactions. In particular, this chapter focuses on the potential activation and detoxication of xenobiotics by metabolising enzymes.

3.1 ACTIVATION AND DETOXICATION OF XENOBIOTICS

In attempting to predict or evaluate the metabolism of a compound, it should be considered that more than one metabolic pathway may contribute towards the ultimate toxic properties of a small molecule. It is often the case that many competing metabolic reactions, some activating and some detoxifying, contribute to the overall fate of a compound. In general, however, it is assumed that metabolism results in the detoxication of compounds and ultimately increases their solubility either by the addition of ionisable groups or by conjugation of the molecule to a more polar compound. If this is the case, then it is purely unfortunate that in some cases metabolism leads to toxicity by activation (by the generation or modification of reactive functional groups) of an initially chemically unreactive xenobiotic. Under 'normal' circumstances an enzyme may activate an endogenous substrate as part of a vital step in a specific, tightly controlled metabolic pathway. In some cases (such as the *O*-demethylation of codeine to morphine and the sulphation of minoxidil to minoxidil sulphate), xenobiotic activation is beneficial in producing an effective drug. However, when concentrations of a xenobiotic (which may act to mimic a 'normal' substrate) are too high, or the balance between activation and detoxication kinetics is affected, then activation mechanisms can predominate and may potentially overload the system with a toxic species.

3.2 FACTORS INFLUENCING THE METABOLISM OF A COMPOUND

Although the precise chemistry of the reactions that are performed by metabolising enzymes is considered to be similar throughout species, the balance and effects of competing metabolic reactions may vary. In particular, this may become an issue when tissue becomes overloaded with a reactive species, some metabolic pathways/enzymes fail or are absent, or enzymes are induced[1] by either endogenous or exogenous agents (including drugs, alcohol, dietary components and smoking). The overall balance of enzymatic reactions in the individual may then determine the resulting toxicity of a compound. Factors that may affect this balance are inherent, acquired or biochemical:

- i inherent factors: sex, age, species or strain, genetic variations in enzyme production, and tissue differences in the production of enzymes;
- ii acquired factors: diet and diseased state of the tissue;
- iii biochemical factors: relative rates of activation vs detoxication pathways, cofactor availability, availability of protective agents, dose, enzyme saturation level, induction or inhibition of enzymes.

It may be necessary in attempting to predict the metabolism of an unknown compound to take into account all of the above factors. With this in mind, studies of inherent inter-individual variability, by detecting the presence of enzymes in different tissues, across species, in males and females of varying ages, is important in attempting to characterise these differences. Such studies may indicate whether a generic classification of a toxic compound is applicable, or whether aspects pertaining to the individual should be taken into account when assessing potential toxicity. For example, a compound may only be toxic in individuals whose age, sex, relative enzyme levels etc., renders them susceptible.

The acquired factors of diet and disease, which may indirectly contribute to metabolism, are more difficult to assess and require bioassays and clinical histories to be evaluated.

In these early days of understanding metabolism, it is a more reasonable undertaking to assess the biochemical factors listed above, by isolating specific reaction systems and performing biochemical assays to provide an insight into distinct metabolic reaction mechanisms and their kinetics. These data, along with three-dimensional pictures of the metabolising enzymes in molecular detail, are the first invaluable ways in which to define the pathways of metabolism. Such biochemical studies have led to the classification of three phases of metabolism defined by enzyme functionality: namely phase I, phase II and phase III metabolism.

3.3 THE THREE PHASES OF METABOLISM

To reiterate, the major purpose of xenobiotic metabolism is to ultimately protect the body from toxic substances by converting them to more water-soluble, therefore more easily excreted compounds. It has historically been hypothesised that there are two major stages of metabolism: phase I metabolism activates or functionalises an initially unreactive endogenous or exogenous substrate in preparation for phase II metabolism, which serves to detoxify the active species by conjugating it to a more water-soluble compound. A third stage, phase III, has been defined for the further metabolism of glutathione-conjugates. As will be seen in the following sections, these hypotheses may be too generalised in attempting to define a purpose for metabolism, as research within the last decade has indicated that both phase I and phase II reactions can lead to both activation and detoxication of xenobiotics. It is more correct to purely regard phase I metabolism as functionalisation and phase II metabolism as conjugation.

3.3.1 Phase I metabolism

General examples of a range of enzymatic biotransformations that have been classified under phase I metabolism are presented in the following sections for a selection of xenobiotics.

3.3.1.1 Oxidation by the microsomal mixed-function oxidase system

The microsomal mixed-function oxidase (MFO) system was first described by Omura and Sato in 1964. Since then, there have been approximately 30 000 papers published on the subject (more than 17 000 of these during the last decade), which is an indication of the importance given to this system. During the 1970s it became clear that the MFO system was not a single enzyme but the product of a pair of enzymes that could exist in multiple forms, which were the products of distinct genetic loci. The MFO system is found in both prokaryotes and eukaryotes, and comprises isoforms of the haem-containing-enzyme cytochrome P450 (CYP), which acts as the terminal oxidase in a complex with the flavoenzyme NADPH-cytochrome P450 reductase. Phospholipids are also involved in maintaining the integrity of the reductase:CYP complex.

It was demonstrated by Smith and co-workers in London (Mahgoub *et al.*, 1977) that certain individuals were poor CYP2D6 metabolisers of debrisoquine and this observation led to the notion that some individuals may have deficiencies in oxidising certain drugs by CYPs. Genetic polymorphisms of CYPs are responsible for these inter-individual variabilities in metabolism and the study of genetic variation in relation to drug metabolising capacity is a field of CYP research that is continuing today (Nebert, 1997). With the advent in July 2000 of the first draft of the human genome, analysis of CYP sequences within the genome has begun (see David Nelson's CYP webpage listed in Appendix 2).

The mammalian MFO system is the most versatile and ubiquitous system involved in the metabolism of endogenous compounds (e.g. steroids, bile acids, prostaglandins, leukotrienes and biogenic amines) and a wide range of xenobiotics, through performing a diverse array of oxidative, peroxidative and reductive biotransformations. To date, 17 families of human CYP isoforms have been identified, covering 39 sub-families of genes (nomenclature reviewed by Nelson *et al.*, 1996 and as presented on the CYP website listed in Appendix 2) of which 53 sequences are known and have been mapped in the draft human genome. There are also 24 CYP pseudogenes present in the human genome. In terms of substrate specificities, the MFO system is the most promiscuous xenobiotic-metabolising system, with the different isoforms of CYPs exhibiting broad-range substrate specificities and different functionalities (Gonzalez and Gelboin, 1994). CYPs are most abundant in the liver but have been found in almost every tissue, with CYP3A being the most abundant constitutive hepatic isoform in humans (Figure 3.1).

At present, there are no known three-dimensional structures of any mammalian CYP enzymes (due to problems in isolating soluble forms of these membrane-bound enzymes) to confirm their active site chemistry (Poulos, 1995). However, the structure of rat liver NAD(P)H CYP-reductase, the partner enzyme of the MFO system, provides an insight into the possible mechanisms of electron transfer between its $NADP^+$ cofactor and the haem moiety of CYP via the FMN and FAD cofactors of the reductase (Wang *et al.*, 1997).

The major human CYPs (belonging to families CYP1 through CYP4) that are known to be involved in xenobiotic metabolism are listed in Table 3.1, along with some common exogenous substrates, inhibitors and inducers (reviewed by Rendic and Di

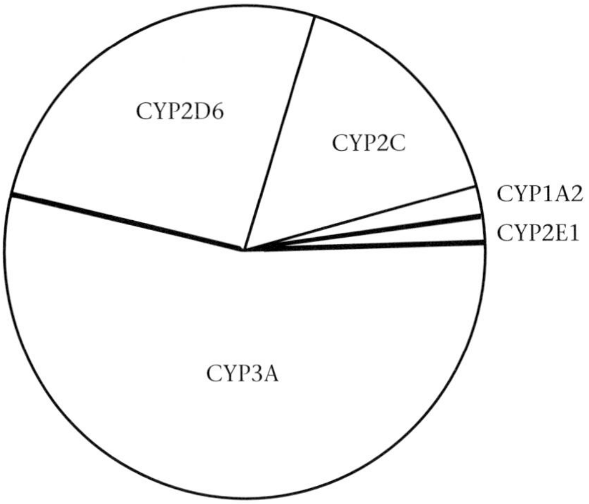

Figure 3.1: Pie chart showing the proportion of xenobiotics metabolised by the major human liver cytochrome P450 (CYPs) isoenzymes.

Carlo, 1997; Guengerich *et al.*, 1998). With the development of mono-specific anti-CYP peptide antibodies against the major xenobiotic metabolising isoforms of CYP, it has been possible to probe the comparative CYP content of 30 human liver microsomal samples (Edwards *et al.*, 1998). CYP3A was seen in 97% of samples. Some CYPs were lacking in a percentage of individuals indicating polymorphic expression: CYP2A6 (7%); CYP2C19 (10%); CYP2D6 (13%); CYP2B6 (80%). No constitutive hepatic CYP1A1 or CYP1B1 expression could be detected by immunochemical methods, in agreement with the known inducible nature of these hepatic enzymes.

In some instances, it could be argued that the diverse CYP functionalisation reactions might contribute to the detoxication of xenobiotics, for example by increasing solubility by hydroxylation or dealkylation. However, in general CYP oxidations are activating reactions and new functional groups are generated that bestow further reactivity. Many of the pathways in which CYPs are involved lead to the formation of reactive intermediates (e.g. epoxides) or allow leakage of highly toxic free radical species (e.g. dehalogenation) (Ortiz de Montellano, 1989). Examples of the various types of oxidative reactions that are catalysed by the MFO system are detailed below. In all of these oxidative reactions it is postulated that molecular oxygen acts as the oxygen atom donor.

3.3.1.1.1 Aliphatic and aromatic hydroxylation

Hydroxylation by the MFO system (Figure 3.2) is postulated to occur via the following multistep mechanism involving the iron centre of the haem moiety of CYP, where RH represents the substrate (Timbrell, 1991):

TABLE 3.1

Major isoforms of human hepatic CYPs involved in xenobiotic metabolism and examples to illustrate the wide variation of known substrates, inhibitors and inducers

Enzyme	Common substrates	Inhibitors	Inducers
CYP1A1	Poly aromatic hydrocarbons (PAHs), e.g. benzo(a)pyrene, ethoxyresorufin, 6-Nitrochrysene, Paracetamol, Quinones	7,8-Benzoflavone, Ellipticine, Phenethylisothiocyanate	Poly aromatic hydrocarbons (PAHs)
CYP1A2	Acetanilide, Caffeine, Estradiol, 7-Ethoxyresorufin, Flutamide, Imipramine, Lignocaine, Mianserin, Mexiletine, Paracetamol, Phenacetin, Propafenone, Theophylline, Verapamil, Warfarin	7,8-Benzoflavone, Fluvoxamine, Furafylline, α-Naphthoflavone,	5-t-Butyl-1,3 benzodioxole, 3,3-Diindolylmethane, Omeprazole, Simazine, 2,3,7,8 Tetrachloro-dibenzo-p-dioxin (TCDD)
CYP2A6	Corticosteroids, Coumarin, Halothane, Nicotine, 4-Nitrophenol, 4-Nitroanisole	Diethyldithiocarbamate, 8-Methoxypsoralen, Tranylcypromine	Barbiturates, Dexamethasone
CYP2B6	Cyclophosphamide, Halothane, Ifosphamide, Lignocaine, Testosterone	Orphenadrine	Unknown
CYP2C8	Carbamazepine, Taxol, Tolbutamide, Warfarin	Quercetin, Sulphaphenazole, Sulfinpyrazone	Unknown
CYP2C9	Diazepam, Diclofenac, Ibuprofen, Phenylbutazone, Phenytoin, Piroxicam, Proguanil, Tenoxicam, Tienilic acid, Tolbutamide, Trimethoprim, Warfarin	Sulphaphenazole, Sulfinpyrazone	Rifampicin
CYP2C19	Citalopram, Clomipramine, Clozapine, Diazepam, Hexobarbital, Imipramine, Lansoprazole, S-Mephenytoin, Omeprazole, Pentamidine, Proguanil, Propranolol	Fluconazole, Omeprazole, Tranylcypromine, Warfarin	Rifampicin
CYP2D6	Amitriptyline, Bufuralol, Cinnarizine, Citalopram, Clomipramine, Clozapine, Codeine, Debrisoquine, Desipramine, Dextromethorphan, Encainide, Flecainide, Fluoxetine, Fluphenazine, Imipramine, Metoprolol, Mexiletene, Mianserin, Nortriptyline, Ondansetron, Paroxetine, Perhexiline, Propafenone, Propranolol, Sparteine, Thioridazine, Timulol, Trifluperidol	Ajmaline, Amiodarone, Clomipramine, Flecainide, Fluoxetine, Paroxetine, Quinidine, Trifluperidol	Unknown

CYP2E1	Aniline, Benzene, Caffeine, Chlorzoxazone, Dapsone, Enflurane, Ethanol, Halothane, Isoflurane, Methylformamide, 4-Nitroanisole, 4-Nitrophenol, Pyridine, Styrene, Theophylline, Toluene	3-Amino-1,2,3-triazole, Diethyldithiocarbamate, Dihydrocapsaicin, Dimethylsulphoxide, Disulfiram, Phenethyl isothiocyanate, 4-Methylpyrazole	Acetone, Ethanol, Isoniazid, 4-Methylpyrazole, Pyridine
CYP3A4	Alfentanil, Amiodarone, Astemizole, Benzphentamine, Budesonide, Carbemazepine, Cyclophosphamide, Cyclosporin, Dapsone, Digitoxin, Diltiazem, Diazepam, Erythromycin, Ethinylestradiol, Etoposide, Ifosphamide, Imipramine, Lansoprazole, Lignocaine, Loratadine, Losartan, Lovastatin, Midazolam, Nifedipine, Omeprazole, Paracetamol, Quinidine, Retinoic acid, Tacrolimus, Taxol, Teniposide, Terfenadine, Tetrahydrocannabinol, Theophylline, Toremifene, Triazolam, Troleandomycin, Verapamil, Warfarin	Clotrimazole, Ethinylestradiol, Gestodene, Itraconazole, Ketoconazole, Miconazole, Naringenin, Troleandomycin	Carbemazepine, Dexamethasone, Omeprazole, Phenobarbital, Phenytoin, Rifampicin, Sulphadimidine, Sulphinpyrazone, Troleandomycin
CYP4	Lauric acid, Leukotrienes, Midazolam, Prostaglandins	None known	Clofibrate

More examples can be seen on the webpage 'Cytochrome P450 Drug Interaction Table' (listed in Appendix 2).

$$Fe^{3+} + RH \rightarrow Fe^{3+}RH$$
$$Fe^{3+}RH + e^{-} \rightarrow Fe^{2+}RH$$
$$Fe^{2+}RH + O_2 \rightarrow Fe^{2+}RH{-}O{-}O$$
$$Fe^{2+}RH{-}O{-}O + e^{-} \rightarrow Fe^{3+} + H_2O + ROH$$

The electrons in this reaction scheme are provided by the MFO system NAD(P)H reductase, which catalyses the oxidation of its NAD(P)H cofactor.

There are hundreds of known substrates for CYP hydroxylation, some of which are shown in Scheme 3.1 as examples (Lessard *et al.*, 1997; Nakajima *et al.*, 1997; Eiermann *et al.*, 1998; Hiroi, Imaoka and Funae, 1998; Yang *et al.*, 1998).

3.3.1.1.2 Alcohol oxidation

Scheme 3.2 illustrates the principle of oxidation of alcohols to aldehydes (for primary alcohols) or ketones (for secondary and tertiary alcohols) by the MFO system (for review see Lieber, 1999). The products are more susceptible to nucleophilic attack than the parent alcohol due to the increased electropositivity of the newly formed carbonyl carbon atom. For example, 2-hexanol is converted to hexan-2,5-diol, which is further converted to the neurotoxin hexane-2,5-dione (Scheme 3.2) (Toftgard *et al.*, 1986).

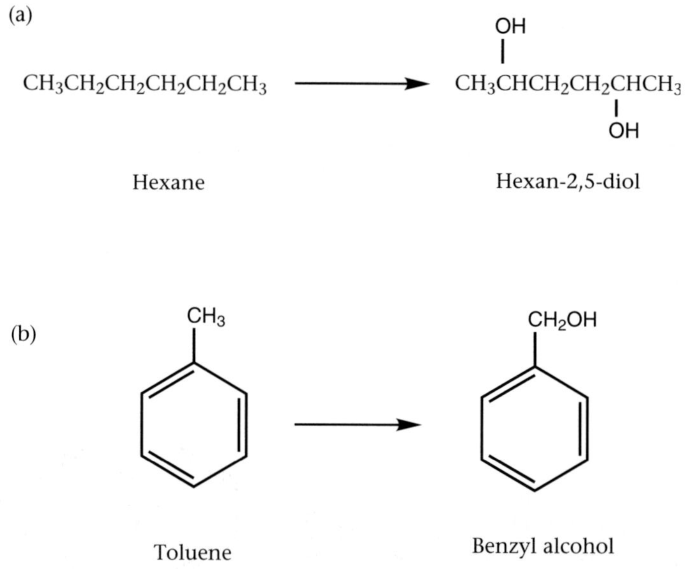

Scheme 3.1: Examples of: (a) aliphatic and (b) aromatic hydroxylation by the MFO system.

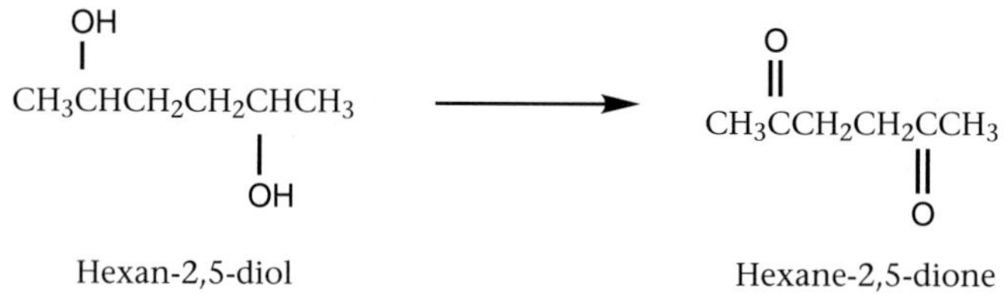

Scheme 3.2: Example of aliphatic alcohol oxidation by the MFO system.

3.3.1.1.3 Epoxidation

Scheme 3.3(a) illustrates how epoxidation can lead to activation of a compound. In this case trichloroethylene is converted firstly to an epoxide, which is formed across the unsaturated C=C bond, and finally to an aldehyde; both of these products are susceptible to nucleophilic attack. Epoxides are particularly short-lived, highly reactive species.

Scheme 3.3(b) illustrates a general unsaturated ring epoxidation that ultimately leads to an increase in solubility for the lipophilic aromatic compound (in this case the pneumotoxin naphthalene) by hydroxylation (England *et al.*, 1998).[2]

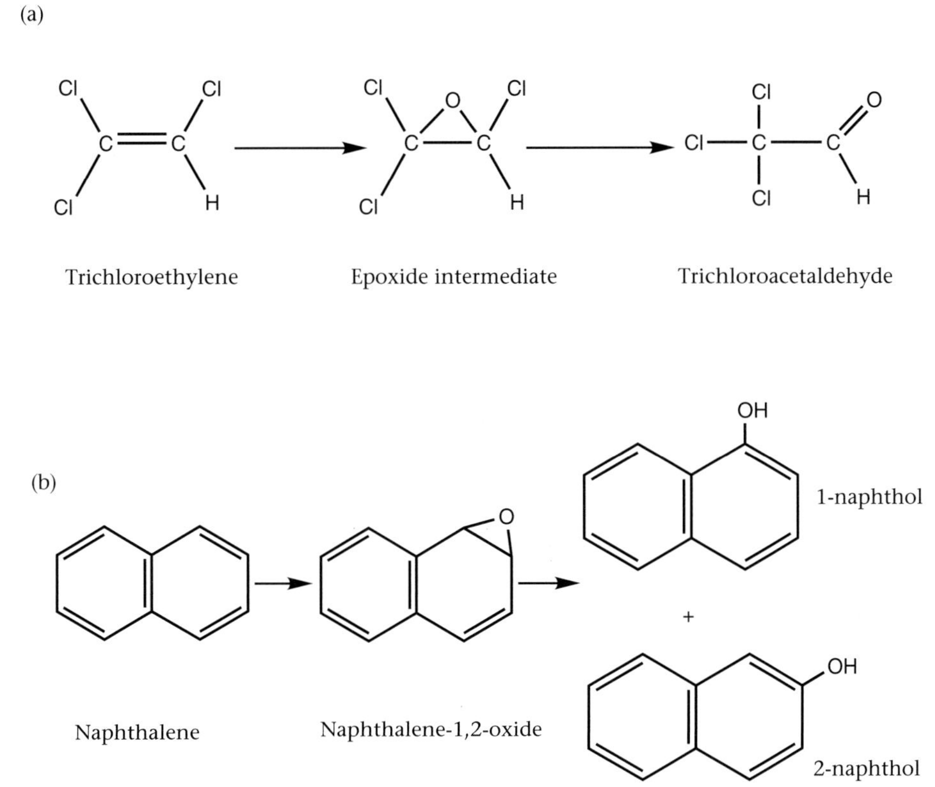

Scheme 3.3: Examples of epoxidation performed by the MFO system for (a) trichloroethylene, which is activated first to epoxide and then to a reactive aldehyde and (b) naphthalene, which is initially activated to an epoxide that is ultimately detoxified to an alcohol.

3.3.1.1.4 N-, O- and S-dealkylation

As can be seen in Scheme 3.4, although dealkylation may lead to an increase in solubility of the substrate by the removal of hydrophobic groups, the generation of a new reactive functional group by deprotection and the potential generation of toxic side products lead these mechanisms to be classed as activations. Demethylation reactions (e.g. Scheme 3.4(a and c)), in oxidising conditions, may lead to the generation of formaldehyde or methyl radicals, both of which could result in toxic effects. N-demethylation of clozapine, an antipsychotic drug, is an example of this (Fang *et al.*, 1998). Chlorimipramine, chlorpromazine and buprenorphine are also classical examples of xenobiotics that can undergo N-dealkylation by CYP (Kobayashi *et al.*, 1998; Valoti *et al.*, 1998).

(a) *N*-dealkylation

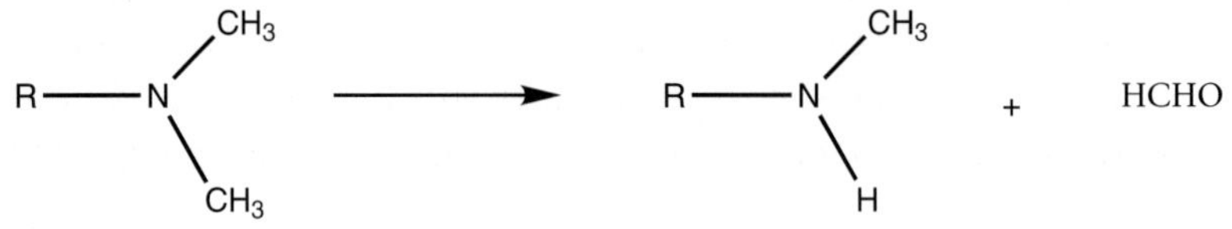

(b) *O*-dealkylation

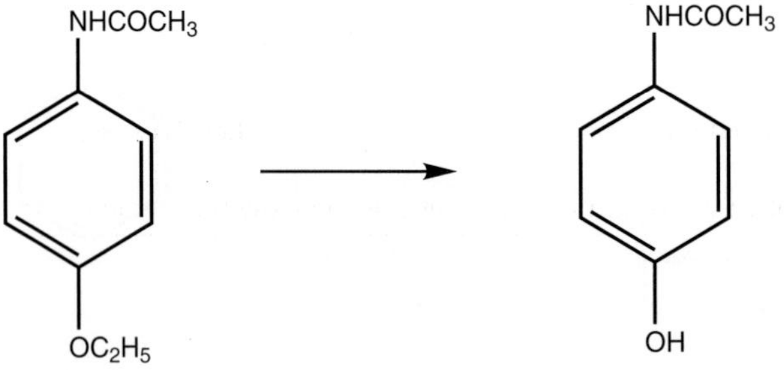

Phenacetin

Paracetamol

(c) *S*-dealkylation

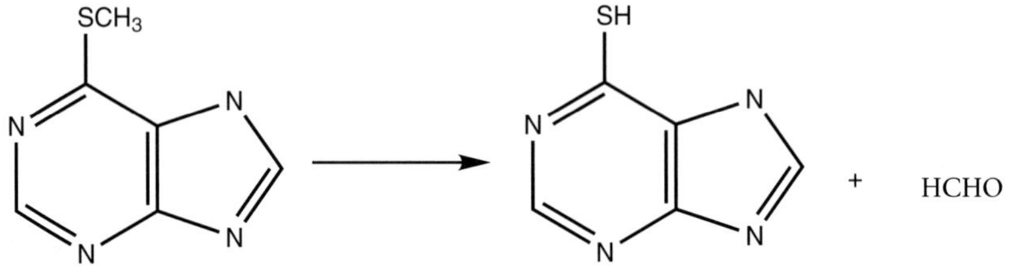

6-methylthiopurine

6-mercaptopurine

Scheme 3.4: Examples of: (a) N-, (b) O- and (c) S-dealkylation performed by the MFO system. Note that in the demethylation reactions shown in (a) and (c), formaldehyde is a potentially toxic by-product of the reaction.

3.3.1.1.5 Oxidative deamination (of amines containing -CH(CH$_3$)-NH$_2$)

When secondary amines, such as in the example in Scheme 3.5, are oxidatively deaminated, the resulting ketone product is more susceptible to nucleophilic attack than the parent amine, therefore the reaction is activating. Ammonia is also generated as a by-product. A typical example of xenobiotic deamination is that of amphetamine (Yamada *et al.*, 1997).

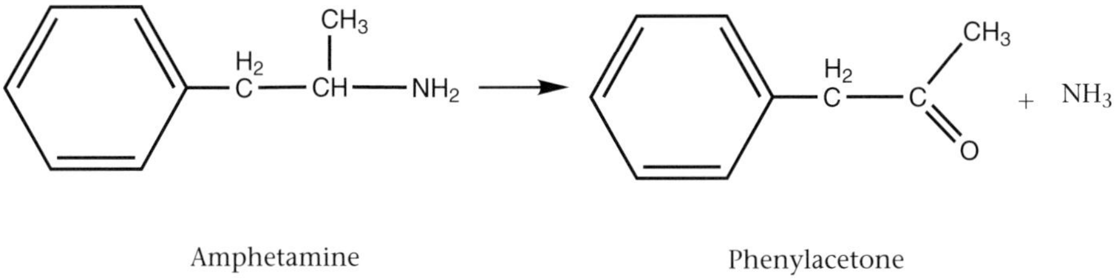

Scheme 3.5: Example of oxidative deamination performed by the MFO system.

3.3.1.1.6 N- and S-oxidation

S-oxidation by CYP is common for phenothiazines such as chlorpromazine (Scheme 3.6), an antidepressant, and mequitazine (i.e. 10-(3-quinuclidinylmethyl)-phenothiazine), which is a long acting selective histamine H1 receptor antagonist (Nakamura *et al.*, 1998). CYP2D6 has been implicated as the major isoform responsible for metabolising phenothiazines.

(a) *N*-oxidation

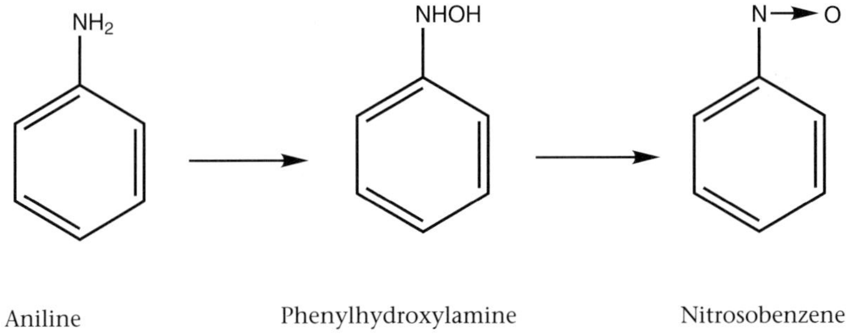

Scheme 3.6: Examples of: (a) N- and (b) S-oxidation performed by the MFO system.

(b) *S*-oxidation

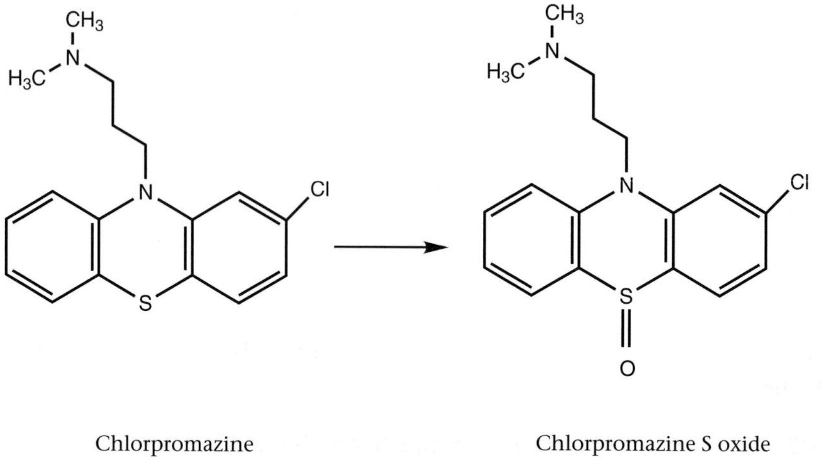

Scheme 3.6: Continued.

3.3.1.1.7 Phosphorothionate oxidation

A typical example of phosphorothionate oxidation is that for the organophosphorus insecticide parathion (Scheme 3.7) (Agyeman and Sultatos, 1998).

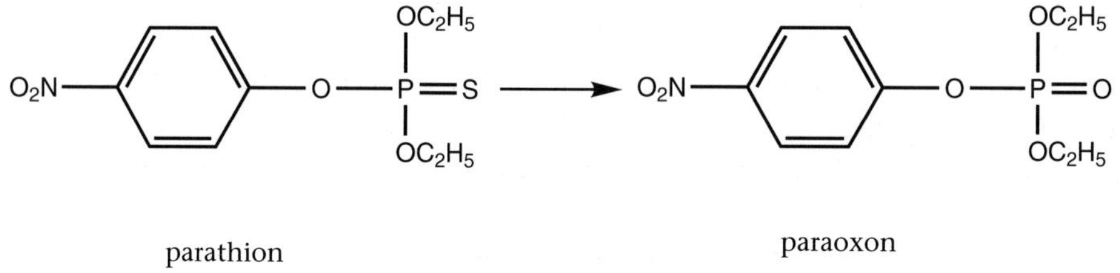

Scheme 3.7: Example of phosphothionate oxidation by the MFO system.

3.3.1.1.8 Dehalogenation

A typical example of xenobiotic oxidative dehalogenation is that for halothane (Scheme 3.8), which has been observed to be principally due to CYP2E1 metabolism (Spracklin *et al.*, 1997).

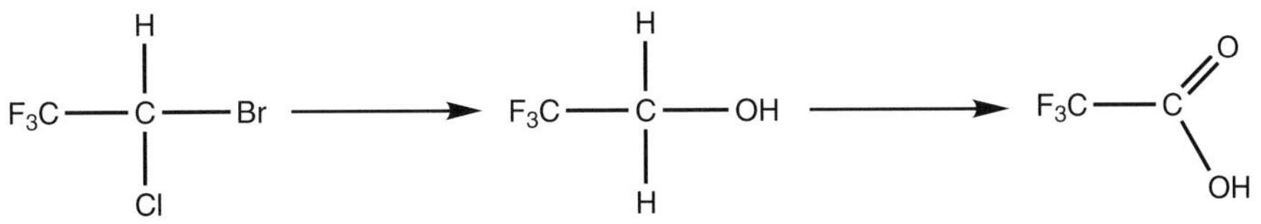

halothane

Scheme 3.8: Example of oxidative dehalogenation performed by the MFO system.

For an overview of the reductive metabolism performed by the MFO system, see section 3.3.1.3 below.

3.3.1.2 Oxidation by enzymes other than the MFO system

Although the MFO system is generally considered to be the main oxidoreductase system involved in xenobiotic metabolism, a range of other oxidoreductase enzymes may also be important (Beedham, 1997). Some of the major classes of alternative oxidoreductases are discussed in more detail below.

3.3.1.2.1 Alcohol dehydrogenase (ADH)

There are six classes of mammalian ADH (classes 1–6) (reviewed by Jornvall *et al.*, 1995 and Duester *et al.*, 1999), which are defined by sequence homology and substrate specificities. Five of these six, classes 1–5, have been identified in humans (see Table 3.2). In general, ADH catalyses the interconversion of alcohols and aldehydes (Scheme 3.9a) using NAD^+/NADH as a cofactor. Alcohols are oxidised to reactive aldehydes that can, amongst other things, covalently bind to macromolecules. However, ADH also has the capacity to act as an aldehyde dismutase by converting aldehydes, in the presence of NAD^+ cofactor, to acids (Scheme 3.9a) (Svensson *et al.*, 1996). Hence, there is a balance between all of the competing activating and detoxifying properties of this enzyme.

The three-dimensional crystal structure of horse liver ADH class I has been well characterised and the active site mechanisms probed using a variety of substrates, including substituted benzyl alcohols and ethanol, with and without the cofactor NAD (Colby *et al.*, 1998; Li *et al.*, 1994; Ramaswamy, Eklund and Plapp, 1994). A structure of human ADH class I $\beta_3\beta_3$ has also been determined with the cofactor NAD^+ and the competitive inhibitor 4-iodopyrazole bound (Davis *et al.*, 1996). A colour ribbon view of the structurally homologous ADH class 1 $\beta_1\beta_1$ dimer with NAD and 4-iodopyrazole in the active site is shown in Figure 3.2 (see colour section). These structures have also been compared with that of the human class IV $\sigma\sigma$ form of ADH (Xie *et al.*, 1997). Human $\chi\chi$ ADH, a glutathione-dependent formaldehyde dehydrogenase, has also been structurally characterised in complex with NAD^+ (Yang, Bosron and Hurley, 1997). These structures

TABLE 3.2
Human ADH isoenzymes: genes, subunits, catalytic forms and substrates

ADH class	1	2	3	4	5
Gene	ADH1 ADH2 ADH3	ADH4	ADH5	ADH7	ADH6
Subunit	α (β_1, β_2, β_3) (γ_1, γ_2)	π	$\chi_1\chi_2$	σ	Unknown
Catalytic forms	Homo- and heterodimers of α, β and γ subunits	$\pi\pi$	$\chi\chi$	$\sigma\sigma$	Unknown
Substrates	Ethanol and primary alcohols (Li & Bosron, 1981)	Primary aliphatic alcohols and aromatic aldehydes (Ditlow *et al.*, 1984; Mardh *et al.*, 1986)	Formaldehyde (Koivusalo, 1989)	Retinol (Haselbeck & Duester, 1997) and aromatic aldehydes (Moreno and Pares, 1991)	Unknown

have confirmed the requirement of a catalytic zinc atom in the active site of the enzyme that is postulated to bind directly to the alcohol/aldehyde substrate in mammalian ADHs. Figure 3.3(a–d) (see colour section) shows overlays of the active site from $\beta1$ with (b) the α, (c) the χ and (d) the σ monomer active sites. It can be seen from these overlays that α, β and σ active sites possess very similar spacial arrangements to one another but that the χ active site is markedly different from the other three.

Pyrazole and 4-methylpyrazole are often the inhibitors of choice in activity studies looking at the substrate metabolising capabilities of ADH. However, these inhibitors are also substrates for CYPs and therefore their use does not entirely prove that ADH alone is responsible for alcohol conversion. Also, these inhibitors are not ADH class-specific.

3.3.1.2.2 Aldehyde dehydrogenase (ALDH)

There are 12 mammalian classes of ALDH that have been classified at the gene level (reviewed by Yoshida *et al.*, 1998; see Table 3.3). ALDHs were originally classified into three different classes: class 1 includes the cytosolic forms; class 2 includes the mitochondrial forms and class 3 comprises the dioxin-inducible ALDH3 enzyme and microsomal ALDHs (Weiner and Flynn, 1989). ALDH catalyses the irreversible conversion of aldehydes to carboxylic acids (Sladek *et al.*, 1989), where the cofactor is NAD^+ and the oxygen donor is water (Scheme 3.9a and b).

TABLE 3.3
Human ALDH isoenzymes

ALDH isoenzyme	Class	Tissue	Subcellular localisation	Major substrate	Subunit no. amino acids
ALDH1	1	liver, stomach, brain, blood, eye lens, hair roots, etc.	cytosolic	retinal	500
ALDH2	2	liver, stomach, etc.	mitochondrial	acetaldehyde	500
ALDH3	3	stomach, lung	cytosolic	fatty and aromatic aldehydes	452
ALDH4	2	liver, kidney	mitochondrial	glutamate γ-semialdehyde	~540
ALDH5	2	testis, liver	mitochondrial	propionaldehyde	500
ALDH6	1	stomach, kidney, salivary gland	cytosolic	aliphatic aldehydes	511
ALDH7	3	kidney, lung	microsomal	aliphatic and aromatic aldehydes	467
ALDH8	3	parotid	microsomal	unknown	450
γABDH	1	liver, kidney, muscle	cytosolic	amine aldehyde	492
FALDH	3	liver, heart, muscle	microsomal	fatty and aromatic aldehydes	484
SSDH	2	brain, liver, heart	mitochondrial	succinic semialdehyde	488
MMSDH	2	kidney, liver, heart	mitochondrial	methylmalonate semialdehyde	503

Data adapted from Yoshida *et al.*, 1998. The class definitions are based on the nomenclature originated by Weiner & Flynn (1989).

The three-dimensional structure of bovine ALDH class 2, which is a mitochondrial enzyme, has been determined in its apo and NAD-bound forms (Steinmetz *et al.*, 1997). This structure suggests that the oxygen donor in the conversion of aldehyde to acid is water and that an active site glutamic acid (Glu) residue acts as the general base in the mechanism. Subsequent site-directed mutagenesis of human liver ALDH class 2 studies

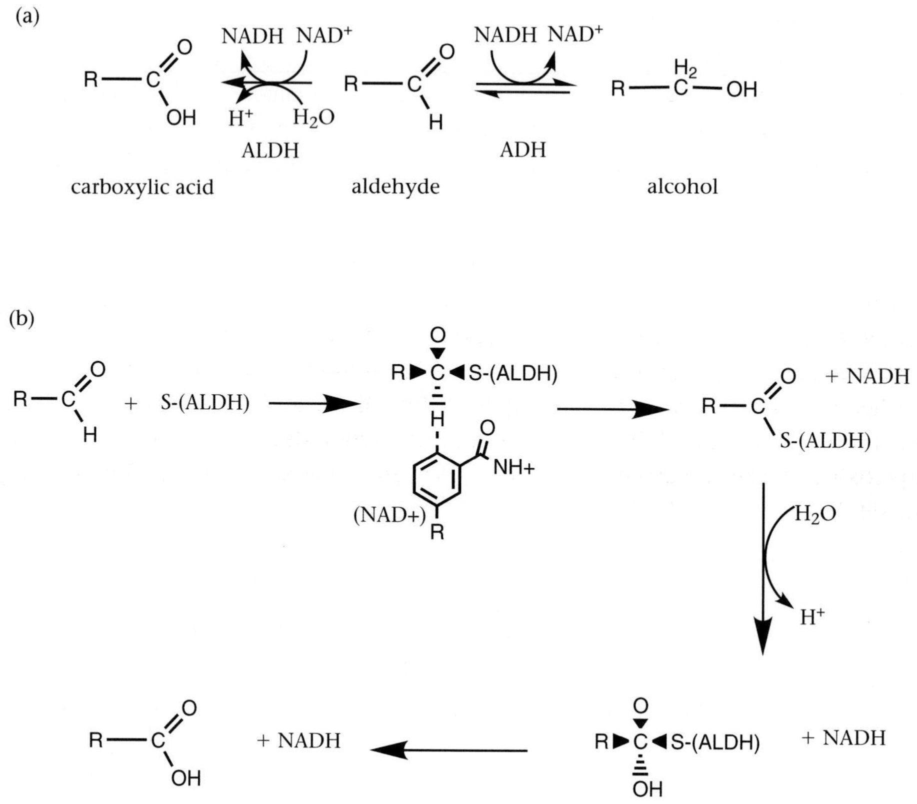

Scheme 3.9: (a) General biotransformation of aldehydes and alcohols by the enzymes alcohol dehydrogenase (ADH) and aldehyde dehydrogenase (ALDH). (b) The postulated mechanism for ALDH class 3 activity via an active site cysteine residue (Liu *et al.*, 1997).

have confirmed that Glu268 is the general base that is necessary to activate an active site cysteine nucleophile that is essential to both dehydrogenase and esterase activities (Sheikh *et al.*, 1997).

A structure of an ALDH class 3 enzyme has also been determined and a mechanism of enzyme specificity and activity has been postulated (Scheme 3.9b) (Liu *et al.*, 1997). The active site from this structure is illustrated in colour in Figure 3.4 (see colour section).

A general inhibitor of ALDH commonly used in activity studies is disulfiram (antabuse), although as different classes of ALDH have different physiological roles it may be more relevant to look at class-specific inhibitors. Russo *et al.* (1995) have identified 4-(N,N-dimethylamino)benzaldehyde as a potent, reversible inhibitor of class 1 ALDH. A study by Kikonyogo (Kikonyogo and Pietruszko, 1997) has shown that the histamine H2-receptor antagonists, cimetidine and tiotidine, are potent competitive inhibitors of human E3 ALDH activity with aldehyde substrates.[3]

3.3.1.2.3 Xanthine oxidase

Xanthine oxidase is a molybdenum containing flavoenzyme that is involved in the metabolism of purines and pyrimidines. Its name derives from the classic conversion of hypoxanthine to xanthine to uric acid (Scheme 3.10). At present, there is no structural information on any mammalian form of the enzyme and in general little is known about xanthine oxidase in humans. It has been detected in the liver and has been identified as a major cytoplasmic source of superoxide radicals and hydrogen peroxide, both of which are highly reactive by-products (Sarnesto, Linder and Raivio, 1996).

There is some evidence from a bacterial form of xanthine oxidase, that a molybdenum bound water molecule acts as the oxygen donor but as yet there is no evidence of this in a mammalian form (Huber *et al.*, 1996). A range of inhibition studies with the purified enzyme have shown that purpurogallin, allopurinol, silymarin, catechins from tea and flavonoids all inhibit activity, and some flavonoids have also been seen to act as superoxide radical scavengers (Cos *et al.*, 1998; Sheu, Lai and Chiang, 1998; Aucamp *et al.*, 1997).

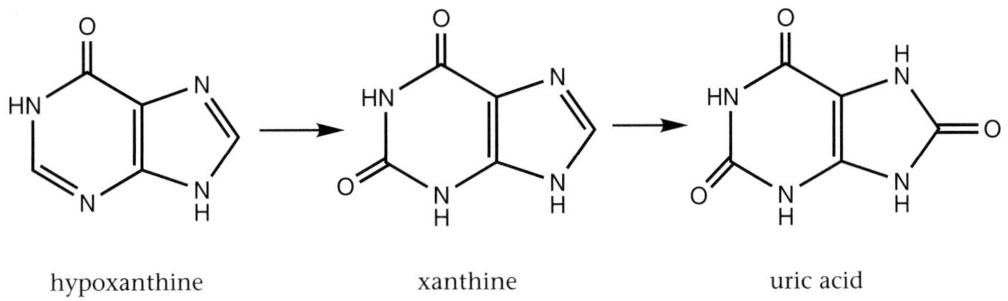

Scheme 3.10: Conversion of hypoxanthine to uric acid by xanthine oxidase.

3.3.1.2.4 Monoamine oxidase (MAO)

Monoamine oxidases (A and B) are typically involved in the conversion of primary amines to aldehydes (Scheme 3.11).

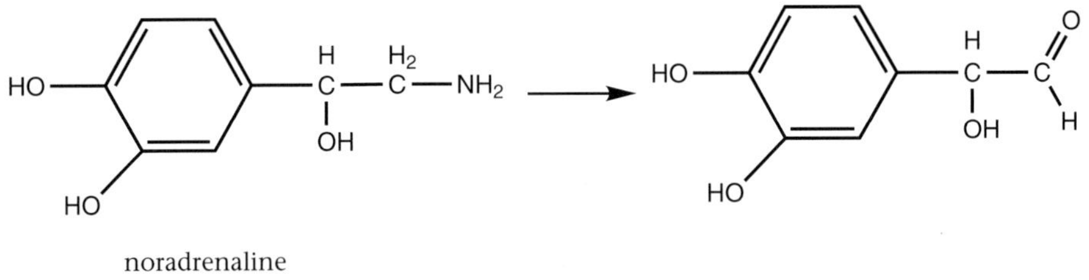

Scheme 3.11: Example of primary amine oxidation by monoamine oxidase.

A partial three-dimensional model of human monoamine oxidase A has been determined and shows the FAD cofactor bound covalently to an active site cysteine residue (Wouters and Baudoux, 1998) (Figure 3.5, see colour section).

A variety of nitrogen-containing inhibitors of monoamine oxidase, which are reversible and selective have recently been identified (reviewed by Wouters, 1998).

3.3.1.2.5 Flavin-containing monooxygenase (FMO)

FAD-containing monooxygenases (FMO) perform a variety of oxidations at N- and S-centres (Ziegler, 1990) (Scheme 3.12). They require NADPH as cofactor and use molecular oxygen as the oxidative species. Five major forms of FMO are known (FMO1–5), classified within mammals by amino acid sequence similarities (Lawton *et al.*, 1994). The cDNA for three classes, FMO1, FMO3 and FMO4 have been observed in humans. However, differential expression is seen between species and organs, e.g. FMO1 is expressed in adult human kidney but not in liver, whereas in other mammals, FMO1 is the major hepatic form (Dolphin *et al.*, 1996).

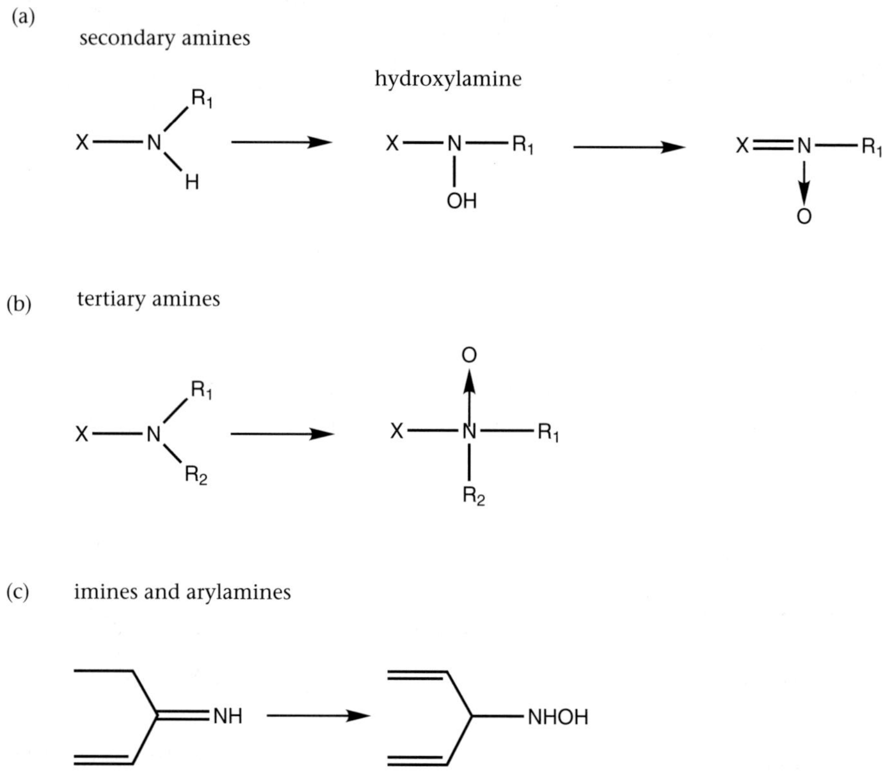

Scheme 3.12: Examples of: (a) secondary amine, (b) tertiary amine and (c) imine and arylamine oxidation by FMOs.

3.3.1.2.6 *Aromatase*

Aromatase (CYP19) is a cytochrome P450 that is involved in the *in vivo* synthesis of oestrogens (Chen, 1998). As this enzyme is principally involved in endogenous metabolism, it has been considered separately here, rather than included in the general discussion of xenobiotic metabolism by CYPs in section 3.3.1.1. However, aromatase activity may have some relevance to the metabolism of steroids when they are administered therapeutically. In particular, steroids and flavones have been seen to act as aromatase inhibitors (Brodie and Njar, 1998; Moslemi and Seralini, 1997). A typical example of how aromatase action may also be applicable to xenobiotics is given in Scheme 3.13 for cyclohexane carboxylic acid. The aromatisation depends upon the presence of FAD and molecular oxygen and the CoA derivatisation of the carboxylic acid group. A theoretical study on the mechanism of aromatase action has concluded that, from a chemically geometric point of view, only a mechanism via a ferroxy radical is feasible (Ahmed, 1997).

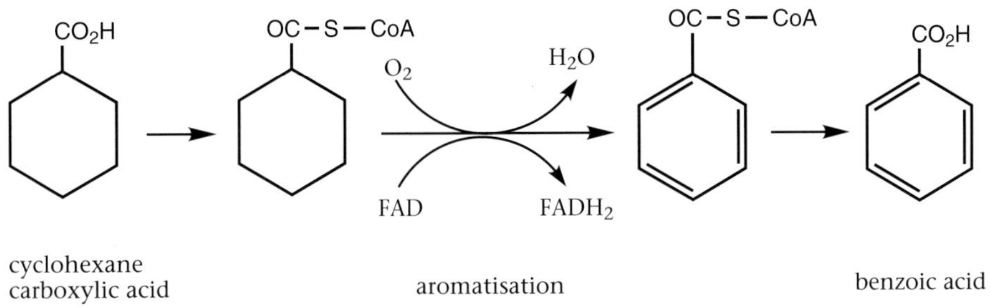

Scheme 3.13: Example of aromatase action.

3.3.1.2.7 *Hydroxysteroid dehydrogenase (HSD)*

Steroid oxidation is an important feature of endogenous metabolism and in general HSDs are substrate specific CYP enzymes that perform specific oxidations at designated

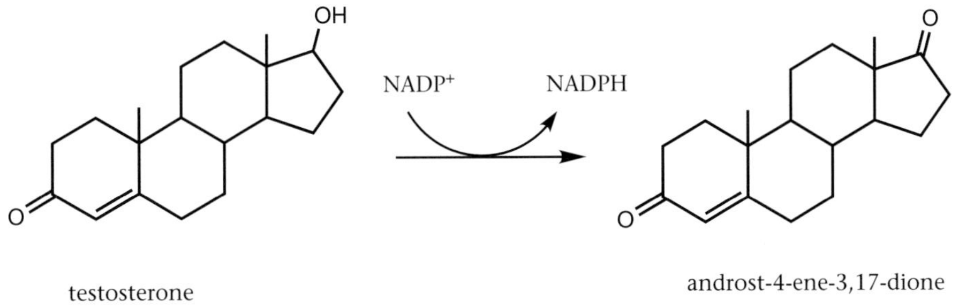

Scheme 3.14: Example of testosterone oxidation at the C17 position by 17-hydroxysteroid oxidoreductase.

atoms on the steroid ring system (Penning, 1997), thus they are named according to these properties. For example, testosterone is specifically oxidised at the C17 atom to androst-4-ene-3,17-dione by the CYP enzyme 17-HSD (Scheme 3.14).

The best characterised of the mammalian HSDs, with respect to chemical reactivity, are rat liver 3α-HSD (Penning *et al.*, 1997) and human oestrogenic 17β-HSD (Lin *et al.*, 1996) in that their three-dimensional structures are known.

3.3.1.2.8 Peroxidases

Peroxidases are an important family of enzymes involved in endogenous metabolism, which include prostaglandin synthases (PGSs), lactoperoxidase and myeloperoxidase. All of these enzymes catalyse the conversion of -OOH to -OH with the possible generation of free-radical intermediates and by-products.

As an example, Scheme 3.15 illustrates:

- a how the final step of the synthesis of prostaglandin H by prostaglandin H synthase (PGHS) can lead to the oxidation of a xenobiotic substrate; and
- b how free radicals are generated on reaction of a substrate with PGS and endoperoxide (see review by Smith, Curtis and Eling, 1991).

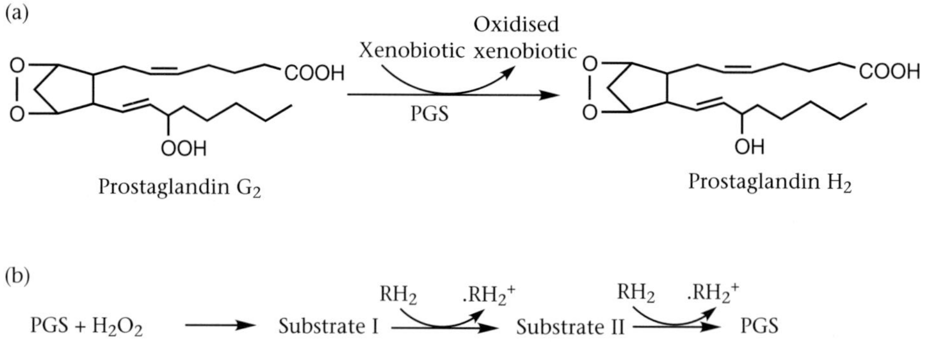

Scheme 3.15: (a) The oxidation of xenobiotics via the reduction of prostaglandin, as catalysed by PGS. The generation of free-radical intermediates by this system is shown in part (b).

For lactoperoxidase and myeloperoxidase, two structurally homologous enzymes, it has been suggested that aromatic substrates (peracids, alcohols or amines) may be the preferred substrates due to the presence of a hydrophobic pocket at the entrance to the haem cavity. EPR spectroscopic studies on myeloperoxidase indicated that the substrates phenol, p-cresol, resorcinol, and 4-amino salicylate all interact with the haem centre of the enzyme (Hori *et al.*, 1994). The nature of inhibitory binding of salicylhydroxamic acid to human myeloperoxidase has been investigated at the atomic level and revealed that the inhibitor was stabilised by hydrogen bonding in the active site but was not coordinated to the haem iron (Davey and Fenna, 1996).

3.3.1.3 Reduction by the MFO system

In addition to the oxidation by the MFO system, which has been described in section 3.3.1.1, the MFO system also performs a range of reductive reactions.

3.3.1.3.1 Azo and nitro compounds

Scheme 3.16 illustrates how the MFO system reduces azo and nitro compounds to primary amines. The electronic aspects of azo dye susceptibility to reduction by the MFO system have been reviewed by Zbaida (1995), who concluded that azo compounds possessing an overall Hammett sigma substituent constant more negative than −0.37, i.e. they have a significant number of electron-donating substituents, will not be reduced by the MFO system.

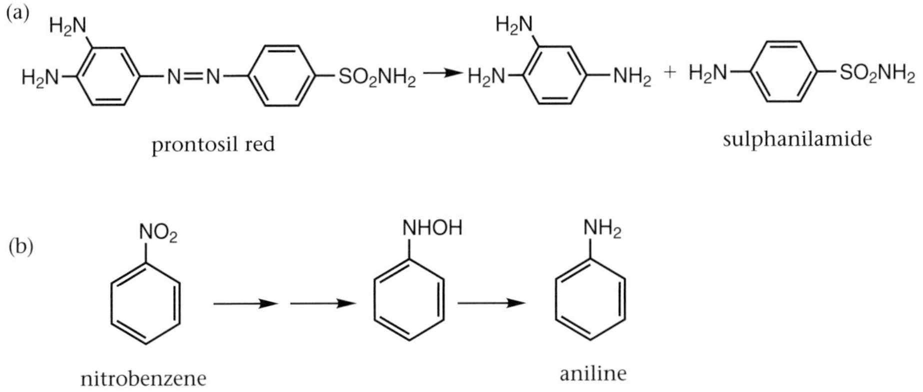

Scheme 3.16: Examples of reduction of: (a) an azo dye and (b) nitrobenzene by the MFO system.

3.3.1.3.2 Heterocyclic ring compounds

Ring cleavage by the MFO system may also activate xenobiotics by generating new functional groups (Scheme 3.17).

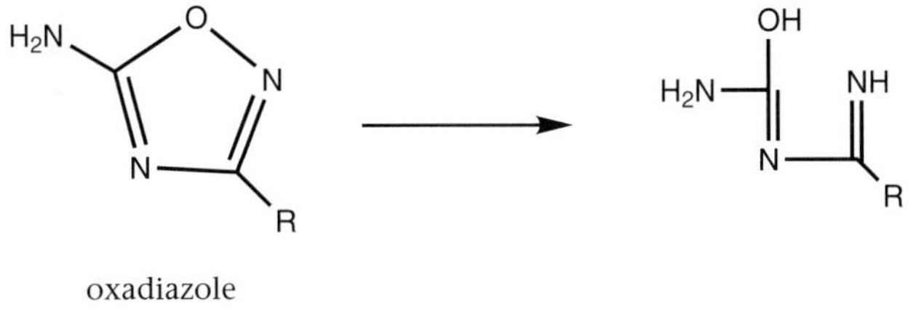

Scheme 3.17: Example of ring cleavage of a heterocyclic ring compound by the MFO system.

3.3.1.3.3 Halogenated hydrocarbons

The reduction of halothane (Scheme 3.18) is the classic example given to illustrate the reduction of halogenated hydrocarbons by the MFO system. The formation of the trifluorochloroacetyl radical is potentially damaging to tissue by covalent binding to macromolecules (Eliasson *et al.*, 1998).

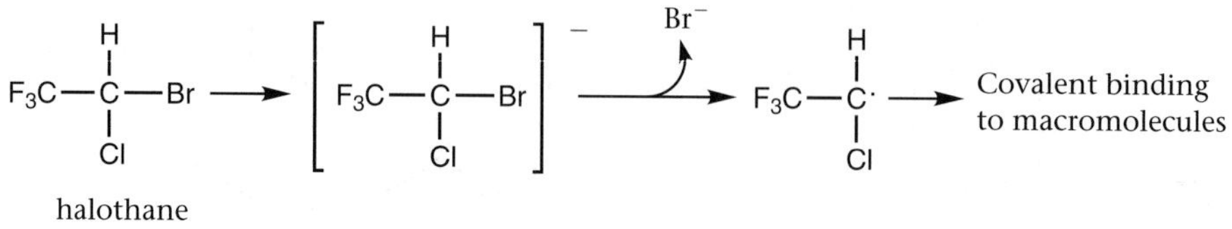

Scheme 3.18: Reductive dehalogenation of halothane by the MFO system.

3.3.1.4 Reduction by enzymes other than the MFO system

This section describes some of the major reductive enzymes other than the MFO system.

3.3.1.4.1 Azo-reductase and nitroreductase

Azo and nitro compounds may also be reduced, in a similar way to that described in section 3.3.3.1, by azoreductases and nitroreductases. In particular, reduction by these enzymes is performed by bacteria in the human intestinal tract (Rafii and Cerniglia, 1995).

3.3.1.4.2 Glutathione reductase and glutathione peroxidase

As well as reducing oxidised glutathione (GSSG) back to GSH, glutathione reductase also has the capacity to play a role in sulphoxide and sulphide reduction.

Intracellular glutathione peroxidase (GSHPx), the first identified mammalian selenium-containing protein, is a cytosolic enzyme (Aumann *et al.*, 1997). GSHPx is important in protecting the body against oxidative damage, by catalysing the reduction of organic hydroperoxides using glutathione as the reducing substrate. In addition to the classical cellular enzyme, there are two other forms of this peroxidase. A gastrointestinal form is hypothesised to be most important in defence against toxicity of ingested lipid hydroperoxides. A form purified from human plasma has been structurally characterised, but its physiological role remains unclear due to the low level of activity observed for this enzyme (Ren *et al.*, 1997). A study by Asahi *et al.* (1997) has shown that GSHPx can be specifically inactivated both by the nitric oxide donor, *S*-nitroso-*N*-acetyl-D,L-penicillamine and peroxynitrite, which suggests that a build-up of nitric oxide *in vivo* would ultimately lead to an increase in damaging intracellular peroxides.

3.3.1.4.3 Steroid reductases

In a similar way to the oxidation of steroids outlined in section 3.3.2, the reduction of steroids occurs by specific CYP enzymes that act at specific positions on the ring system (e.g. Scheme 3.19). The enzymes are named according to the specific reduction that they perform i.e. 5α-reductase performs its reduction at the C5 atom of a steroid.

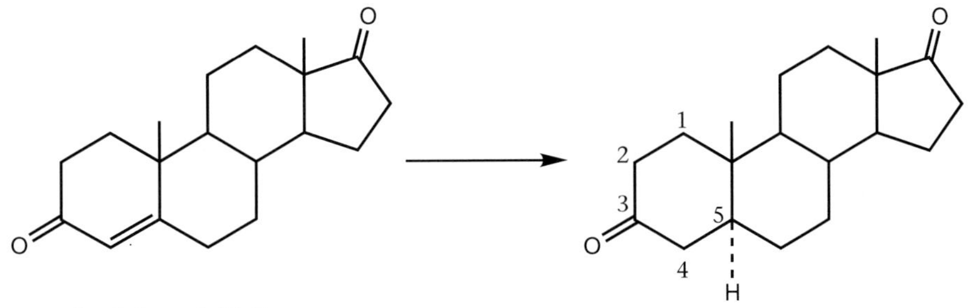

Scheme 3.19: Example of steroid reduction by 5α-reductase.

3.3.1.5 Hydrolysis

Hydrolysis is the term given to a reaction that involves cleavage of a substrate by the action of water.

3.3.1.5.1 Esterases

Esterases are the family of enzymes that hydrolyse esters and are important in the detoxication of xenobiotic esters (which may be commonly encountered as pesticides). The number of known esterase sequences is greater than 100 (Anthonsen *et al.*, 1995), which suggests a high degree of substrate selectivity is found with these enzymes, although the ester cleavage mechanisms are expected to be similar throughout. As a brief overview, there are three classes of esterase as defined by their interaction with organophosphates: A-esterases (e.g. arylesterase and phosphotriesterase) hydrolyse organophosphates; B-esterases (e.g. carboxylesterase, cholinesterase and arylamidase) are inhibited by organophosphates; C-esterases (e.g. acetylesterase) do not interact with organophosphates. Lipases, the enzymes that hydrolyse fatty acid esters, may also be termed as esterases.

Microsomal, cytosolic and plasma esterases have been identified, but the action of all esterases is typified by the examples for acetylcholine and procaine hydrolysis given in Scheme 3.20.

A few examples of *in vivo* studies illustrate the broad significance of esterase activity in metabolism. Carboxylesterases and lipases have been implicated in the hydrolysis of retinyl ester, which is the major storage form of vitamin A and is primarily found in the liver (Harrison, 1998). Retinyl esters are transported to peripheral tissues where they can be cleaved to release active vitamin A by a local esterase. The pesticides, fluazifop-butyl, carbaryl and paraoxon are all hydrolysed to differing extents in the liver, lung, blood

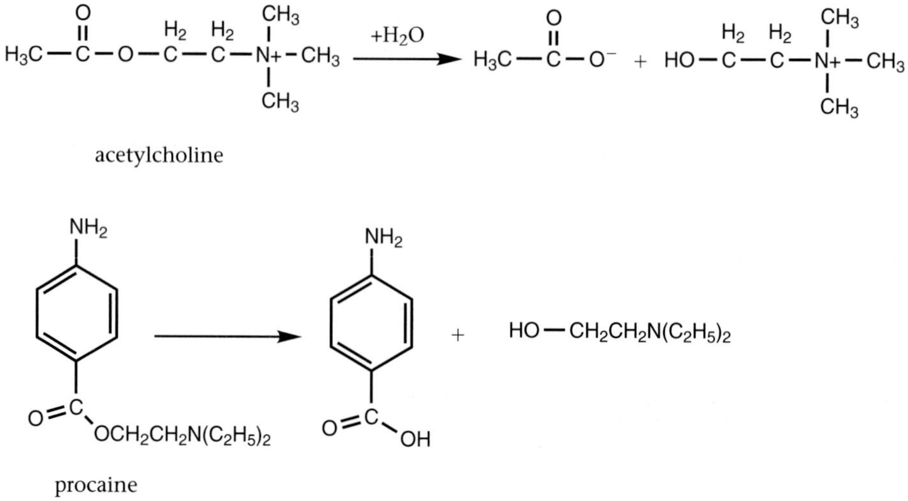

Scheme 3.20: Examples of esterase action on: (a) acetylcholine and (b) procaine.

and skin by esterases: fluazifop-butyl and carbaryl by carboxylesterases and paraoxon by plasma and microsomal arylesterases (McCracken, Blain and Williams, 1993).

Inhibition of arylesterase by aliphatic alcohols has been investigated empirically in human serum and theoretically by QSAR analysis and both methods indicated that as the length of the alkyl chain of the alcohol increased, inhibition increased (Debord *et al.*, 1998).

The classical inhibitors of esterases are: mercuric chloride (A-esterases, which contain an active site for cysteine); paraoxon (B-esterases); bis-nitrophenol phosphate (carboxylesterases) and physostigmine (cholinesterase) (Gaustad, Johnsen and Fonnum, 1991).

3.3.1.5.2 Amidase

The name amidase (amidohydrolase) is given to any enzyme that performs amide hydrolysis (Scheme 3.21). In mammalian systems, amidases are particularly important in:

a the breakdown of glycosylated proteins by cleaving the amide linkage formed between amino acids and oligosaccharides; and
b in the hydrolysis of bioactive fatty acid amides and esters, which is a process involved in neuromodulation.

Human lysosomal aspartylglucosaminidase, which specifically cleaves asparagine-oligosaccharide linkages, has been structurally characterised (Tikkanen *et al.*, 1996a, b) and provides some insight into the active site capabilities of glycoprotein amidases.

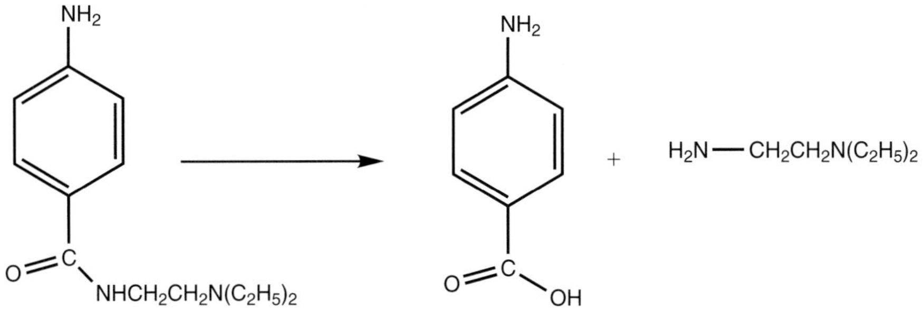

procainamide

Scheme 3.21: Example of amide hydrolysis by amidases.

Human, mouse and rat liver amidase activities have been identified for a specific membrane-bound fatty-acid amide hydrolase (FAAH) that hydrolyses cis-9-octadecenamide (oleamide) and N-arachidonoyl ethanolamine (anandamide), which are substrates of cannabinoid receptor (Cravatt *et al.*, 1996; Giang and Cravatt, 1997). The inactive metabolites of these two substrates are oleic acid and arachidonic acid, respectively. It has therefore been hypothesised that the main function of amidases is to inactivate bioactive signalling molecules such as fatty acid amides. Inhibitors of FAAH are known and include grenadadiene, arachidonoylethylene glycol and arachidonoyl serotonin (Bisogno *et al.*, 1998).

In rabbit liver, it has also been observed that metabolism of *N*-(3,5-dichlorophenyl)succinimide to 3,5-dichloroaniline and succinic acid was predominantly amidase-mediated (Griffin *et al.*, 1996).

It is also possible that amidases may catalyse hydrazide hydrolysis (Scheme 3.22).

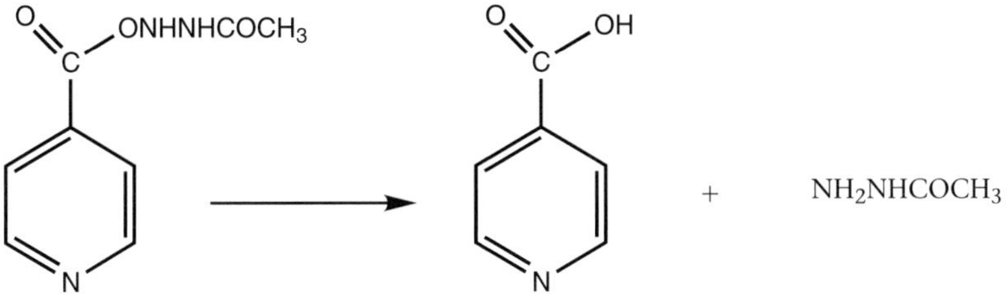

acetylisoniazid | isonicotinic acid | acetylhydrazine

Scheme 3.22: Potential hydrolysis of an example hydrazide by amidase.

3.3.1.6 Quinone:semiquinone redox cycling

A general scheme for quinone:semiquinone redox cycling by the MFO system is shown in Scheme 3.23. Quinones occur ubiquitously in biological membranes at low levels and play an essential role in the mitochondrial electron transport chain by generating oxidative species such as superoxide and hydroxyl radicals. Quinones are highly protein-reactive compounds that produce free radicals when they are metabolised, but enzymes such as superoxide dismutase and catalase exist *in vivo*, which control the production of damaging radicals. However, if a quinone is administered (for example, daunomycin and related compounds which are used as anticancer therapies), these endogenous enzymes that control the by-products of quinone metabolism are swamped with high

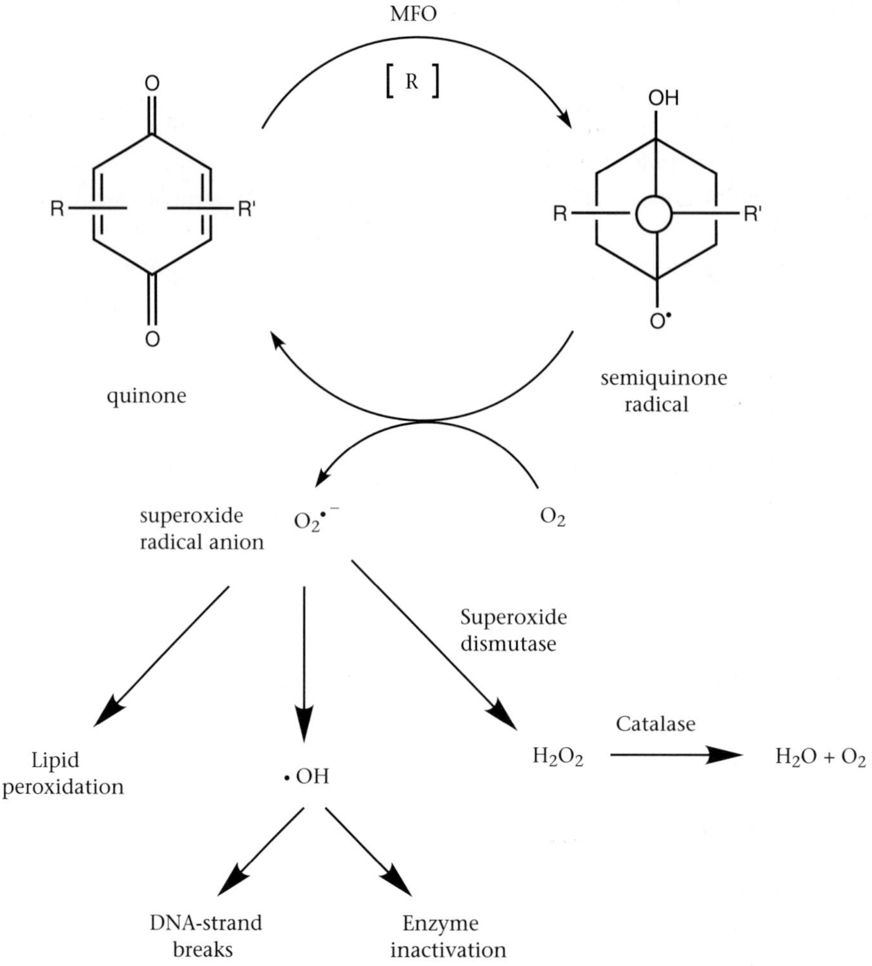

Scheme 3.23: General quinone redox cycling catalysed by NADH dehydrogenase and resulting potential toxicity from radical species.

local concentrations, which can result in the formation of high levels of cytotoxic radicals.

Quinones also bind to non-protein sulphhydryls, the major one being glutathione. This area is discussed in more detail under phase II metabolism (section 3.3.2).

3.3.1.7 Hydration

3.3.1.7.1 Epoxide hydrolase

Hydration mechanisms serve to add water to a compound to increase its solubility without causing dissociation of the compound. One important metabolic reaction where this occurs is the detoxication of epoxides by conversion to diols as performed by the enzyme epoxide hydrolase (Scheme 3.24). Enzymatic hydration is essentially irreversible and in general leads to metabolites that are more polar and less reactive than the parent compound (Seidegard and Ekstrom, 1997).

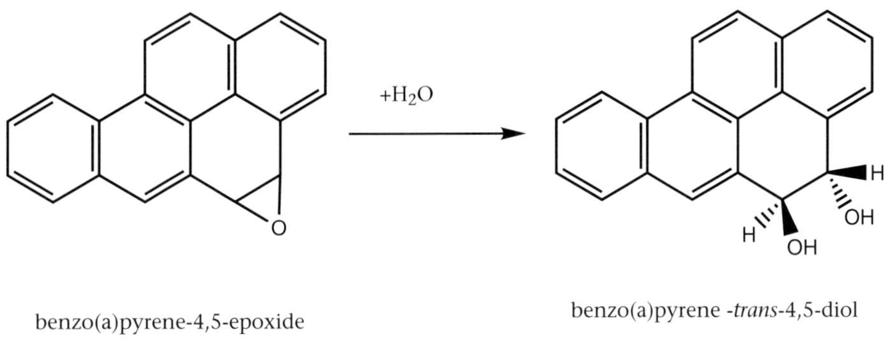

Scheme 3.24: Hydration of the epoxide group in benzo(a)pyrene-4,5-epoxide by epoxide hydrolase.

3.3.1.8 Miscellaneous non-enzymatic phase I reactions

The following reactions may occur non-enzymatically and cannot be classified into any of the above categories but may contribute in some cases of xenobiotic metabolism:

- i Ring cyclisation;
- ii N-carboxylation;
- iii Dimerisation;
- iv Transamidation;
- v Isomerisation;
- vi Decarboxylation;
- vii Dethioacetylation.

3.3.2 Phase II metabolism

Phase II metabolism involves the enzymes that perform conjugation reactions which, in general, have historically been designated as detoxication reactions. However, it is evident from research performed within the last decade that conjugation reactions can also lead to activation of xenobiotics, therefore the definition of phase II reactions purely leading to detoxication becomes untenable and over-simplistic (Olson *et al.*, 1992; Burchell and Coughtrie, 1997). In reality, a molecule that can be conjugated can also be deconjugated and the balance of these processes will contribute to the ultimate fate of the xenobiotic. Table 3.4 lists the major biotransformations that have been classified as phase II metabolism.

TABLE 3.4
Phase II enzymes and conjugation reactions

UDP-glucuronosyltransferase	– glucuronidation at -OH, -COOH, NH_2 and -SH
Sulphotransferase	– sulphation at $-NH_2$, $-SO_2NH_2$ and OH
Methyltransferase	– methylation at -OH and $-NH_2$
Acetyltransferase	– acetylation at $-NH_2$, $-SO_2NH_2$ and -OH
Glutathione S-transferase	– glutathione conjugation at epoxides and halides
Miscellaneous reactions	– amino acid conjugation at -COOH
	– condensation

3.3.2.1 Glucuronidation: glucuronosyltranferase vs glucuronidase

Glucuronide formation occurs via the action of microsomal UDP-glucuronosyltransferase isoforms typically with alcohols, phenols, hydroxylamines, carboxylic acids, amines, sulphonamides and thiols as substrates and uridine diphosphate glucuronic acid (UDPGA) as cofactor. Examples of glucuronide conjugation with chloramphenicol, sulphanilamide and disulfiram (antabuse) are shown in Scheme 3.25.

Although glucuronide conjugation has typically been regarded as a detoxication mechanism by increasing the solubility of the xenobiotic, it has recently been discovered that the production of glucuronide conjugates may contribute to the net drug effects of some xenobiotics (reviewed in Kroemer and Klotz, 1992). For example, morphine-6-glucuronide has a direct analgesic effect when administered. Also, some active compounds may be regenerated by cleavage of glucuronides via the enzyme glucuronidase, as has been observed for clofibric acid conjugates. Glucuronides also have the ability to covalently bind to protein, which leads to toxicity and immune responses; acyl glucuronides in particular are resistant to degradation by glucuronidases once they have undergone intramolecular rearrangement and may lead to toxicity (Spahn-Langguth and Benet, 1992). All of these cases illustrate possible activation by glucuronidation.

Systemically, it may be hypothesised that xenobiotic glucuronidation forms a more soluble metabolite that aids its transportation to a target tissue where, on arrival, the

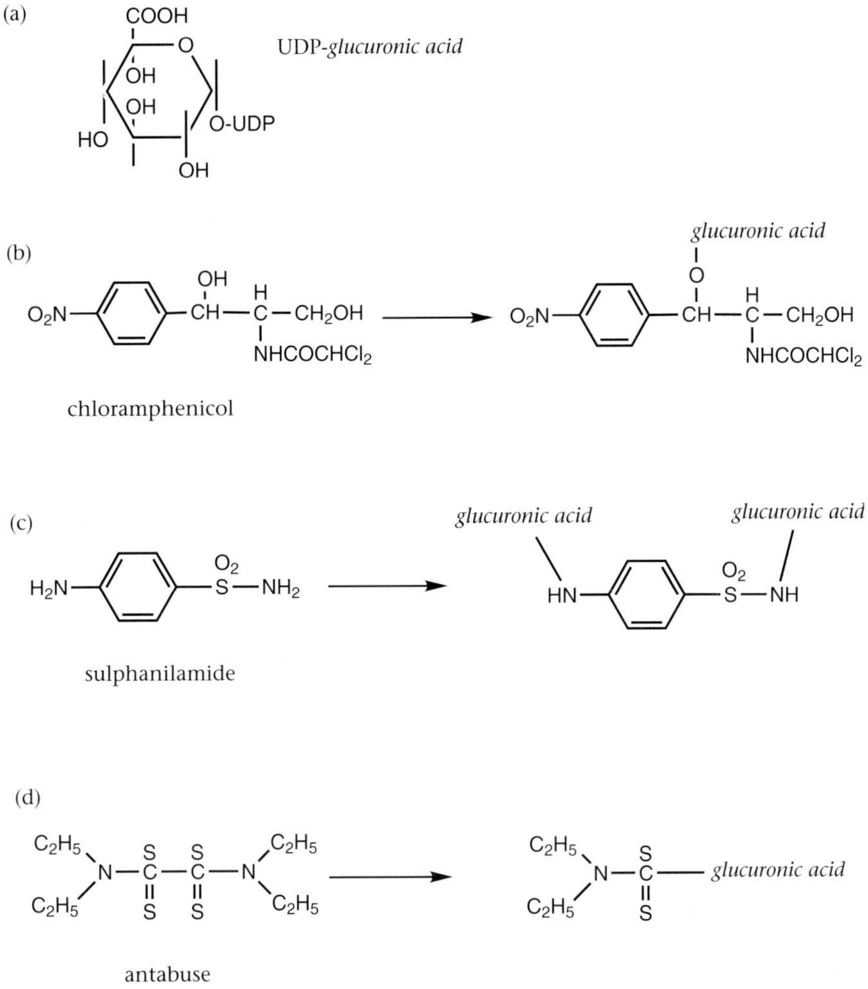

Scheme 3.25: Schematic of glucuronic acid (a) and examples of glucuronide conjugation of (b) chloramphenicol, (c) suphanilamide and (d) antabuse.

conjugate is reactivated enzymatically to the parent xenobiotic. Such may be the case for the *N*-glucuronidation of carcinogenic arylamines (and their *N*-hydroxylated metabolites), which can either lead to inactive metabolites or labile conjugates (Green and Tephly, 1998).

One particular area of glucuronidation, the importance of which has not been pharmacologically investigated, is the production of quaternary ammonium N^+-glucuronides via conjugation with tertiary amines (Hawes, 1998). This class of compounds includes, amongst others, the marketed drugs cyclizine, cyclobenzaprine, dothiepin, mianserin, tioconazole etc. and other antidepressants.

3.3.2.2 Sulphation: sulphotransferase vs sulphatase

Sulphation occurs via sulphotransferases, which use 3′-phosphoadenosine-5′-phosphosulphate (PAPS) as the sulphate donor (Scheme 3.26).

In general, sulphation leads to the detoxication of most xenobiotics, but there are some cases where sulphation leads to activation, for instance with aromatic amines, safrole, benzylic alcohols and polycyclic aromatic hydrocarbons (Coughtrie, 1996; Coughtrie *et al.*, 1998). In particular, activation may lead to DNA adduct formation resulting in tumourigenesis.

Sulphatase is the enzyme that potentially removes sulphate groups from sulphated conjugates and may regenerate active species.

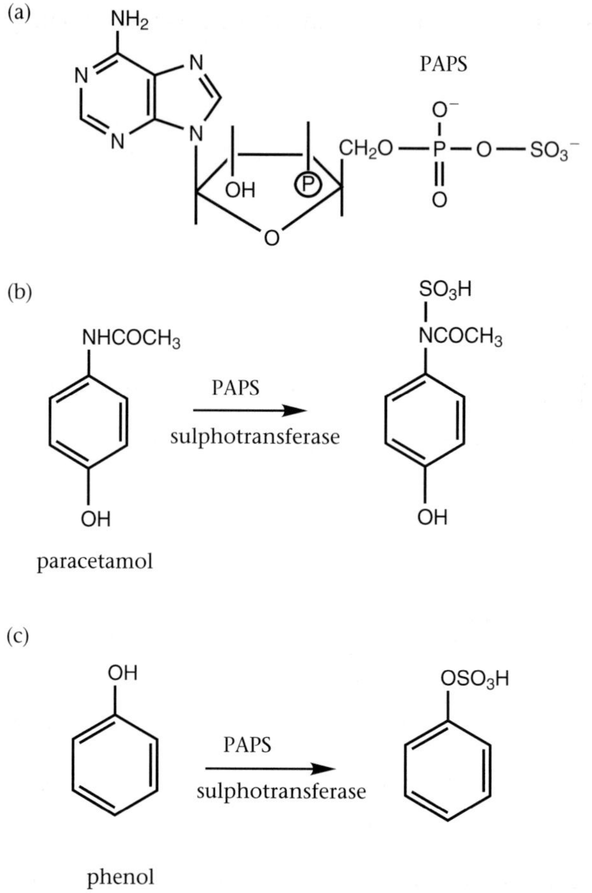

Scheme 3.26: Schematic of: (a) 3′-phosphoadenosine-5′-phosphosulphate (PAPS) and examples of sulphation via sulphotransferases for (b) paracetamol and (c) phenol.

3.3.2.3 Methylation: methyltransferase vs demethylase

Methylation at amino, hydroxyl and thiol groups may lead to a small increase in lipophilicity of a xenobiotic but in general serves to detoxify by protecting/deactivating functional groups. Methyltransferases use S-adenosylmethionine as the methyl group donor (Scheme 3.27).

Oxidative demethylation (dealkylation) has been discussed earlier in section 3.3.1.4 and is performed by certain CYP enzymes, which act as dealkylases.

3.3.2.4 Acetylation: acetyltransferase

Acetylation is performed by the two classes of polymorphic enzymes N-acetyltransferase 1 (NAT1) and N-acetyltransferase 2 (NAT2) (for nomenclature see Vatsis *et al.*, 1995). The acetyl group is donated by the co-factor acetyl-CoA (Scheme 3.28a).

Again, this area of phase II metabolism is duplicitous, and acetylation has particular importance in both the activation and detoxication of arylamines which, when oxidised may act as toxins and carcinogens. In terms of the observed genetic polymorphisms for

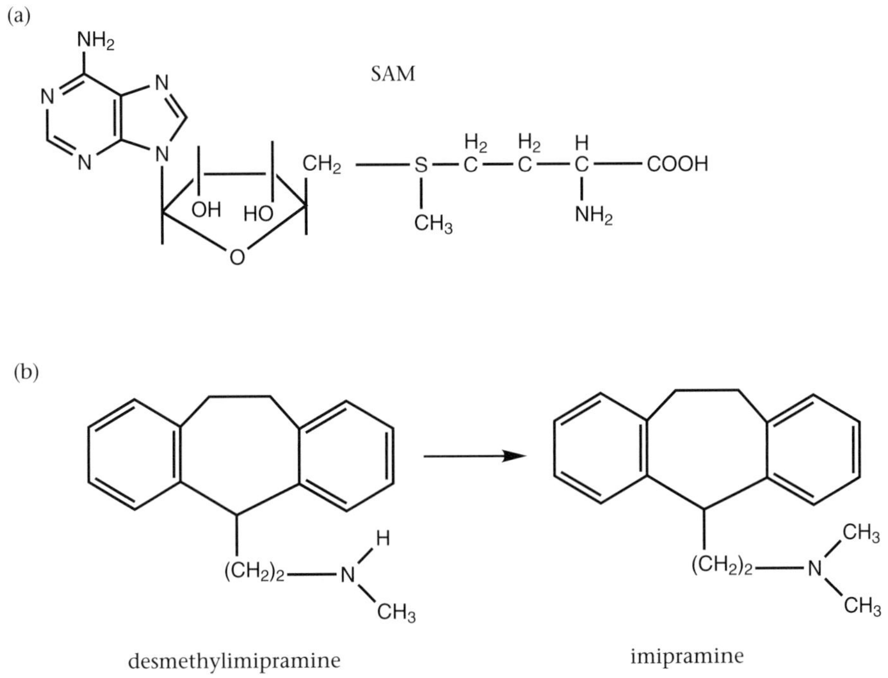

Scheme 3.27: Schematic of: (a) S-adenosylmethionine (SAM) and an example of methylation by methyltransferases for (b) desmethylimipramine.

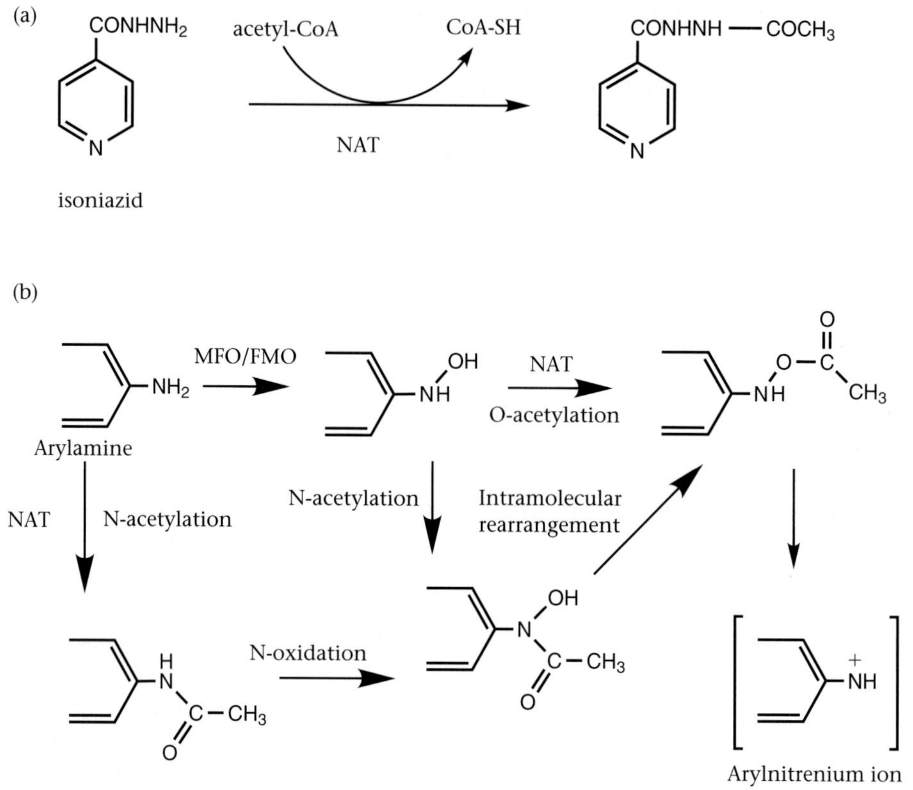

Scheme 3.28: Examples of: (a) N-acetylation for isoniazid, (b) N- and O-acetylation of arylamines by acetyltransferase using acetyl CoA as a cofactor.

NAT1 and NAT2, sets of individuals have been characterised as rapid, intermediate and slow acetylators with respect to arylamine metabolism (Hein *et al.*, 1992). Direct O-acetylation of an N-hydroxyarylamine (i.e. a phase I oxidised arylamine) generates an unstable acetoxyarylamine that breaks down to yield the highly reactive carcinogenic arylnitrenium ion (Scheme 3.28b). In contrast, N-acetylation of arylamines initially forms a non-toxic amide derivative, but this product can undergo intramolecular rearrangement to yield the same unstable acetoxyarylamine (Scheme 3.28b).

3.3.2.5 Glutathione conjugation: glutathione S-transferase

Phase I metabolism of xenobiotics can lead to the generation of potent electrophilic compounds, which can bind to macromolecules and result in toxic or immunogenic complexes. In general, xenobiotic conjugation (via multiple isoforms of glutathione S-transferase (alpha, mu, pi, theta and sigma forms) (Seidegard and Ekstrom, 1997)), to the abundant cellular tripeptide glutathione (Gly-Cys-Glu; GSH) (Scheme 3.29a) has been identified as one of the major ways through which they can be detoxified. Epoxides, halo- and nitroalkanes, alkenes and aromatic halo- and nitro-compounds are typical electrophilic molecules that conjugate GSH. An example of detoxifying GSH conjugation to the strong sensitiser 2,4-dinitrochlorobenzene (DNCB) is shown in Scheme 3.29b.

In addition to the extensive level of detoxication resulting from this area of phase II metabolism, GSH conjugation can also lead to the generation of toxic species (Monks and Lau, 1994). In particular, toxic GSH S-conjugates are formed with haloalkanes, haloalkenes, hydroquinones and aminophenol (Dekant and Vamvakas, 1993). The breakdown of S-(chloromethyl)-GSH conjugates generated from dichloromethane eventually results in the production of formaldehyde (Scheme 3.29c). GSH conjugation is also responsible for the ultimate generation of sulphur half-mustards and episulphonium ions from dihaloalkanes (Scheme 3.29d). These metabolites go on to form DNA-adducts that induce genotoxicity (van Bladeren *et al.*, 1980). The production of GSH conjugates of polyhalogenated alkenes also ultimately leads to protein-reactive metabolites (after phase III metabolism; see section 3.3.3 and Scheme 3.32 below) (Anders and Dekant, 1998).

Hydroquinones and aminophenols (which are converted to benzoquinone imines by CYP) may also be metabolised to toxic GSH-conjugates (quinone-thioethers), the general reaction for which is illustrated in Scheme 3.29e. Quinone-thioethers are capable of

(a)

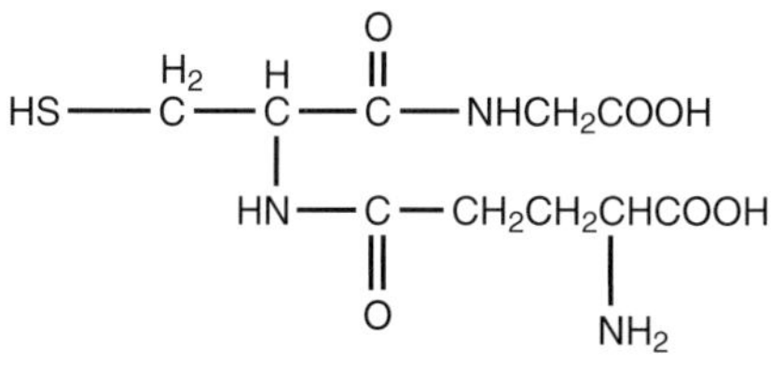

GSH - γ-glutamylcysteinylglycine

(b)

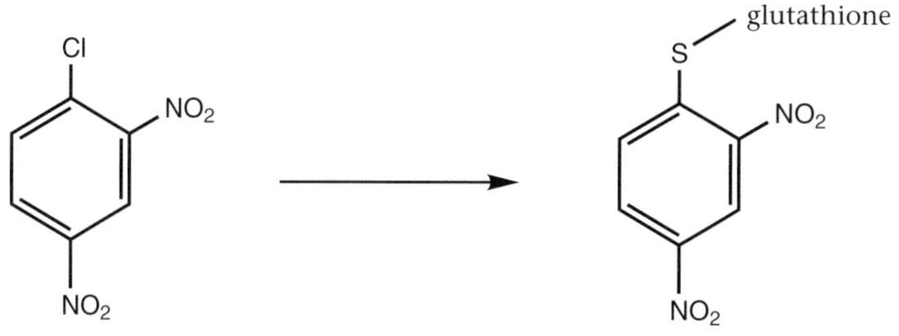

2,4-dinitrochlorobenzene

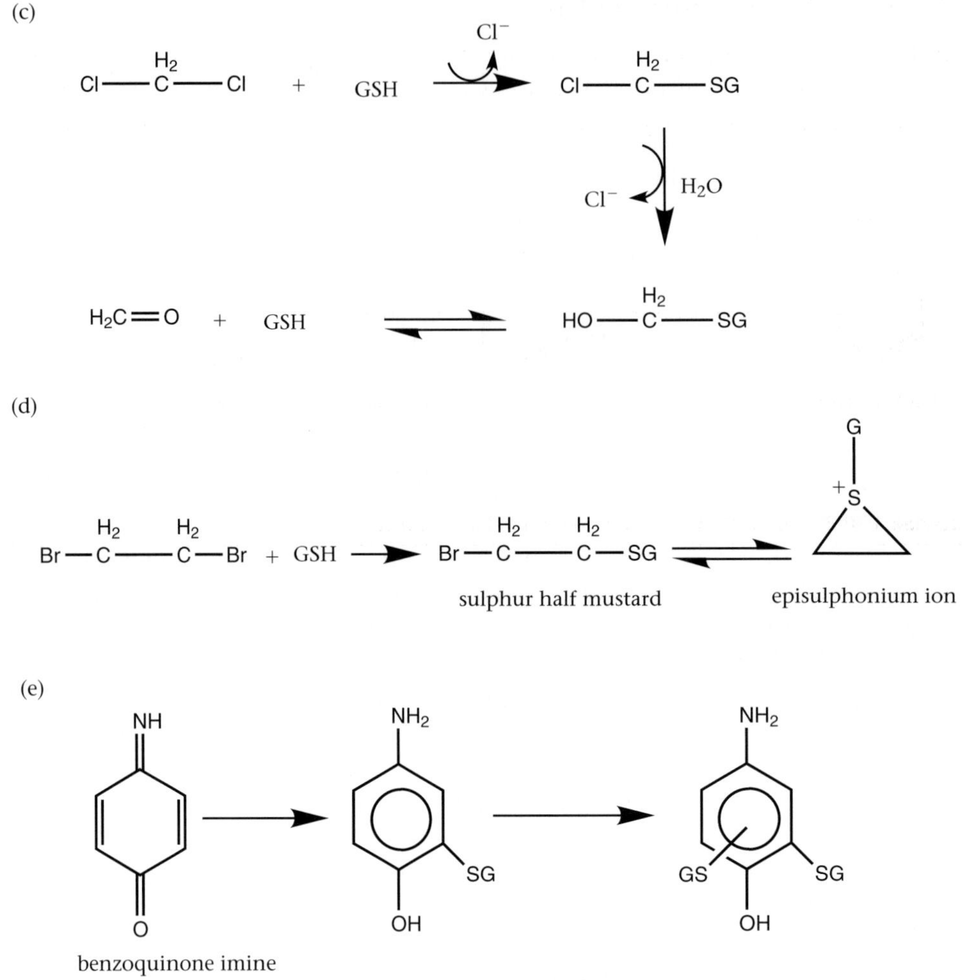

Scheme 3.29: Schematic of: (a) glutathione (GSH) and examples of GSH conjugation for (b) 2,4-DNCB, (c) dichloromethane, (d) 1,2-dibromoethane and (e) benzoquinone imines.

redox cycling in a similar way to that shown in Scheme 3.23 and are also capable of binding covalently to macromolecules (Monks and Lau, 1992).

It has been hypothesised that GSH-conjugation may aid in the transport of a lipophilic xenobiotic to a target tissue distal to the site of conjugation (Monks and Lau, 1994), by increasing its solubility, in a similar way to that suggested for glucuronide-conjugation in section 3.3.2.1 above. This further supports the idea that conjugation reactions do not exist purely for the purpose of detoxication.

3.3.2.6 Amino acid conjugation

Glycine, glutamine, ornithine, arginine and taurine are typically the amino acids that form conjugates of increased solubility with CoA derivatised carboxylic acids. A representative example for glycine conjugation to benzoic acid is given in Scheme 3.30.

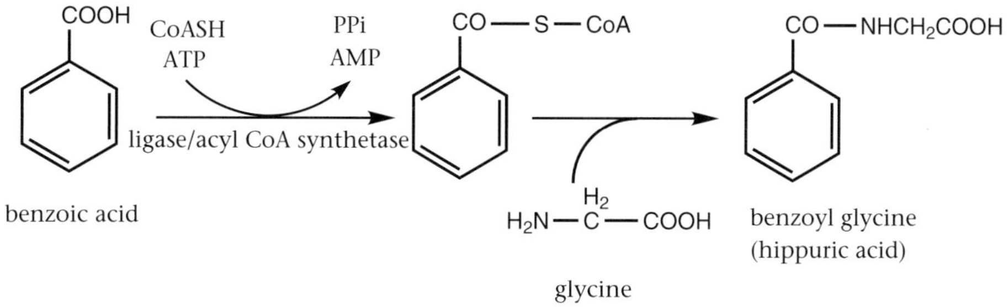

Scheme 3.30: Example of glycine conjugation to benzoic acid.

3.3.2.7 Condensation

Condensation is a non-enzymatic reaction that has been observed between amines and aldehydes (Scheme 3.31) and is essentially a detoxication reaction, eliminating the potential reactivity of the amine and aldehyde groups, although the overall lipophilicity of the product may be greater than the individual compounds.

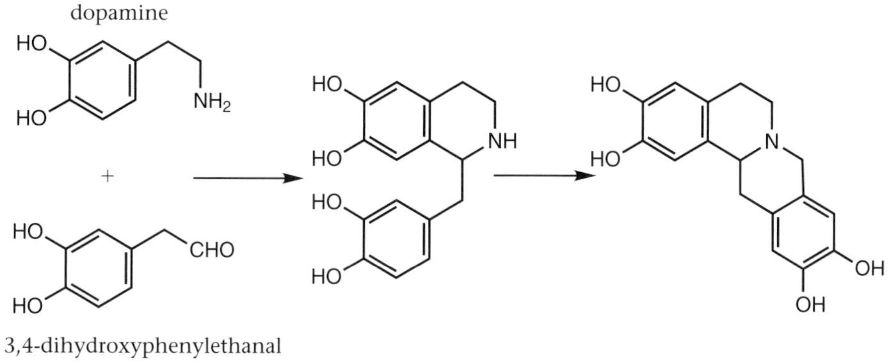

Scheme 3.31: Example of a condensation reaction between dopamine and 3,4-dihydroxyphenylethanal.

3.3.3 Phase III metabolism

It is possible for sulphur containing conjugates, such as GSH-conjugates, to undergo further metabolism by an enzyme that has been identified in the gut called cysteine-conjugate β-lyase (C-S lyase) and such further metabolism has been termed as phase III metabolism. The initial conjugation of GSH serves in general as a detoxication mechanism for xenobiotic phase I metabolites but it has been shown earlier in section 3.3.2.5 that activation by GSH conjugation should also be considered. Further phase III metabolism of cysteine conjugates resulting from a GSH-conjugate may lead to ultimate protein-reactive products. Examples of reactivating phase III metabolism for the 2,4-dinitrochlorobenzene-GSH-conjugate and polyhalogenated alkene-GSH-conjugates (as generated by the phase II metabolism illustrated in Scheme 3.29) are given in Schemes 3.32a and b, respectively.

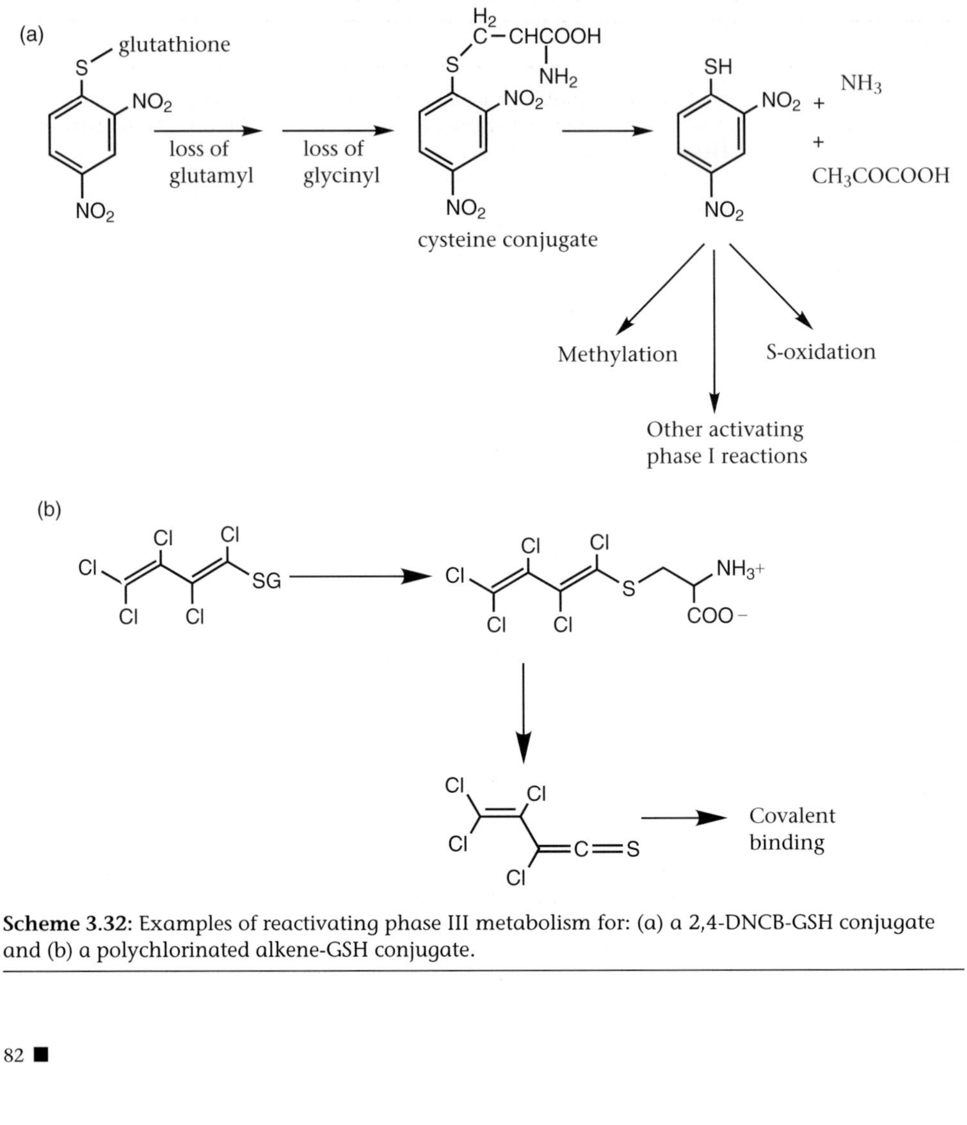

Scheme 3.32: Examples of reactivating phase III metabolism for: (a) a 2,4-DNCB-GSH conjugate and (b) a polychlorinated alkene-GSH conjugate.

3.4 PROTEIN PROCESSING ENZYMES

As well as considering xenobiotic-metabolising enzymes in isolation, it is also of importance to mention in brief, the potential roles of other *in vivo* protein processing enzymes that regulate cellular processes and hence may indirectly have a bearing on the balance of activating and detoxicating xenobiotic biotransformations. Many of the metabolising enzymes presented above, once expressed *in vivo,* may need to be processed into active forms by enzymatic post-translational modification, e.g. by removal of carbohydrates (deglycosylation) or removal of a terminal peptide etc. The potential scope for

TABLE 3.5
Protein processing enzymes — their functions and relevant reviews

Enzyme	Function	References
Phosphatases and phosphotransferases	Many cell signalling processes *in vivo* are regulated by reversible protein phosphorylation. Phosphatases perform the dephosphorylation reactions, often at specific amino acids, and phosphotransferases transfer a phosphate group from an NTP cofactor to the substrate.	Barford, Das & Egloff, 1998. Oliver & Shenolikar, 1998. Zhang, 1998.
Sulphatases and sulphotransferases	Sulphatases remove sulphate groups and sulphotransferases transfer sulphate from a PAPS cofactor to the substrate.	Coughtrie *et al.*, 1998.
Proteases and peptidases	Proteases and peptidases cleave proteins and peptides, often at specific types of residues. Often enzymes may be initially expressed as proenzymes, which may require cleavage of a terminal peptide before they can become active. Proteases have also been implicated in cell signalling by cleaving and triggering proteinase-activated receptor molecules. Proteolysis in general is important in cell cycle control and apoptosis.	Dery *et al.*, 1998. Santella *et al.*, 1998. Solary *et al.*, 1998.
Glycosidases and glycosyl transferases	In order for some enzymes to become active it may be necessary for them to be deglycosylated, i.e. have their surface bound carbohydrates removed. Levels of glycosylation may also be important in regulating cytokines and matrix proteases.	Crout & Vic, 1998. Henrissat, 1998. Van den Steen *et al.*, 1998.

discussing the types of processing enzyme is enormous, therefore only the major types of enzyme in this category are outlined in Table 3.5 along with a comment on their function and a selection of review articles relevant to each enzyme family.

In some cases, where inter-individual variability may be a factor in xenobiotic metabolism, it may not necessarily be the case that a particular metabolising enzyme is lacking but that the processing enzyme, which converts proenzyme into an active enzyme, is the missing factor.

3.5 SUMMARY

The above chapter has reviewed the major metabolising enzymes, in terms of their generic classifications and general functionalities, but many other specific enzyme pathways exist that are too diverse to discuss here. Indeed, it is not definite as to how far further research into identifying hepatic and extrahepatic metabolic enzymes has to go, i.e. how many more enzymes are as yet unidentified? It is in no way intended that this overview should be regarded as a fully comprehensive guide to xenobiotic metabolism but it hopefully provides an overall impression of the types of diverse chemistry that a selection of the major xenobiotic-metabolising enzymes can perform.

It has hopefully been emphasised throughout this chapter that once a xenobiotic enters the body, a whole host of biotransformations may occur, given the right conditions. The metabolism of xenobiotics is complex and the prediction of the ultimate fate of a compound relies on a careful consideration of the kinetics of all possible simultaneous competing biotransformations that each molecule may undergo, rather than focusing on one specific pathway for an explanation of toxicity.

Whilst it is generally accepted that phase I metabolism leads to activation, it is also the case that phase II conjugation is not only a detoxication mechanism but may also facilitate in the activation of xenobiotics distal to the site of exposure by aiding their transport to target organs. This area in particular requires further research to provide conclusive evidence that the historical definitions of phase I and phase II metabolism may be too general.

Interindividual variability of xenobiotic-metabolising enzymes is another key area that requires further research for all enzymes. Not only in relation to activating and detoxifying enzymes relating directly to biotransformations of a xenobiotic, but also in identifying, in some individuals, inefficient levels of enzymes that cope with the production of potentially toxic by-products, i.e. nitric oxide, superoxide, hydroxyl radicals, hydrogen peroxide etc. As we are increasingly developing the tools for phenotyping and genotyping individuals, it is possible that more widespread variability between individuals in the expression and activity of xenobiotic-metabolising enzymes will be revealed.

An area that is also in its infancy is the role of free-radical formation in metabolism. Free radicals are notoriously toxic species in that they irreparably damage intracellular macromolecules (i.e. proteins, lipids and DNA) and particularly in the case of the phase I oxidoreductive enzymes, the regulation of radical species may be crucial to the levels of toxicity observed with some of their substrates. The generation of toxicity from a substrate may not necessarily be as a direct result of its activation but by the overproduction of damaging free-radicals in the presence of high substrate concentrations. This area is too large to discuss within the scope of this review but is also worthy of consideration when attempting to predict toxicity. (Toxicity resulting from free-radical production in biological systems has been reviewed in Wallace (1997).)

As the extent of data for liver enzymes increases, it is becoming necessary to assess the extent to which the same enzymes also occur in extrahepatic tissues. With respect to this review, the detailed study of skin metabolism is still in its very early stages. In theory, there should be no reason why similar enzyme functionalities to those seen in liver and other tissues should not be seen in the skin, but at different levels, in a more reductive environment and with different kinetics. Research within the last decade has identified a significant number of cutaneous metabolising-enzymes, although their specific activities have not been thoroughly analysed in all cases. The following chapter illustrates how far research has come to date in identifying skin counterparts of the enzymes discussed above.

NOTES

1 This chapter is principally concerned with illustrating enzyme mechanisms. For a review of the toxicological relevance of induction of human drug-metabolising enzymes see Park *et al.* (1996).

2 Of interest, is the potential application of 1- and 2-naphthol metabolite detection in urine as a biomarker of exposure to airborne polycyclic aromatic hydrocarbons (Yang *et al.*, 1999a).

3 It is interesting to point out at this juncture that even in the case where only two enzymes are considered in predicting aldehyde metabolism (i.e. alcohol dehydrogenase and aldehyde dehydrogenase are competing for the same aldehyde substrate), it would be difficult to estimate the levels of reactive aldehyde that may be produced in an *in vivo* system, without knowing details of the kinetics (i.e. the Michaelis-Menten rate constant K_m and initial maximal rate V_{max}) of these competing mechanisms.

CHAPTER 4

Enzymes and Pathways of Xenobiotic Metabolism in Skin

Contents

Following on from the previous chapter on general xenobiotic metabolism, this chapter focuses initially on the basic understanding of skin as a metabolising organ and continues with an overview of the major metabolising enzymes that have been detected in skin to date. Towards the end of the chapter, some general principles are addressed, that may apply when considering the roles cutaneous xenobiotic metabolism could play in contact sensitisation.

4.1 SKIN AS A METABOLISING ORGAN

For centuries it was thought that the skin acted as purely an inert structural barrier between the body and the environment and that it was composed principally of dead cells. It is only in relatively recent times, within the last two centuries, that the skin has been regarded as not only a barrier but as a living, metabolically active organ and is indeed the largest organ of the human body. It was in 1775, when the English doctor Sir Percivall Pott observed an increased incidence of scrotal cancer in chimney sweeps, that skin exposure to soot was first reported to be a cause of cutaneous toxicity. It was later discovered that the chemicals in soot responsible for this toxicity were polyaromatic hydrocarbons (PAHs) (Clonfero *et al.*, 1986; Mukhtar *et al.*, 1986; Schoket *et al.*, 1988). This provided primary evidence that some property of the skin was activating these relatively inert PAHs into toxic species. It is now known that this 'property' is cutaneous metabolism and in the main, activation of PAHs results from oxidation by the inducible enzyme cytochrome P450 1A (CYP1A) (see sections 3.3.1.1 and 4.2.1.1.1). This represents just one early finding relating to cutaneous metabolism, but during this century it has been established that many metabolising enzymes are present in the skin and are the likely catalysts of xenobiotic biotransformations, potentially playing roles in generating reactive species (see review by Hotchkiss, 1998). The first direct study on xenobiotic metabolism in skin can be traced back to Norden (1953), who observed the appearance, metabolism and disappearance of 3,5-benzopyrene in mouse skin epithelial tissue. However, many of the detailed enzyme-mediated reaction pathways in skin, which result in the metabolism of both endogenous chemicals (for example hormones, steroids and inflammatory mediators) and exogenous compounds (xenobiotics including drugs, pesticides, industrial and environmental chemicals) remain to be determined. For the purposes of this review, with respect to the role of metabolism in the manifestation of allergic contact dermatitis, the following chapter concentrates on human and rodent skin enzymes that have been identified and are known to be involved in xenobiotic metabolism. There are many skin enzymes that metabolise endogenous substrates but as mentioned in Chapter 3, it may be the case that xenobiotic-metabolising and endogenous substrate-metabolising enzymes are one and the same.

4.2 ENZYMOLOGY OF THE SKIN

In recent years, studies with mammalian skin have focused on determining the presence and localisation of skin counterparts of many of the metabolising-enzymes that have already been found in other organs, in particular, the liver. It is assumed that much of the fundamental biochemistry of xenobiotic metabolism, which has been derived from studies of hepatic enzymes (discussed in Chapter 3), is applicable to skin metabolism, where the same enzymes have been identified (see reviews by Hotchkiss, 1998; Steinstrasser and Merkle, 1995; Kao and Carver, 1990; Bickers and Mukhtar, 1990; Finnen *et al.*, 1985). However, differences in enzyme expression levels and substrate activities have been observed between analogous hepatic and cutaneous enzymes, which may reveal important tissue specific differences that could contribute to differences in target organ and/or systemic toxicity.

4.2.1 Overview of enzymes identified in skin

Table 4.1 summarises the breadth of enzymes that have been detected in a variety of skin samples to date. The enzymes are listed according to their roles in phase I or phase II metabolism, comparable to the discussion presented in Chapter 3. In each case, details of the analysed substrate activity, species, localisation in skin, whether the enzyme has been detected at the mRNA or protein level, the method used and appropriate references for relevant studies on each enzyme, are given. In many cases, substrate activity and/or inhibition studies have been used to identify the presence of a particular enzyme isoform. Such studies do not positively confirm the presence of a specific isoform but provide evidence to infer its presence. Likewise, immunochemical and molecular biological studies have detected mRNA or identified a specific protein in skin. The identification alone, however, does not signify the presence of active protein. Therefore, Table 4.1 provides information on whether activity, protein expression and mRNA studies have been performed to identify different skin enzymes. Together, all three types of studies for an enzyme provide strong evidence that it exists and is active in skin.

4.2.1.1 Phase I enzymes in skin

4.2.1.1.1 Mixed function oxidase system — cytochrome P450 (CYPs)

It is generally considered that the most ubiquitous and broad-ranging metabolising enzymes in the skin are (as in the liver) the cytochrome P450s (CYPs) (see reviews by Mukhtar and Khan (1989) and Hotchkiss (1998) and also see section 3.3.1.1 for descriptions of oxidative mechanisms). New CYP isoforms are continually being discovered and defined by the nomenclature derived by Nelson *et al.* (1996). Of the 17 mammalian families of CYPs, four (CYPs 1–4) are involved in xenobiotic metabolism (see Table 3.1).[1] To date, several isoforms from CYP families 1–3 have been identified in skin, both directly, at the mRNA[2] and protein levels or indirectly from substrate activity assays (see Table 4.1). Of the major xenobiotic-metabolising isoforms listed in Table 3.1, CYPs 2A6, isoforms of the 2C and 2D sub-families (most notably 2D6) and isoforms of CYP4 have not yet been detected in skin. Studies relating to those isoforms that have been detected in skin are discussed in more detail below.

4.2.1.1.1.1 CYP1A

CYP1A1 (arylhydrocarbon hydroxylase) is the CYP isoform that has been most studied in skin (see reviews by Hotchkiss, 1998; Ahmad *et al.*, 1996; Vecchini and Michel, 1994). To date, there are no known endogenous substrates for this enzyme. The most notable xenobiotic substrates of cutaneous CYP1A1 are PAHs, such as benzo(a)pyrene and benz(a)anthracene, which are known to be mutagenic in animals and humans (Mukhtar *et al.*, 1986; Schoket *et al.*, 1988; van Pelt, 1990; Hecht *et al.*, 1985; Allen-Hoffmann and Rheinwald, 1984; Amin *et al.*, 1981). It is thought that CYP activation of PAHs to diol-epoxides, which can form adducts with protein and DNA, is the pathway responsible for the ultimate mutagenicity and toxicity of PAHs.

Constitutive expression levels of CYP1A1 are too low to be observed in skin by immunohistochemistry without the action of inducers (Bickers and Mukhtar, 1990; Pham *et al.*, 1989). Numerous studies using human and rodent skin have shown that CYP1A1 activity is inducible by the PAHs and β-naphthoflavone (Mukhtar and Bickers, 1981, 1983; Ichikawa *et al.*, 1989; Khan *et al.*, 1989a, 1989b; Berghard *et al.*, 1990; Raza *et al.*, 1992; Einolf *et al.*, 1997). More recently, PCR and Northern blot analysis have shown the induction of CYP1A1 mRNA expression in cultured human epidermal keratinocytes by these compounds (Khan *et al.*, 1992).

Western blot analysis (which is a more sensitive immunochemical technique than immunohistochemistry) was performed by Jugert *et al.* (1994) who showed low level constitutive presence of CYP1A1/2 enzymes in human keratinocytes. This supports results from PCR analysis, which has been used to show the constitutive presence of CYP1A1/2 mRNA in human keratinocytes (Mercurio *et al.*, 1995; Khan *et al.*, 1992; Omiecinski *et al.*, 1990). Baron *et al.* (1998) have also reported constitutive expression of CYP1A1 (as detected by the more sensitive technique of RT-PCR) in particular in skin-derived T cells and endothelial cells.

Li *et al.* (1995) concluded that retinoic acid was also a substrate for CYP1A1 in human skin. These authors also reported the presence of CYP1A2 in rat and human epidermis, but activity for this isoform has not been shown in skin to date.

4.2.1.1.1.2 CYP1B

The recently discovered CYP1B1 isoform (Sutter *et al.*, 1994) is a dioxin-inducible form and has been observed predominantly in tumour-related tissue (Reiners *et al.*, 1998). One recent study, however, has reported the detection of constitutive CYP1B1 mRNA and protein expression in human epidermal keratinocytes, skin-derived monocytes and macrophages by RT-PCR and Western blot analysis (Baron *et al.*, 1998).

4.2.1.1.1.3 CYP2A

No isoforms of the CYP2A family have been observed in skin to date, although investigations have been performed. CYP2A6 in the liver performs efficient 7-hydroxylation of coumarin. Such metabolism was not observed for coumarin neither in metabolically viable human, rat and mouse skin in flow-through diffusion cells, in skin homogenates

TABLE 4.1

Enzymes in skin: detection (protein/mRNA), localisation and examples of substrate activity

Phase I Mixed function oxidase system	Substrate activity	Species	Activity	Protein	mRNA	Localisation	Method	Reference
Cytochrome P450s (CYPs)								
CYP1A1	benzo(a)pyrene	human	+			E/micro		Chapman *et al.*, 1979
	"	human	+			E/micro		Bickers *et al.*, 1984
	"	human	+			HF		Merk *et al.*, 1984
	"	human	+			E		Kuroki *et al.*, 1989
	"	human/g-pig/mouse	+			micro		Storm *et al.*, 1990
	"	human	+		+	kerat	NB/RT-PCR	Khan *et al.*, 1992
	"	rat	+		+	E	NB/RT-PCR	Khan *et al.*, 1992
	"	rat	+			micro		Williams & Woodhouse, 1995
	"	mouse	+			sebo		Coomes *et al.*, 1983
	"	mouse	+			E/micro		Das *et al.*, 1986
	"	rat	+	+		E/micro	WB	Raza *et al.*, 1992
	7-ethoxyresorufin	rat	+	+		micro	WB	Pham *et al.*, 1989
	"	mouse	+	+	+	micro	WB/NB	Jugert *et al.*, 1994
CYP1A1	"	human/rat/mouse	+			E		Pendlington *et al.*, 1994
		human		+	+	kerat/TC/EC	WB/NB/RT-PCR	Baron *et al.*, 1998
	benzo(c)phenanthrene	mouse	+			micro		Einolf *et al.*, 1997
CYP1A1/2B	7-ethoxycoumarin	mouse	+			E/kerat		Bickers *et al.*, 1982
	"	rat/mouse	+			E		Moloney *et al.*, 1982
	"	g-pig/mouse	+			micro		Storm *et al.*, 1990
	"	human	+			RHE		Cotovio *et al.*, 1996
CYP1A2		mouse		+		E/micro	WB/IHC	Venkatesh *et al.*, 1992
CYP1B1		human			+	kerat	NB	Sutter *et al.*, 1994
		human		+	+	kerat/mon/mac	WB/NB/RT-PCR	Baron *et al.*, 1998
	Tumour-related	mouse			+	skin tumours	RT-PCR	Reiners *et al.*, 1998
CYP2B	7-pentoxyresorufin	rat	+	+		micro	WB	Pham *et al.*, 1989
CYP2B1/2		mouse		+		E/HF/micro	IHC/WB	Jugert *et al.*, 1994
CYP2B1/2	7-pentoxyresorufin	human/rat/mouse	+			E		Pendlington *et al.*, 1994
CYP2B1		human		+	+	kerat	WB/NB/RT-PCR	Baron *et al.*, 1998
CYP2B6		human		+	+	kerat/mon/mac	WB/NB/RT-PCR	Baron *et al.*, 1998
CYP2B12		rat			+	SG	NB	Friedberg *et al.*, 1992
	arachidonic acid	rat	+		+	sebo	NB/IS/RT-PCR	Keeney *et al.*, 1998
CYP2E1	ethanol	mouse	+	+	+	E/HF/SG	ISH/WB	Ashcroft *et al.*, 1997
		mouse		+		micro	WB	Sampol *et al.*, 1997

TABLE 4.1
Continued

Phase I	Substrate activity	Species	Activity	Protein	mRNA	Localisation	Method	Reference
		human		+	+	kerat/mon/mac	WB/NB/RT-PCR	Baron *et al.*, 1998
		mouse		+	+	micro	WB/NB	Jugert *et al.*, 1994
CYP3A	erythromycin	mouse	+	+		micro	WB	Jugert *et al.*, 1994
	testosterone	human	+			whole skin		Beckley-Kartey *et al.*, 1997
		mouse		+		micro	WB	Cheung *et al.*, 2000a
		human		+		E	WB	Wolkenstein *et al.*, 1998
		human		+	+	kerat	IHC/NB/RT-PCR	Baron *et al.*, 1998
CYP3A5		human		+		E	WB	Li *et al.*, 1994b
		human			+	E	PCR	Mercurio *et al.*, 1995
CYP 2B/3A	aldrin	rat	+			micro		Graham *et al.*, 1991
CYP Aromatase	testosterone	human	+			DF		Stillman *et al.*, 1991
		human			+	DF	RT-PCR	Harada, 1992
		human		+		HF/SG	IHC	Sawaya & Penneys, 1992
NADPH cytochrome	cytochrome c	rat	+			micro		Mukhtar & Bickers, 1981
c reductase	"	human	+			RHE		Pham *et al.*, 1990
NADPH cytochrome P450 reductase		rat		+		E	WB/IHC	Takahara *et al.*, 1993
Other oxidoreductases								
Alcohol dehydrogenase (ADH)	primary aliphatic alcohols	human	+					Wilkin & Stewart, 1987
	thiodiglycol	human	+			cytosol		Brimfield *et al.*, 1998
classes 1, 2 and 3		human		+		E/HF/SG	WB/IHC	Cheung *et al.*, 1999
		human			+	whole skin	NB	Engeland & Maret, 1993
classes 1 and 3 (2 absent)		rat/mouse/g-pig		+		E/HF/SG	WB/IHC	Cheung *et al.*, 2000b
class 1	ethanol	human	+					Li & Bosron, 1981
class 3	long chain aliphatic	mouse	+					Haselbeck & Duester, 1997
	and aromatic alcohols,	rat	+					Boleda *et al.*, 1989
class 4	e.g. retinol	mouse	+					Haselbeck & Duester, 1997
		rat	+					Boleda *et al.*, 1989
Aldehyde dehydrogenase (ALDH)								
classes 1, 2 and 3		human		+		E/HF/SG	WB/IHC	Cheung *et al.*, 1999, 2000b
classes 1 and 2		rat/mouse/g-pig		+		E/HF/SG	WB/IHC	Cheung et al., 2000b
class 3		rat/mouse		+		E/HF/SG	WB/IHC	Cheung *et al.*, 2000b
Monoamine oxidase (MAO)	Hydroxytryptamine	human	+	+		kerat/M	IHC	Schallreuter *et al.*, 1996
A and B forms	hydrocortisone	human	+			DF		Edelstein & Breakefield, 1986

TABLE 4.1
Continued

Phase I	Substrate activity	Species	Activity	Protein	mRNA	Localisation	Method	Reference
Flavin-containing	nucleophilic N- or S- centres	pig	+			E		Dannan & Guengerich, 1982
monooxygenase (FMO)	thiobenzamide/ methimazole	mouse	+	+		E/micro	WB/IHC	Venkatesh *et al.*, 1992
3-α-Hydroxysteroid dehydrogenase	dihydrotestosterone	rat	+			cyto/micro		Pirog & Collins, 1994
3-β-Hydroxysteroid dehydrogenase	3-β-hydroxy-5-ene steroids	human	+			SG/HF		Itami & Takayusu, 1982
		human		+		SG	IHC	Dumont *et al.*, 1992
11-β-Hydroxysteroid dehydrogenase	cortisol	human	+			SG		Kenouch *et al.*, 1994
17-β-hydroxysteroid dehydrogenase	17-β-estradiol	human	+			E		Weinstein *et al.*, 1968
types I, II and III		human			+	kerat	NB/RT-PCR	Hughes *et al.*, 1997
types II and IV		human			+	SG	NB	Thiboutot *et al.*, 1998
types I–IV		human			+	SG	RT-PCR	Thiboutot *et al.*, 1998
Prostaglandin H synthase-2	linoleic acid	human	+	+		DF	WB	Godessart *et al.*, 1996
Glutathione peroxidase		human			+	DF	RT-PCR	Keogh *et al.*, 1996
Lipoxygenase	fatty acids	rat	+			micro/cyto		Kim *et al.*, 1998
12-lipoxygenase	arachidonic acid	human	+			E		Bar-Natan *et al.*, 1996
Cyclooxygenase (COX1 and COX2)		human/mouse		+		E/kerat	IHC	Leong *et al.*, 1996
Azoreductase	1-phenylazophenol or 1-phenylazo-2-naphthol	human/mouse/g-pig	+			E/cyto/micro		Collier *et al.*, 1993
NAD(P)H:quinone reductase	dichlorophenol indophenol	rat/mouse	+			E		Khan *et al.*, 1987
	dichlorophenol indophenol	human	+			E		Merk & Jugert, 1991
5α-reductase	testosterone	human	+			RHE		Pham *et al.*, 1989
	"	human	+			LSE		Tamura *et al.*, 1996
5α-reductase type 1		human		+		sebo/cyto	IHC/WB	Chen *et al.*, 1998
Thioredoxin reductase		rat		+		LC, M, HF, SG	IHC	Rozell & Hansson, 1985
		human		+		DF/M/kerat	WB	Rafferty *et al.*, 1998
Hydrolases								
Esterases								
Acetylcholinesterase	acetylcholine	pig	+			E		Meyer & Neurand, 1976
	"	human	+	+		E/kerat	IHC	Grando *et al.*, 1993

TABLE 4.1

Continued

Phase I	Substrate activity	Species	Activity	Protein	mRNA	Localisation	Method	Reference
Butyrylcholinesterase	butyrylcholine	pig	+			E		Meyer & Neurand, 1976
Carboxylesterases	carboxylic acid esters	pig	+	+		E/HF/SG	IHC	Meyer & Neurand, 1976
		human/rat/pig	+	+		EBM	IHC	Clark *et al.*, 1993
	fluazifop butyl or carbaryl	rat	+			cyto/micro		McCracken *et al.*, 1993
	fluoroxypyr methylheptyl ester	human/rat	+			whole skin		Hewitt *et al.*, 2000a, 2000b
Cholinesterase	5′esters of 5′I-2′-dU	mouse	+			whole skin		Ghosh & Mitra, 1990
Esterase	benzyl acetate	human	+			whole skin		Garnett, 1992
	corticosteroid 21-monoesters	human/g-pig/rat	+			E/D		Tauber & Rost, 1987
	dialkylphthalate	human/rat	+			whole skin		Mint, 1995
	glyceryl trinitrate	human/mouse	+			whole skin		Santus *et al.*, 1987
	salicylic acid esters	g-pig	+			whole skin		Boehnlein *et al.*, 1994
	viprostol	human/rat	+			whole skin		Nicolau & Yacobi, 1990
Epoxide hydrolase	benzo(a)pyrene epoxides	rat	+			whole skin		Del Tito *et al.*, 1984
	cis or trans-stilbene oxide	rat	+			E/micro		Pham *et al.*, 1989
Tyrosine hydroxylase	dopamine	human	+			kerat		Ramchand *et al.*, 1995
Dopamine beta hydroxylase	dopamine	human	+			kerat		Ramchand *et al.*, 1995
UDP-Glucuronosyl transferases	1-naphthol/7-hydroxy-coumarin/bilirubin	rat/mouse	+			EBM/SG		Coomes *et al.*, 1984
	1-naphthol, bilirubin	rat	+	+		micro	WB	Pham *et al.*, 1989
	4-nitrophenol/bilirubin	human	+	+		SC	IF	Peters *et al.*, 1987
Sulphotransferases	cholesterol	human	+			E		Epstein *et al.*, 1988
	5-hydroxymethylchrysene	mouse	+			E		Okuda *et al.*, 1988
	minoxidil	rat		+		HF	IHC	Dooley *et al.*, 1991
	"	stumptailed macaque	+			HF		Baker *et al.*, 1994
	"	rat	+			cyto		Wong *et al.*, 1993
	1-naphthol	rat	+			whole skin		Macpherson *et al.*, 1991
	4-nitrophenol	mouse	+			E		Epstein *et al.*, 1984
Methyltransferases								
Catechol O-methyltransferase	adrenaline, dopamine	human	+			M		Le Poole *et al.*, 1994
	dopamine	human	+			kerat		Ramchand *et al.*, 1995
O6-alkylguanine-DNA-alkyltransferase	alkylated DNA	human	+			E/D		Wani & Dambrosio, 1995

TABLE 4.1
Continued

Phase I	Substrate activity	Species	Activity	Protein	mRNA	Localisation	Method	Reference
Acetyltranferases								
Choline acetyltransferase	acetylcholine	human	+			kerat/E		Grando *et al.*, 1993
N-acetyltransferase	p-aminobenzoic acid (PABA)	mouse	+			whole skin		Chung et al., 1993
	aniline	human/mouse	+			whole skin		Collier *et al.*, 1993
	benzocaine	human	+			whole skin		Kraeling *et al.*, 1996
(NAT1)	tryptamine, PABA	hamster	+			whole skin		Gaudet *et al.*, 1993
(NAT2)	dopamine, serotonin	hamster	+			whole skin		Gaudet *et al.*, 1993
		mouse		+		E/SG/HF	IHC	Stanley *et al.*, 1997
(NAT1)	sulfamethoxazole	human			+	kerat	RT-PCR	Reilly *et al.*, 2000
Glutathione S-transferases								
α, μ, π, θ, σ	conjugation of epoxides, quinones, alkenes, alkyl halides, aryl halides to GSH	human	+					Campbell *et al.*, 1991
α, π		human		+		HF	IHC	Campbell *et al.*, 1991
	cis-stilbene oxide	human	+			RHE		Pham *et al.*, 1990
		rat	+			E		Pham *et al.*, 1989
	Dinitrochlorobenzene (DNCB)	mouse	+			kerat/SG		Coomes *et al.*, 1983
	"	mouse	+			cyto		
	"	human	+	+			WB	Singhal *et al.*, 1993
GST								
π, α, μ	DNCB	human/rat/mouse	+	+		micro/cyto	WB	Raza *et al.*, 1991
	benzo(a)pyrene-4,5 oxide	"	+			"		"
	styrene-7,8-oxide	"	+			"		"
	leukotriene A4	"	+			"		"
	ethacrynic acid	"	+			"		"
π, μ		mouse		+		SG/HF	IHC	"
	butachlor	human	+			micro/cyto		Ademola *et al.*, 1993
π	DNCB	human	+			kerat		Blacker *et al.*, 1991
Glycine conjugation	benzoic acid	human/rat	+			kerat		Nasseri-Sina *et al.*, 1997
Phosphatases								
Phosphorylphosphatase	organophosphates	human/guinea pig	+			whole skin		Van Hooidonk *et al.*, 1980
	"	human	+			whole skin/E		Loden 1985

Abbreviations

AA – amino acid
cyto – cytosolic
D – dermis
DF – dermal fibroblast
E – epidermis
EC – endothelial cells
EBM – epidermal basement membrane
g-pig – guinea pig
HF – hair follicle
IF – immunofluorescence
IS – in situ hybridisation
kerat – keratinocytes
L – Langerhans' cell
LSE – living skin equivalent
M – melanocytes
mac – macrophage
micro – microsomes
mon – monocytes
NB – Northern blot
RHE – reconstructed human epidermis
RT-PCR – reverse transcriptase polymerase chain reaction
SC – stratum corneum
sebo – sebocytes
SG – sebaceous glands
TC – T cells
WB – Western blot

nor in cultured human keratinocytes (Beckley-Kartey *et al.*, 1997). A low level of coumarin 7-hydroxylation was observed in BALB/c mouse skin microsomes after a 20-minute incubation, suggesting that if CYP2A6 is present in skin, it is expressed in much lower levels than the other CYPs (Rettie *et al.*, 1986).

4.2.1.1.1.4 CYP2B

The O-dealkylation of 7-pentoxyresorufin has been observed in mouse epidermal microsomes, which is indicative of CYP2B activity in skin (Jugert *et al.*, 1994). However, a similar study in cultured human keratinocytes failed to see such activity (Raffali *et al.*, 1994). Expression of CYP2B1 and 2B6 mRNA has been detected in human epidermal keratinocytes by RT-PCR (Baron *et al.*, 1998). These authors also report the constitutive expression of CYP2B6 mRNA in skin-derived monocytes and macrophages.

One particular 2B isoform, CYP2B12, has been named as the first skin-specific CYP due to its high constitutive level of expression in sebaceous glands, as determined by Northern blot analysis, *in situ* hybridisation and PCR (Keeney *et al.*, 1998). Recombinant CYP2B12 epoxidises arachidonic acid to 11,12- and 8,9-epoxyeicosatrienoic acids, therefore it has been suggested by Keeney *et al.* that this enzyme may play specific roles in the bioactivation of lipids and intracellular signalling mechanisms in skin.

4.2.1.1.1.5 CYP2C and CYP2D

No isoforms of either of these families have been observed in skin to date. One of the most promiscuous polymorphic isoforms, CYP2D6 (see Table 3.1) has not yet been seen in human skin.

4.2.1.1.1.6 CYP2E

CYP2E1 is the major ethanol-inducible isoform of the CYP2E family. Constitutive mRNA expression for CYP2E1 has been detected in mouse skin by Northern blot analysis (Jugert *et al.*, 1994) and by *in situ* hybridisation (Ashcroft *et al.*, 1997); the latter technique localised CYP2E1 to the epidermis and dermal appendages. Low level *p*-nitrophenol metabolism has also been observed indicating CYP2E1 activity in skin (Jugert *et al.*, 1994). Comparative induction studies in liver and skin have indicated that cutaneous CYP2E1 induction by dexamethasone is a skin-specific induction (Sampol *et al.*, 1997).

4.2.1.1.1.7 CYP3A

The CYP3A family is the most prevalent of all the hepatic CYP isoforms in humans but it remains to be proven as to whether this is also the case amongst cutaneous CYPs. CYP3A has been observed in human keratinocytes by Western blot analysis using rabbit polyclonal antisera to rat liver CYP3A (Jugert *et al.*, 1994). CYP3A activity has been observed in mouse skin for aldrin and erythromycin (Jugert *et al.*, 1994; Finnen, 1987) and in human skin for testosterone (Beckley-Kartey *et al.*, 1997). More specifically, mRNA for the CYP3A3 isoform has been detected by PCR analysis in normal human skin (Mercurio *et al.*, 1995). Sampol *et al.* (1997) could not detect protein or mRNA expression for CYP3A in NMRI mouse skin. However, CYP3A protein was detected in Balb/c mouse skin using an anti-CYP-peptide antibody in Balb/c mouse skin (Cheung *et al.*, 2000a), which may suggest a strain difference.

4.2.1.1.1.8 CYP4A

CYP4A, the peroxisome proliferator-inducible CYP isoform, predominantly metabolises endogenous substrates such as fatty acids, however it is suspected that CYP4A also metabolises exogenous leukotrienes (which are endogenous products of arachidonic acid metabolism) and lauric acid. The conversion of exogenous leukotrienes A4 and B4 to unidentified polar metabolites has been observed in cultured human keratinocytes (Morelli *et al.*, 1990; Iversen *et al.*, 1994) and in particular CYP-dependent 20-hydroxylation and 20-carboxylation of leukotriene B4 has been shown (Mukhtar *et al.*, 1989). However, the presence of CYP4A in skin remains to be proven conclusively.

N.B. One recently developed method of localising different CYP isozymes in intact skin and skin homogenates is by the use of commercially available specific anti-CYP antibodies in immunochemical studies. A range of CYP-specific monoclonal antibodies raised against N-terminal peptides of several different human CYP isoforms are now available for such studies (Edwards *et al.*, 1998).

4.2.1.1.2 Mixed function oxidase system — NADPH cytochrome P450 reductase

The partner enzyme of the MFO system, NADPH cytochrome P450 reductase has been detected in mouse and rat skin and in reconstructed human epidermis (Pohl *et al.*, 1976; Mukhtar and Bickers, 1981; Pham *et al.*, 1990). More recently, this reductase has been shown to be present in rat epidermis by immunochemical detection and was purified in an active form (Takahara *et al.*, 1993). The purified protein in the presence of CYP, effected benzo(a)pyrene hydroxylation *in vitro*. Cross-reactivity was observed between rat epidermal and liver forms of the enzyme by Western blot analysis in this study. Immunohistochemistry localised the enzyme predominantly to the epidermis. On treating the rat skin with β-naphthoflavone, which induces CYP1A1 activity, no change in staining intensity or tissue distribution was seen for the reductase.

4.2.1.1.3 Alcohol dehydrogenase (ADH)

Wilkin and Stewart (1987) have shown substrate-usage in human skin of a selection of primary aliphatic alcohols (ethanol, propanol, butanol, pentanol, 2-methylpropanol, 3-methylbutanol and 2,2-dimethyl-propanol); they concluded that cutaneous ADH was responsible for converting these alcohols to the corresponding aldehydes. More recently, human skin cytosol was shown to oxidise 2,2′-thiobis-ethanol (thiodiglycol), a hydrolysis product of sulphur mustard, in an NAD-dependent manner (Brimfield *et al.*, 1998). This activity was inhibited by the ADH inhibitor 4-methylpyrazole, suggesting that ADH was responsible for this oxidation.

In terms of specifically identifying the five known human classes of ADH (see Table

3.2), three (ADH classes 1–3) have been conclusively identified in human skin both at the mRNA (Engeland and Maret, 1993) and protein (Cheung *et al.*, 1999, 2000b) levels. Cheung *et al.* performed semi-quantitative densitometric analysis of human skin cytosol (n = 28 humans) analysed by Western blotting (Figure 4.1a–c, see colour section), and observed that levels of ADH class 1 and ADH class 2 protein in breast and abdomen skin were significantly higher than those in foreskin ($P < 0.001$), per milligram of total protein. Also, Western blot analysis for ADH class 3 revealed a doublet band at ~40 kDa, which may indicate that cutaneous ADH class 3 is proteolytically cleaved. Alternatively, the doublet may be due to cross-reactivity of the antisera with an unrelated protein in the human skin sample; however, the antisera specifically recognises a single band at ~40 kDa in human liver. In comparison to the protein levels observed in human liver for ADH classes 1, 2 and 3, the mean cutaneous levels were 30-, 80- and 22-fold less, respectively. Immunohistochemistry showed that ADH class 1 and ADH class 3 were predominantly localised in the epidermis with some staining in the dermal appendages, whereas ADH class 2 was only seen in the epidermis (Figure 4.1d–g) (Cheung *et al.*, 1999).

A subsequent study has also shown species differences between the class-specific expression of ADHs (Cheung *et al.*, 2000b). All classes (ADH1–3) are present in human skin. However, ADH class 2, although present in rodent liver, was not detected in rat, mouse or guinea-pig skin by immunochemical methods employing anti-human ADH class 2 antisera. ADH class 2 is either insufficiently homologous to cross react with this sera or ADH class 2 is absent in rodent skin. This suggests that, whether absent or different with respect to human ADH class 2, metabolism of ADH class 2 substrates in rodents may be different from metabolism in humans.

ADH class 4 mRNA has been detected in the skin, which is the most efficient hepatic ADH to metabolise retinol to retinoic acid *in vitro* (Zgombic-Knight *et al.*, 1995; Haselbeck *et al.*, 1997). Retinol metabolism is known to be important in skin (Vanden Bossche *et al.*, 1988; Bailly *et al.*, 1998; Hodam and Creek, 1998) and has been linked with the ageing process, but as yet no specific ADH class 4 inhibitors are known to identify specific activity of this enzyme in skin. Immunochemical methods have revealed the presence of this class in the basal layer of mouse epidermis using class-specific antisera (Yokoyama *et al.*, 1996; Haselbeck *et al.*, 1997). Also, Handschin *et al.* (1997) have observed ADH4 protein and activity in rat skin homogenates using electrophoresis with substrate (ethanol and crotyl alcohol) activity staining. The presence of ADHs 1, 2 and 3 were not observed in rat skin using this method.

4.2.1.1.4 Aldehyde dehydrogenase (ALDH)

The putative presence of ALDH activity has been shown in human skin absorption experiments by the conversion of cinnamaldehyde to cinnamic acid (Weibel and Hansen, 1989b; Smith *et al.*, 2000a). It is also known that retinol via retinal can be converted to retinoic acid within the skin (Duell *et al.*, 1996a, b; Bailly *et al.*, 1998). It is possible however, that such conversions of aldehydes to acids may also be effected by non-enzymatic oxidative pathways or by the dismutase action of ADH with NAD as a cofactor (Svensson *et al.*, 1996). Therefore, ALDH substrate-specific activity in skin remains to be proven conclusively.[3]

Of the 12 human ALDH genes known to date (see Table 3.3) (reviewed by Yoshida *et al.*, 1998), three have been conclusively identified in human skin. Highly specific single bands have been observed in human skin cytosol for ALDH classes 1, 2 and 3 by Western blot analysis (Figure 4.2a–c, see colour section) (Cheung *et al.*, 1999; 2000b). Densitometric analysis of Western blots revealed significantly higher levels of expression for these ALDHs in foreskin than their respective levels in breast or abdomen skin ($P < 0.001$). Immunohistochemistry showed that ALDH classes 1, 2 and 3 are predominantly localised to the epidermis (Figure 4.2d–g). ALDH 1, 2 and 3 proteins were also detected in rodent skin, although ALDH 3 was absent in guinea-pig skin (Cheung *et al.*, 2000b).

4.2.1.1.5 Xanthine oxidase (XO)

It has been hypothesised that XO may play a role in skin necrosis and tumour-formation resulting from the generation of oxygen-derived free radicals (Athar *et al.*, 1987; Gossrau *et al.*, 1990; Reiners *et al.*, 1991; Picard-Ami *et al.*, 1992; Rees, 1994). However, no studies have detected the constitutive presence of this enzyme in human skin to date. In fact, studies on the activity of cutaneous XO in humans, pigs and rodents have revealed a putative species difference. Picard-Ami *et al.* observed a lack of XO activity in human and pig skin as compared with rat skin. Allopurinol, an XO inhibitor, has been seen to have a beneficial effect on rat skin ischemia, which is presumed to be due to the blockage of XO-generated free radicals, but no effect on pig skin ischemia (Picard-Ami *et al.*, 1992). In addition, XO activity was seen to increase during the ontogeny of chemically-induced murine tumours. After 24-hour topical application of 1 μg of 12-O-tetradecanoylphorbol-13-acetate to the dorsal skin of SENCAR mice, the level of XO activity increased by 350% as compared to the level in skin adjacent to the tumour (Reiners *et al.*, 1991). Moriwaki *et al.* (1996) have analysed a range of rat tissues by immunohistochemistry using polyclonal antisera against XO, but skin was not evaluated. An *in vitro* study using human keratinocyte cytosol that had been exposed to UVB radiation showed XO-derived superoxide generation, which can be inhibited by oxypurinol, suggesting that photo-induced XO free radical formation in humans may play a role in sunburn erythema and inflammation (Deliconstantinos *et al.*, 1996). It has also been suggested that XO may play a role in ageing of the skin (see review by Emerit, 1992).

4.2.1.1.6 Monoamine oxidase (MAO)

MAO types A and B activities have both been observed in human fibroblast cultures as determined by substrate preferences and differential inhibition by clorgyline and deprenyl (Groshong *et al.*, 1977; Edelstein and Breakefield, 1986). It has been observed that the level of MAO-A activity in human fibroblasts can differ by up to 500-fold in unrelated donors, and it is hypothesised that such extreme differences may reflect genuine individual, genetic variation in the regulation of MAO-A (Denney, 1998; Denney *et al.*, 1999). MAO-A activity, using 5-hydroxytryptamine as a substrate, has also been seen in human keratinocytes and melanocytes; immunohistochemical staining of human skin with a mouse monoclonal antibody supported this observation (Schallreuter *et al.*, 1996).

4.2.1.1.7 Flavin-containing monooxygenase (FMO)

FMOs are microsomal enzymes that catalyse the monooxygenation of a range of xenobiotic substrates containing soft nucleophilic N-, S-, P- and Se-centres (Ziegler, 1990; Hodgson and Levi, 1992). In a similar way to the MFO system involving CYPs, oxidation is performed in an NADPH-dependent manner, with molecular oxygen acting as the oxygen donor. It has been suggested that FMO activity assumes a greater relative role in extrahepatic tissues in comparison to MFO activity. For example, Venkatesh *et al.* (1992) found that, in mouse skin microsomes, 66–69% of phorate sulphoxidation activity was due to FMO and the remainder due to CYP, although the rate of sulphoxidation for this substrate in skin was only 3–4% of the rate seen in the liver. Using methimazole and thiobenzamide as substrates, FMO activity in skin was seen to be 10% and 19% respectively, of the activities seen in mouse liver for these substrates. Venkatesh *et al.* (1992) also performed Western blot analysis and immunohistochemistry in mouse and pig skin using an antibody raised against mouse liver FMO, indicating that FMO is present in skin and localised in the epidermis.[4]

4.2.1.1.8 Aromatase

Aromatase (CYP19) principally catalyses the formation of endogenous aromatic C18 oestrogenic steroids from C19 androgens. However, exogenous androgens such as testosterone and mibolerone (a synthetic androgen) can also stimulate aromatase activity in genital skin fibroblasts from normal males (Stillman *et al.*, 1991). The induction of mRNA for aromatase in human skin fibroblasts has also been observed with dexamethasone (a glucocorticoid) treatment (Berkovitz *et al.*, 1992; Harada, 1992).

Immunohistochemistry has revealed that aromatase is located in hair follicles and sebaceous glands in human skin, from both males and females, and it is hypothesised that this enzyme may be involved in the hair follicle cycle by regulating the formation of local androgens (Sawaya and Penneys, 1992). The presence and distribution of aromatase in this study was not seen to vary with body site or gender.

4.2.1.1.9 Hydroxysteroid dehydrogenase (HSD)

Although hydroxysteroid dehydrogenases (HSDs) are principally involved in oxidative endogenous steroid metabolism, they may also play a role in xenobiotic steroid metabolism. Glucocorticoids (GCs), such as cortisol, are used widely as immunosuppressants to treat skin dermatoses that derive from inflammatory or immune responses (Ahluwalia, 1998; Hennebold and Daynes, 1998); hence GCs may be substrates for cutaneous HSDs. Specific forms of HSDs that have been identified in human and rodent skin are 3-α-HSD (Pirog and Collins, 1994), 3-β-HSD (Itami and Takayasu, 1982; Dumont *et al.*, 1992; Toth *et al.*, 1997), 11-β-HSD (Kenouch *et al.*, 1994) and 17-β-HSD (Hughes *et al.*, 1997; Thiboutot *et al.*, 1998).

3-α-HSD activity, as determined by the NADPH-dependent reduction of dihydrotestosterone to 5-α-androstane-3-α-17-β-diol (inhibited by indomethacin), was present in cytosolic and microsomal fractions of rodent skin (Pirog and Collins, 1994).

3-β-HSD (δ5-δ4 isomerase) catalyses the conversion of 3-β-hydroxy-5-ene steroids to 3-keto-4-ene steroids and such activity has been observed in the sebaceous glands and hair follicles of human skin, with negligible activity in the epidermis or dermis (Itami and Takayasu, 1982). Such activity is in agreement with Dumont *et al.* (1992), who observed 3-β-HSD in sebaceous glands by immunohistochemistry. cDNA (coding for 372 amino acids) for 3-β-HSD has been isolated from human skin and transfected into HeLa cells for protein expression (Dumont *et al.*, 1992). The expressed enzyme has been shown to be catalytically active for pregnenolone, dihydropiandrosterone and dihydrotestosterone.

11-β-HSD converts active 11-hydroxy GCs to inactive 11-keto-GCs. Hence, GCs used topically to suppress the elicitation of ACD may be minimally effective due to such inactivation in the skin. Cortisol has been used to probe 11-β-HSD activity in human skin (Kenouch *et al.*, 1994). Significant activity was seen in sweat gland ducts (5 fmol/3 mm length, 10 min incubation with 10 nmol substrate), with negligible activity in the epidermis. Hence, the skin does have the ability to inactivate cortisol. Hennebold and Daynes (1998) have shown that only a combined topical treatment of specific 11-β-HSD inhibitors and low doses of GCs is capable of potentiating the effects of cortisol to provide effective treatment against ACD elicitation.

Three isoforms of 17-β-HSD (types I–III) have been detected at the mRNA level in human keratinocytes by RT-PCR and Northern blotting (Hughes *et al.*, 1997). In addition, RT-PCR analysis of human sebaceous glands showed transcripts for types I–IV but only types II and IV could be detected by Northern analysis (Thiboutot *et al.*, 1998). These isoenzymes convert active estradiol to inactive estrone and may be involved in regulating sebum production in different areas of the body and in sex hormone regulation.

Courchay *et al.* (1996) performed semi-quantitative RT-PCR on the expression of all of the aforementioned forms of HSD in individual components of the pilosebaceous units of human skin including anagen hairs, sebaceous glands and dermal papilla. This study showed varying levels of HSDs in keratinocytes derived from the inner and outer root sheaths of human hair, in comparison to the control levels seen in other organs such as liver, testis, placenta, prostate, ovary, uterus and adrenal glands. High levels of type 2 17-β-HSD, moderate levels of type 1 17-β-HSD and low levels of 3-β-HSD were seen in human hair; 11-β-HSD mRNA was found in primary cultures of dermal papilla.

4.2.1.1.10 Peroxidase

Two peroxidases have been studied in human skin, namely prostaglandin H synthase (PGHS) and glutathione peroxidase. PGHS has been implicated in the bioactivation of PAHs and aromatic amines (see review by Smith, Curtis and Eling, 1991), some of which are contact sensitisers and carcinogens. Oxidation of xenobiotics by PGHS often leads to metabolites that can form covalent adducts with cellular macromolecules. PGHS-2 has been identified by Western blot analysis in human dermal fibroblasts and this expression was seen to be upregulated, in a time-dependent manner, when cells were stimulated by interleukin-1 (Godessart *et al.*, 1996). It was also shown in this study that linoleic acid was converted to octadecanoids in fibroblasts and the authors postulate that this conversion is catalysed by PGHS-2.

Glutathione peroxidase mRNA has been identified in human fibroblasts from donors of different ages (14 gestational weeks to 94 yrs). Levels of mRNA were higher in postnatal donors than in fetally derived samples, however, no age-related differences were observed in the postnatal donors (Keogh *et al.*, 1996).

4.2.1.1.11 Lipoxygenase

Lipoxygenase activity has been found in rodent epidermis, in both microsomal and cytosolic fractions, as determined by the analysis of eicosanoids generated from polyunsaturated fatty-acid metabolism (Lomnitski *et al.*, 1995; Kim *et al*, 1998). There are four distinct genes of murine lipoxygenases: 5-lipoxygenase, platelet-type 12-lipoxygenase and leukocyte-type 12-lipoxygenase and epidermal lipoxygenase (Funk *et al.*, 1996). In human epidermal homogenates, the presence of eicosanoids derived from exogenous arachidonic acid indicates the presence of 12-lipoxygenase (Anton *et al.*, 1995; Bar-Natan *et al.*, 1996). Bar-Natan *et al.* (1996) showed that beta-carotene (a common ingredient of skin care therapies) affects lipid peroxidation in human skin: linoleic acid metabolism to 13-hydroxy-cis-9-trans-11-octadecadienoic acid was inhibited by 80%. It is hypothesised that beta-carotene acts either as a radical scavenger or as a specific lipoxygenase inhibitor (Lomnitski *et al.*, 1997). As far as is known, no study has specifically detected the presence of the epidermal lipoxygenase gene or gene product in humans.

4.2.1.1.12 Cyclooxygenase

Cyclooxygenase activity, with respect to arachidonic acid metabolism (see review by Vane *et al.*, 1998), has been assessed in human skin (Atkins *et al.*, 1995). The nonsteroidal antiinflammatory drug tenidap sodium was seen to inhibit the production of cyclooxygenase-generated metabolites in human skin, but this inhibitor had no effect on skin prick tests to allergens. Hence, the authors concluded that cyclooxygenase-derived arachidonic acid metabolites are not important in the development of cutaneous allergic reactions.

Immunohistochemistry has revealed that prostaglandin H-generating cyclooxygenases (COX-1 and COX-2) are present in human epidermis and human keratinocyte cultures (Leong *et al.*, 1996). In neonatal foreskin, COX-1 immunostaining was observed throughout the epidermis, whereas COX-2 was seen to be differentially located more in suprabasal keratinocytes. Constitutive COX-1 and COX-2 expression was also observed in human keratinocyte cultures. Expression of COX-2 was seen to increase but COX-1 expression was unaltered when the extracellular level of calcium was raised. Calcium is a known stimulant for keratinocyte differentiation and calcium-regulated COX-2 expression is thus believed to play a role in the normal differentiation of human keratinocytes. In contrast, low constitutive COX-1 and only induced COX-2 expression has been seen in normal mouse skin (Leong *et al.*, 1996).

4.2.1.1.13 *Azo-reductase*

Azo dyes are known carcinogens and toxins, which are commonly used in the foods, cosmetics, textiles and printing industries. Dyes such as phenylazo-2-naphthol (Sudan I), 5-(phenylazo)-6-hydroxynaphthalene-2-sulfonic acid and phenylazophenol (Solvent Yellow 7) undergo activating azoreduction to aniline in the cytosolic and microsomal fractions of mouse, guinea-pig and human epidermal homogenates (Collier *et al.*, 1993).[5] The aniline produced is further acetylated to acetanilide. The production of reactive arylamines, such as aniline, upon azoreduction has been implicated in the carcinogenic action of some azo dyes (Chung, 1983; Nakayama *et al.*, 1983), although it may be the case that free radicals are also generated during azo reduction (Mason *et al.*, 1977).

4.2.1.1.14 *Glutathione reductase*

Glutathione reductase activity, by analysis of glutathione depletion, has been assessed in human skin fibroblast cell lines derived from donors aged 14 gestational weeks to 94 years (Keogh *et al.*, 1996). No age-related differences were seen for the activity of this enzyme in fibroblasts.

4.2.1.1.15 *NADPH:quinone reductase*

NADPH:quinone reductase (DT diaphorase), which catalyses the two-electron reduction of quinones to hydroquinones, has been seen to be active in rodent epidermis at higher levels than in the liver (specific activities in liver, epidermis and dermis were 53.5 ± 4.1, 63.5 ± 4.2, 10.0 ± 1.3 nmol 2,6-dichlorophenol indophenol (DCPIP) reduced/min/mg protein, respectively) (Khan *et al.*, 1987). In this study, this enzyme was also seen to be inducible by 3-methylcholanthrene and crude coal tar. Studies have also shown that NADPH:quinone reductase activity (also using DCPIP as a substrate) in mouse skin and human keratinocytes is inhibited by dicoumarol, rutin and indomethacin, but not by pyrazole, progesterone or phenobarbitol and induced by anthralin and naphthoflavone (Merk and Jugert, 1991; Merk *et al.*, 1991).

4.2.1.1.16 *Steroid reductase*

The most important steroid reductase that has been studied in skin is 5α-reductase, which is involved in the reduction of testosterone to dihydrotestosterone and hence is believed to be important in androgen physiology (Slivka, 1992; Eicheler *et al.*, 1998; Fritsch *et al.*, 1998). In particular, 5α-reductase activity for testosterone and its 17-O-acyl derivatives has been seen in organotypic coculture of human dermal fibroblasts (living skin equivalent) (Tamura *et al.*, 1996). The presence of two isoenzymes of 5α-reductase (types 1 and 2) have been detected by immunohistochemical analyses using antisera generated to corresponding synthetic C-terminal peptides (Aumuller *et al.*, 1996). Chen *et al.* (1998) found that the type 1 isoenzyme exists mainly in the skin, whereas type 2 is predominantly found in the prostate. This study also showed by immunocytochemistry that 5α-reductase is present in the cytoplasm of human sebocytes, keratinocytes, fibroblasts, dermal microvascular endothelial cells, hair dermal papilla cells and melanocytes, with the strongest expression seen in sebocytes. This differential localisation in sebocytes correlates with studies on the localisation of hydroxysteroid dehydrogenase (see section 4.2.1.1.9 above). A double band corresponding to the expected molecular weight of 28–29 kDa was seen for type 1 5α-reductase in human cytosol by Western blot analysis (Chen *et al.*, 1998). The authors conclude that this phenomenon is unlikely to be due to cross reactivity of the antisera with the type 2 isoform. It is more likely that the type 1 isoform exists in two different states: active and inactive, phosphorylated and dephosphorylated, or possibly partially denatured. One study in rats has shown the presence of two different forms of mRNA for type 1 5α-reductase (Lopez-Solache *et al.*, 1996), therefore the authors favour that the enzyme exists in distinct active and inactive forms.

4.2.1.1.17 Thioredoxin reductase

Epidermal thioredoxin reductase (~60 kDa) has been seen to reduce nitroxide radicals (Schallreuter and Wood, 1986; Schallreuter *et al.*, 1986, 1987). However, a study in mouse epidermis revealed that thioredoxin reductase activity alone (0.1–1.0 pmol enzyme per mg tissue reducing 0.58–5.8 pmol substrate/min) accounts for a relatively insignificant amount of the total nitroxide reducing activity observed in skin (~20 pmol substrate/min/mg epidermal homogenate) (Fuchs *et al.*, 1989). Immunohistochemical analyses have localised thioredoxin reductase in Langerhans' cells, melanocytes, hair follicles and sweat glands (Rozell *et al.*, 1985). Rafferty *et al.* (1998) reported differential thioredoxin reductase expression in human skin cell types by Western blot analysis: relative expression levels were in the order fibroblasts > melanocytes > keratinocytes.

4.2.1.1.18 Esterase

Many studies during the past two decades have shown significant levels of cutaneous esterase activity with a broad range of substrates (V_{max} values ~5–11% of those in liver) (Tauber and Rost, 1987; McCracken, Blain and Williams, 1993; Hotchkiss, 1998). The different forms of esterases (see section 3.3.1.5.1) in skin may activate or detoxify xenobiotic esters. For example, many drugs, such as topically applied corticosteroid esters, are esterified to protect chemically labile hydroxyl groups (Higuchi and Yu, 1987; Lamb *et al.*, 1994). Esterified corticosteroids have higher lipophilicities than the corresponding parent steroid and hence can partition more readily in the skin. Once absorbed, however, there is significant evidence that human skin esterases hydrolyse the ester group to regenerate the parent steroid, which binds more strongly to corticosteroid receptors (Tauber and Rost, 1987). This is an example of esterase activation. Conversely, esters such as fluazifop butyl, carbaryl and paraoxon, which are absorbed into the skin as components in pesticides, have been seen to be detoxified in rat skin during *in vitro* percutaneous absorption (Clark *et al.*, 1993; McCracken, Blain and Williams, 1993). Fluazifop butyl is converted to fluazifop acid, which is excreted in urine; carbaryl is hydrolysed to 1-naphthol, which is then glucuronidated or sulphated; and paraoxon, the oxidated form of the organophosphate pesticide parathion, is hydrolysed to diethylphosphoric acid and *p*-nitrophenol. McCracken, Blain and Williams (1993) confirmed that these esterase activities in rat skin were predominantly in the cytosolic fraction.

Other xenobiotic esters are also detoxified to corresponding acids in human and rodent skin during *in vitro* percutaneous absorption studies, including benzyl acetate (Garnett, 1992), phthalic acid esters (e.g. dimethyl-, diethyl-, and dibutyl- phthalates) (Mint, 1995), fluoroxypyr methyl- and methylheptyl- esters (Hewitt *et al.*, 1996; Hewitt *et al.*, 2000a, b), viprostol (Nicolau and Yacobi, 1990), salicylic acid esters (Guzek *et al.*, 1989; Boehnlein *et al.*, 1994) and glyceryl trinitrate (Santus *et al.*, 1987). Ghosh and Mitra (1990) also showed ester hydrolysis of 5′-esters of 5-iodo-2′-deoxyuridine in hairless and athymic nude mouse skin homogenates. Inhibition of esterase activity with these substrates can be effected by diisopropylfluorophosphate (Bando *et al.*, 1997), phenylmethylsulphonylfluoride (Guzek *et al.*, 1989) and bis-*p*-nitrophenyl phosphate (Hewitt, 1995).

A study by Boehnlein *et al.* (1994) has focused on the human cutaneous metabolism of retinyl palmitate, a common ingredient in skin care products. This study showed that 44% of the absorbed retinyl palmitate was hydrolysed to retinol (vitamin A) by cutaneous esterases; the metabolite is believed to be the active ingredient. Retinol is known to be metabolised to retinoic acid, which can go on to be further metabolised to retinol ester (Duell *et al.*, 1996a, b; Randolph and Simon, 1997; Bailly *et al.*, 1998).

Recently, a reproducible assay has been developed, which will be of use in determining the levels of esterase activity in keratinocyte cultures derived from different individuals. The model substrate used in this assay is 4-methyl umbelliferyl heptanoate, which is hydrolysed in human keratinocyte cultures to the fluorescent metabolite 4-methyl umbelliferone (Barker and Clothier, 1997).

Esterase, in particular carboxylesterase, has been detected in human, pig and rat skin by immunohistochemistry and has been predominantly localised in the epidermis and dermal appendages (hair follicles and sebaceous glands) (Meyer and Neurand, 1976; Clark *et al.*, 1993). The presence of esterases in the epidermis, along with the significant number of studies on esterase activity corroborates the hypothesis that the epidermis is the major site of cutaneous xenobiotic metabolism.

Immunohistochemistry has also been used to detect the presence of the acetylcholine degrading enzyme acetylcholinesterase (AChE) in normal human cultured keratinocytes and cryostat sectioned epidermis (Grando *et al.*, 1993). AChE was predominantly seen in the vicinity of cell membranes. The activity of AChE (1.13 ± 0.15 μmoles acetylcholine iodide hydrolysed per mg protein in whole human skin homogenate) was also assayed in this study by spectrophotometric methods.

4.2.1.1.19 Epoxide hydrolase

Epoxide hydrolase activity has been identified in skin using a small selection of substrates: typical levels of activity in skin microsomes ranged from 3–28% of hepatic values (Mukhtar and Bickers, 1981; Pham *et al.*, 1989). Benzo(a)pyrene-4,5-epoxide and benzo(a)pyrene-7,8-epoxide are rapidly converted to their corresponding diols in neonatal rat skin microsomes (Del Tito *et al.*, 1984). Studies with *cis*- and *trans*-stilbene oxide have shown that epoxide hydrolase is present in both cytosolic and microsomal fractions of rat skin homogenates, with the specific activity of the microsomal form being three- to six-fold higher than the cytosolic form (Pham *et al.*, 1989).

4.2.1.1.20 Tyrosine and dopamine hydroxylases

It has been hypothesised that human keratinocyte cultures could be used in *in vitro* models to study dopamine metabolism relevant to schizophrenia, as activities for tyrosine hydroxylase, dopamine β-hydroxylase and catechol-o-methyltransferase have been observed in such cultures (Ramchand *et al.*, 1995).

4.2.1.2 Phase II enzymes in skin

4.2.1.2.1 UDP-glucuronosyltransferase (GT) and glucuronidation

Glucuronidation of a number of xenobiotic substrates has been observed in rodent skin, including 2- and 4-amino- and nitro-phenols, benzo(a)pyrene-7,8-dihydrodiol, 3-hydroxybenzo(a)pyrene, bilirubin and 1-naphthol (Rugstad and Dybing, 1975; Bock *et al.*, 1980; Lilienblum *et al.*, 1986; Pham *et al.*, 1989; Henrikus *et al.*, 1991; Macpherson *et al.*, 1991; see also review by Hotchkiss, 1998). Relative activities of cutaneous GTs range from 0.6–50% of hepatic levels for these substrates (see Table 4.2). Benzo(a)pyrene and 7-ethoxycoumarin are metabolised to phenols by CYP and these phenolic metabolites have also been seen to be glucuronidated in both rat and mouse skin (Mukhtar and Bickers, 1981; Moloney *et al.*, 1982; Coomes *et al.*, 1984; Finnen and Shuster, 1985a; Finnen, 1987). The sex difference that is apparent with liver GT activity has also been observed for cutaneous GT with activity being higher in both organs in male rats (Pham *et al.*, 1989).

In human skin, GT activity for 4-nitrophenol and bilirubin conjugation to glucuronic acid has been observed in the stratum corneum by immunofluorescence (Peters *et al.*, 1987). Pham *et al.* (1989) detected the presence of two of the major hepatic forms of GT, the phenol- and bilirubin-metabolising forms respectively, in rat skin by immunochemical characterisation. They also found that the isoform responsible for conjugation of testosterone to glucuronic acid was absent in skin, which agreed with the lack of GT activity observed for this substrate. Morphine is also a substrate that does not appear to undergo ‘first-pass’ glucuronidation during skin absorption, despite a comparatively high level of GT activity for other substrates (Matsuzawa *et al.*, 1994).

It is widely believed that glucuronidation of a xenobiotic increases its solubility and aids in its excretion. A recent study has compared the absorption, metabolism and excretion of topically applied all-trans-retinoic acid (RA, which produces toxic skin responses) and all-trans-retinoyl beta-glucuronide (RAG, which is non-toxic) in rat (Barua and Olson, 1996). These authors showed that both RA and RAG were absorbed, metabolised and excreted in a similar way overall and therefore toxicity of RA in rat skin could not be attributed to major differences in these properties.

4.2.1.2.2 Sulphotransferase (ST) and sulphation

It has been known for more than three decades that human skin has the capacity to sulphate the steroids dehydroepiandrosterone and androstene-3β,17β-diol (Gallegos and Berliner, 1967; Berliner *et al.*, 1968; Faredin *et al.*, 1968). Other xenobiotics that have been shown to be sulphated in skin are 4-nitrophenol (in mouse and rabbit: Epstein *et al.* (1994) and Henrikus *et al.* (1991), respectively), cholesterol (in human) (Epstein *et al.*, 1988),

5-hydroxymethyl chrysene (in mouse) (Okuda *et al.*, 1988), 1-naphthol (in rat) (Macpherson *et al.*, 1991) and minoxidil (in stumptailed macaques) (Baker *et al.*, 1994). Table 4.2 lists specific activity of cutaneous ST in relation to hepatic ST for selected substrates.

Sulphation often activates xenobiotic substrates, for example 5-hydroxymethyl chrysene is activated to 5-hydroxymethyl chrysene sulfate, which is a mutagenic sulphate ester (Okuda *et al.*, 1988). ST activates the hair growth stimulant drug, minoxidil, to minoxidil sulphate, which takes place in the scalp and the enzyme minoxidil ST is predominantly expressed in hair follicles (Baker *et al.*, 1994; Hamamoto and Mori, 1989; Dooley *et al.*, 1991). Dooley *et al.* (1991) showed, by immunohistochemistry, that MST was present in rat anagen hair follicles in the region of the lower outer root sheath. It is therefore hypothesised that STs play a role in hair growth in mammals.

4.2.1.2.3 Methyltransferase and methylation

Xenobiotic methylation has not been extensively studied in the skin. Studies in the 1960s reported the methylation of the neurotransmitter noradrenaline, which is suspected to be catalysed by catechol-*O*-methyltransferase (COMT), in human, rat, rabbit and mouse skin (Hakanson and Moller, 1963; Bamshad, 1969). More recently, COMT activity (using dopamine and dihydroxyindole (DHI) as substrates) has been reported to be present in cultured human keratinocytes and in human epidermal homogenates (Ramchand *et al.*, 1995; Le Poole *et al.*, 1994). Le Poole *et al.* postulated that COMT plays a regulatory role in melanin synthesis. In particular, COMT catalysed methylation of the hydroxy groups of the melanin precursor molecule, DHI, inhibits the synthesis of melanin and hence, COMT may be involved in the aetiology of vitiligo. Epidermal punch biopsies were taken from normal and vitiliginous individuals and it was found that the levels of COMT activity in patients with vitiligo was significantly higher ($P < 0.05$). Methylated metabolites of DHI, at the hydroxy groups, were also detected in human epidermal homogenates by HPLC analysis.

Activities for other methyl-conjugating enzymes, such as nicotinamide N-methyltransferase (Aksoy *et al.*, 1994), thiopurine methyltransferase (Weinshilboum, 1992) and thiol methyltransferase (Otterness *et al.*, 1986; Glauser *et al.*, 1992) have been seen in liver, kidney and red blood cells, but the presence of these and other xenobiotic-metabolising methyltransferases has not been investigated in skin.

A recent report on the metabolism of diethanolamine (DEA), a major industrial chemical that causes significant cumulative toxicity in a range of tissues (including liver and kidney) on repeat exposure, may also be of interest in terms of skin metabolism. Mathews *et al.* (1995) found that the N-methyl and N,N-dimethyl metabolites of DEA were incorporated into DEA-derived phospholipids, which in turn increased the methylation and accumulation of aberrant sphingomylenoid lipids in a variety of tissues. These authors propose that such incorporation of methylated xenobiotics into the headgroups of natural ceramides and phospholipids may account for cumulative toxicity of DEA. Such metabolism and lipid incorporation may also occur in skin but it has not been investigated to date.

In addition to xenobiotic methylation, protein methylation has been observed in human skin fibroblasts; the methyl-accepting capacity of proteins was seen to be increased in the presence of the methylation inhibitor, adenosine dialdehyde, in this study (Najbauer *et al.*, 1992).

4.2.1.2.4 N-acetyltransferase (NAT) and acetylation

A number of studies have shown that the skin has N-acetylating capacity. NAT activity has been observed in human skin in the form of carcinogenic arylamine and N-hydroxylamine acetylation (Kawakubo *et al.*, 1988, 1990). *p*-Aminobenzoic acid (PABA) and 2-aminofluorene are both acetylated in mouse skin (Chung *et al.*, 1993); PABA and benzocaine are both acetylated during percutaneous absorption across hairless guinea-pig skin and human skin *in vitro* (Nathan *et al.*, 1990; Bronaugh *et al.*, 1994a; Kraeling *et al.*, 1996); aniline, derived from azo dye reduction, is N-acetylated in mouse, guinea-pig and human skin *in vitro* (Collier *et al.*, 1993); and 2-nitro-para-phenylenediamine is N-acetylated at the amine group following percutaneous absorption through human and fuzzy rat skin *in vitro* (Yourick and Bronaugh, 2000). Activity for the individual NAT1 and NAT2 isoforms has been detected in Syrian hamster skin cytosol for a range of substrates including the aromatic amines serotonin, dopamine, methoxytryptamine, tryptamine, *p*-phenetidine, PABA and sulfamethazine (Gaudet *et al.*, 1993; Slominski *et al.*, 1996). Expression of NAT2 has been localised by immunohistochemical analysis to the outer layers of the epidermis, sebaceous glands and hair shafts in mouse skin (Stanley *et al.*, 1997).

Both NAT1 and NAT2 isoforms exhibit genetic polymorphisms in mammals that result in individuals being 'slow' or 'rapid' acetylators for specific substrates. Low constitutive N-acetylating capacity may be a genetic factor in some individuals that predisposes them to develop adverse reactions to xenobiotics. A recent study has investigated the levels of N-acetylation of 2-aminofluorene in human skin obtained from patients with the severe skin conditions of Stevens-Johnson syndrome (SJS) and toxic epidermal necrolysis (TEN) (Dietrich *et al.*, 1995). This study found patients with SJS or TEN had lower N-acetylating capacity than normal individuals (0.85 nmol/mg/min compared to 2.21 nmol/mg/min in normal humans, $p < 0.05$). In adult and neonatal human keratinocytes, the presence of NAT1 mRNA (but not NAT2) was observed by RT-PCR and has been implicated in sulfamethoxazole acetylation (Reilly *et al.*, 2000). Sulfamethoxazole also causes the severe hypersensitivity SJS in some individuals.

4.2.1.2.5 Glutathione S transferase (GST) and glutathione conjugation

Activity for GST has been found in the soluble cell fraction of intact human skin and human keratinocytes but not in the microsomal cell fraction (Blacker *et al.*, 1991). Also, GST activity, with cis-stilbene oxide as substrate, is present in reconstructed human epidermis from the outer root sheath cells of human hair follicles (Pham *et al.*, 1990). Table 4.2 lists comparative hepatic and cutaneous GST activities for selected substrates. Of the five different isoforms of GST (alpha, mu, pi, theta and sigma), the pi form predominates in human and rodent skin: this was the finding by Western blot analysis using specific polyclonal antibodies to the alpha, mu and pi classes (Raza *et al.*, 1991; Singhal *et al.*, 1993) and by N-terminal sequence analysis of human keratinocyte cytosol-derived

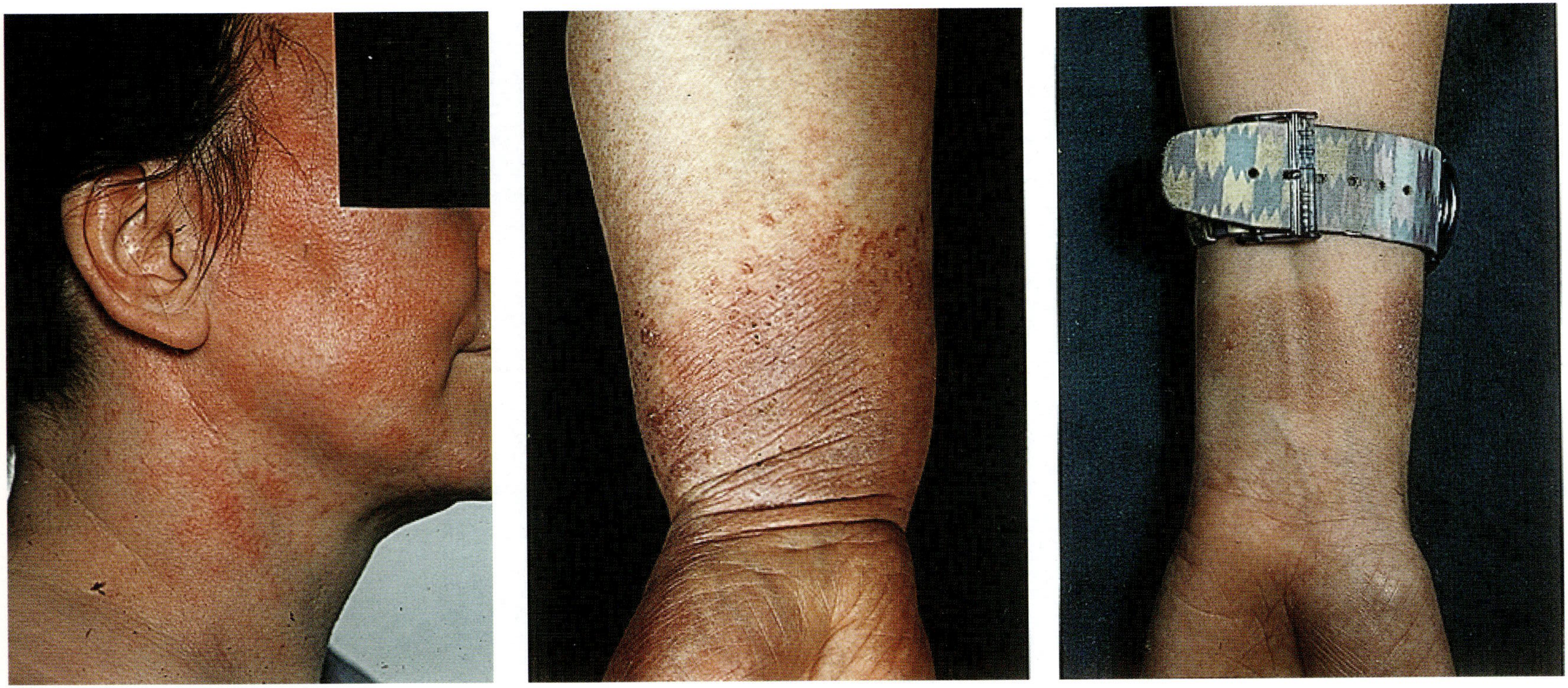

Figure 1.1: Clinical appearance of allergic contact dermatitis (ACD). In these individuals, ACD resulted from topical exposure to: (a) para-phenylene diamine in a hair dye, (b) sesquiterpene lactones in chrysanthemums and (c) epoxy resins in a synthetic watch strap. (Photographs were reproduced, with permission, from the audio-visual department archives at Imperial College School of Medicine, St. Mary's hospital campus, Paddington, London UK.)

(a) (b) (c) (d)
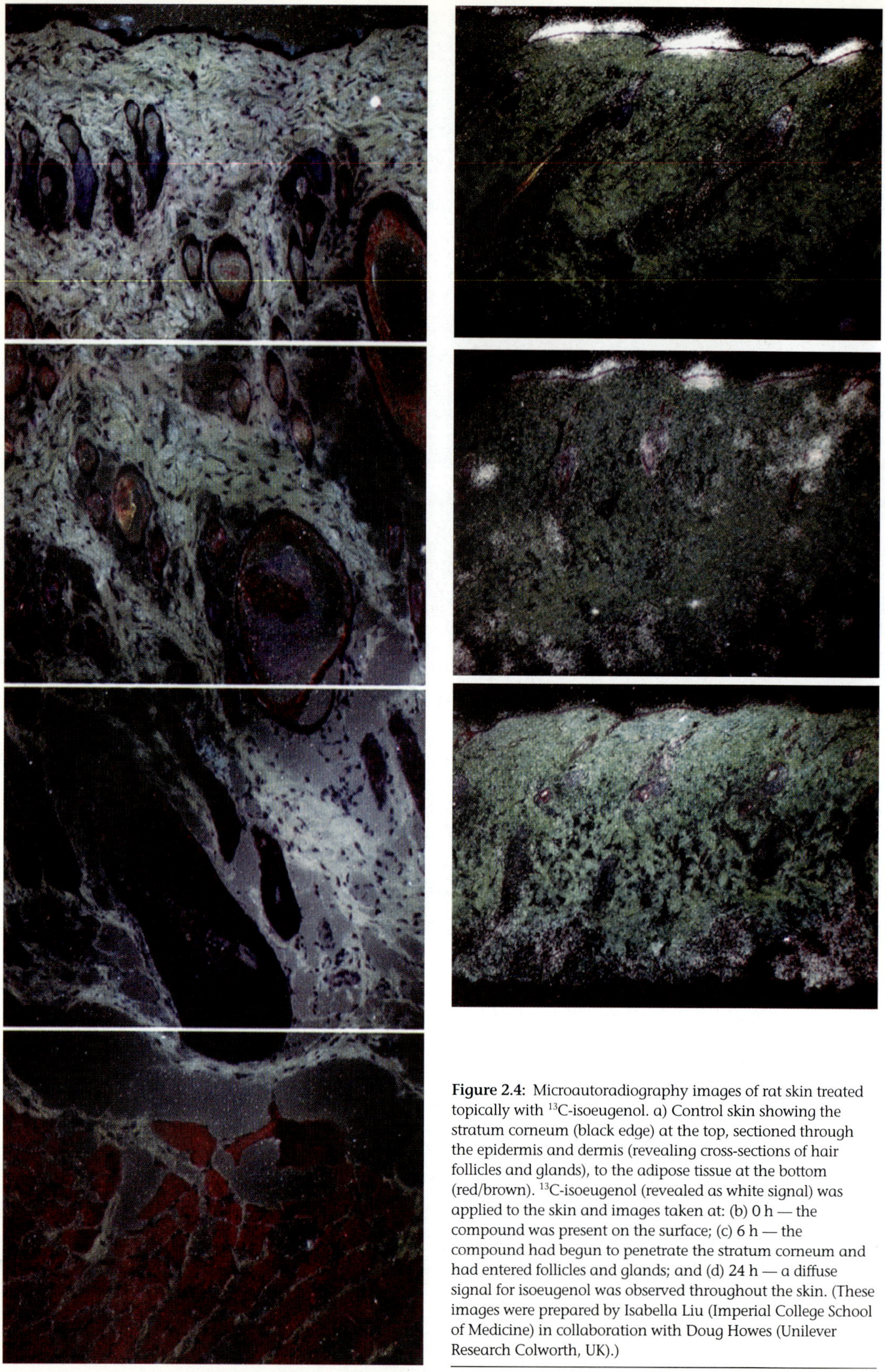

Figure 2.4: Microautoradiography images of rat skin treated topically with ^{13}C-isoeugenol. a) Control skin showing the stratum corneum (black edge) at the top, sectioned through the epidermis and dermis (revealing cross-sections of hair follicles and glands), to the adipose tissue at the bottom (red/brown). ^{13}C-isoeugenol (revealed as white signal) was applied to the skin and images taken at: (b) 0 h — the compound was present on the surface; (c) 6 h — the compound had begun to penetrate the stratum corneum and had entered follicles and glands; and (d) 24 h — a diffuse signal for isoeugenol was observed throughout the skin. (These images were prepared by Isabella Liu (Imperial College School of Medicine) in collaboration with Doug Howes (Unilever Research Colworth, UK).)

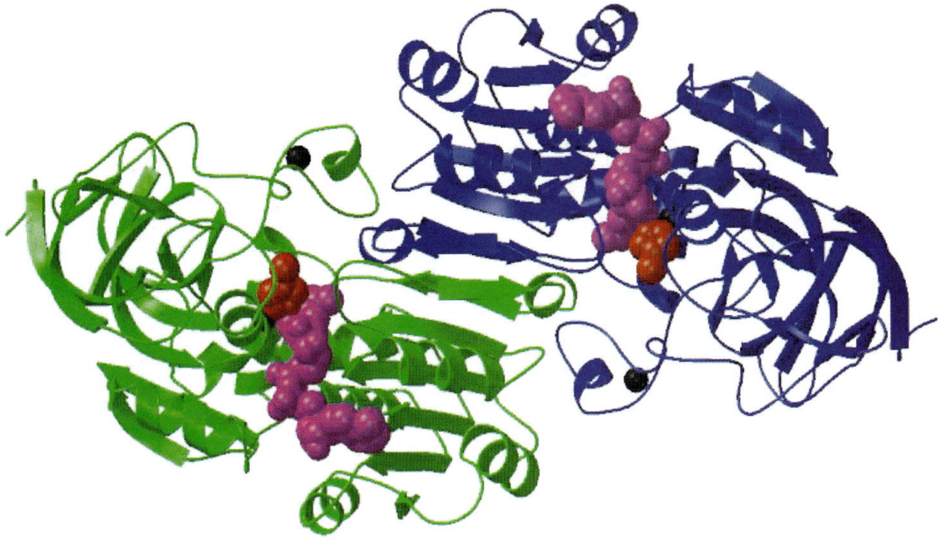

Figure 3.2: Ribbon view of the human class 1 ADH $\beta_1\beta_1$ active dimer. One β_1 subunit is shown in green and the other in blue. The cofactor NAD is shown in pink, in the active site, and the 4-iodopyrazole substrate/inhibitor is shown in red. The catalytic zinc ions are shown as black spheres (one per monomer). (Original figure produced by Dr Thomas Hurley, Indiana University Purdue University Indianapolis (IUPUI), USA.)

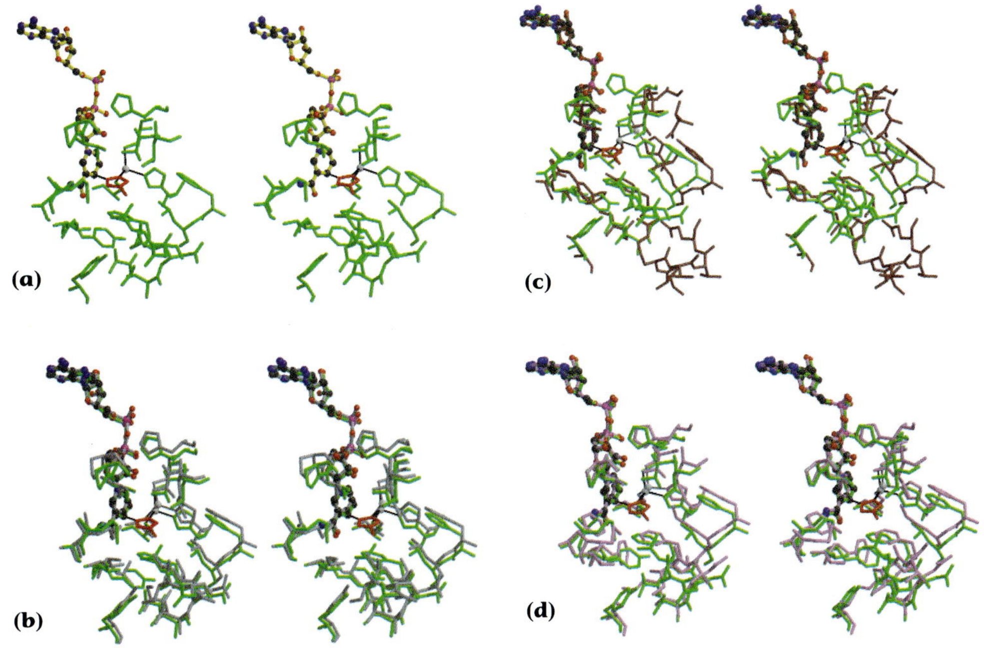

Figure 3.3: Stereoviews of the active sites of the α, β, χ and σ subunits of human alcohol dehydrogenase (ADH). (a) The active site of the β_1 monomer is shown as stick format in green, the NAD cofactor is shown in multicoloured ball and stick format, 4-iodopyrazole is shown in red stick format and the zinc ion is shown as a grey sphere. Overlays are shown between the β_1 monomer active site (green) and (b) the α monomer of class 1 ADH (grey), (c) the χ monomer of class 3 ADH (brown) and (d) the σmonomer of class 4 ADH (lilac). A structure of class 2 ADH was not available for comparison. (Original figure produced by Dr Thomas Hurley, Indiana University Purdue University Indianapolis (IUPUI), USA.)

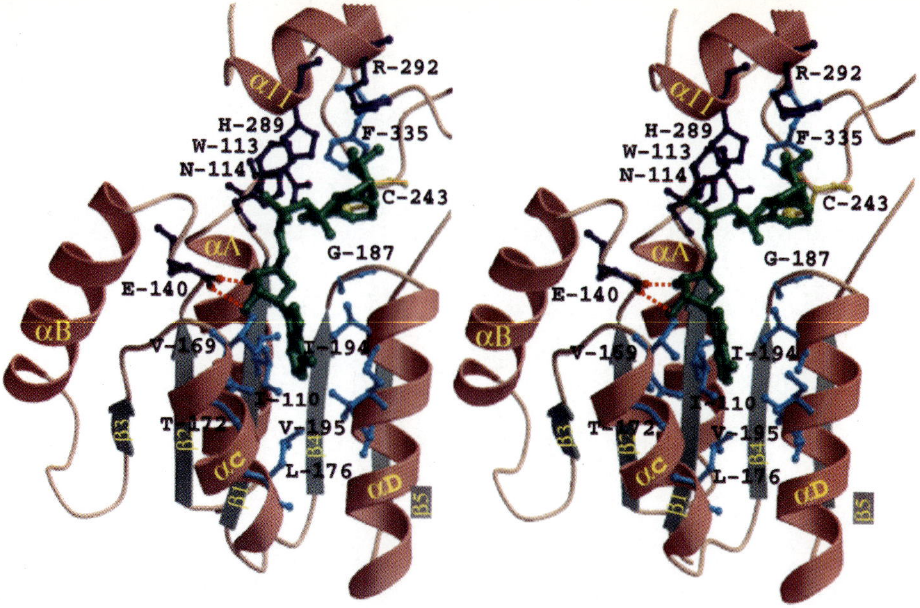

Figure 3.4: Ribbon stereoview of the NAD-binding site in the crystal structure of human aldehyde dehydrogenase class 3. α-Helices are coloured in pink, β-sheet regions are shown as blue arrows. Residues that contact the NAD molecule in the active site are shown in blue and purple stick format and labelled by their single letter amino acid code and residue number. The NAD molecule is shown in green stick format. (Original figure produced by Prof. Bi-Cheng Wang, University of Georgia, USA.)

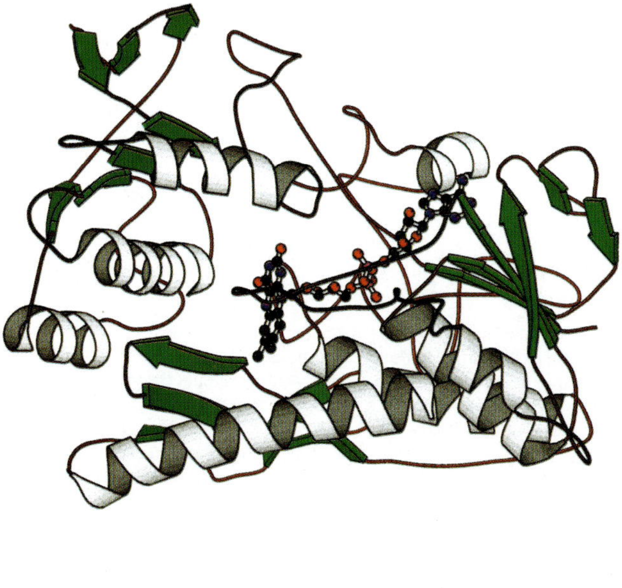

Figure 3.5: Ribbon view of the human monoamine oxidase monomer. α-Helices are drawn in white and green, β-sheets are illustrated as green arrows. The NAD molecule in the active site is drawn in ball-and-stick format. (Original figure produced by Dr Johan Wouters, Facultes Universitaires Notre-Dame de la Paix, Namur, Belgium.)

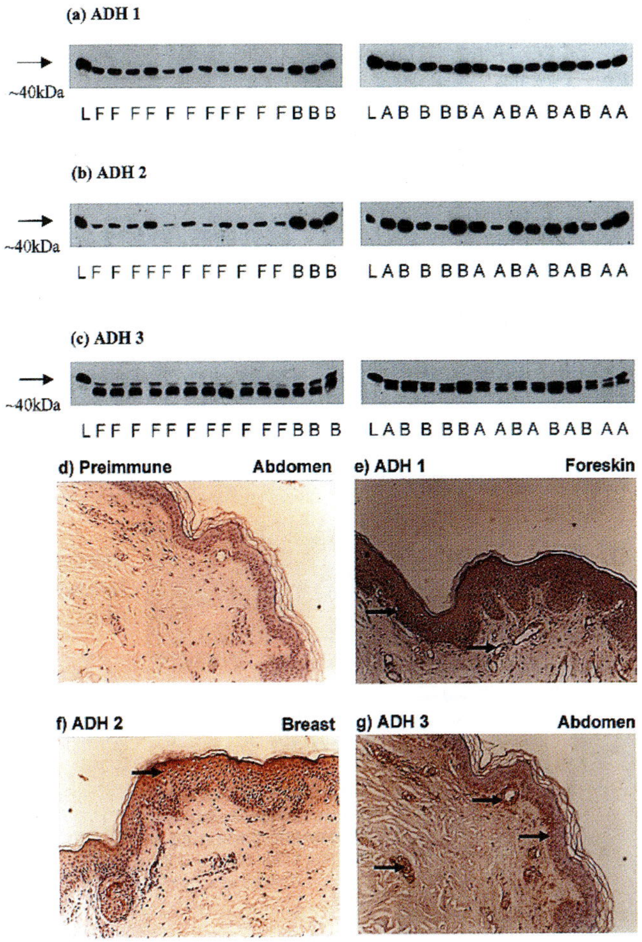

Figure 4.1: Expression and localisation of ADH1 (a and e), ADH2 (b and f) and ADH3 (c and g) in human skin. Figures (a–c): Western blot analysis of ADH enzymes in human skin cytosol fractions. Nitrocellulose membranes were probed with antisera containing class-specific antibodies to (a) ADH 1 (diluted 1:22,000), (b) ADH 2 (diluted 1:5000) and (c) ADH 3 (diluted 1:12,000). L = human liver cytosol sample (1 μg protein loaded except for (b) 0.2 μg loaded), F = foreskin cytosol sample (20 μg protein loaded, age range 1 to 11 years with median age 5, n = 11), B = breast skin cytosol sample (20 μg protein loaded, age range 23 to 59 years with median age 35.5, n = 10) and A = abdomen skin cytosol sample (20 μg protein loaded, age range 30 to 78 years with median age 43, n = 7). Figures (d–g): human skin sections (5 μm) were probed with antisera containing antibodies specific to different ADH classes. Section (d) was incubated with pre-immune sera as a control. Sections were incubated with antisera to (e) ADH 1 (diluted 1:400); (f) ADH 2 (diluted 1:250); (g) ADH 3 (diluted 1:400). Sections (d) and (g) were taken from a 78-year female abdomen skin sample; section (e) was taken from a 5-year male foreskin sample; section (f) was taken from a 24-year breast skin sample. All immunostaining was from diaminobenzidine (DAB) development (brown colour) and all sections were counterstained with Gill's haemtoxylin. Magnification ×125. Arrows on all sections indicate specific immunostaining. For experimental details relating to this work, please see Cheung *et al.*, 1999. (Original figure produced by Connie Cheung, Imperial College School of Medicine, London, UK.)

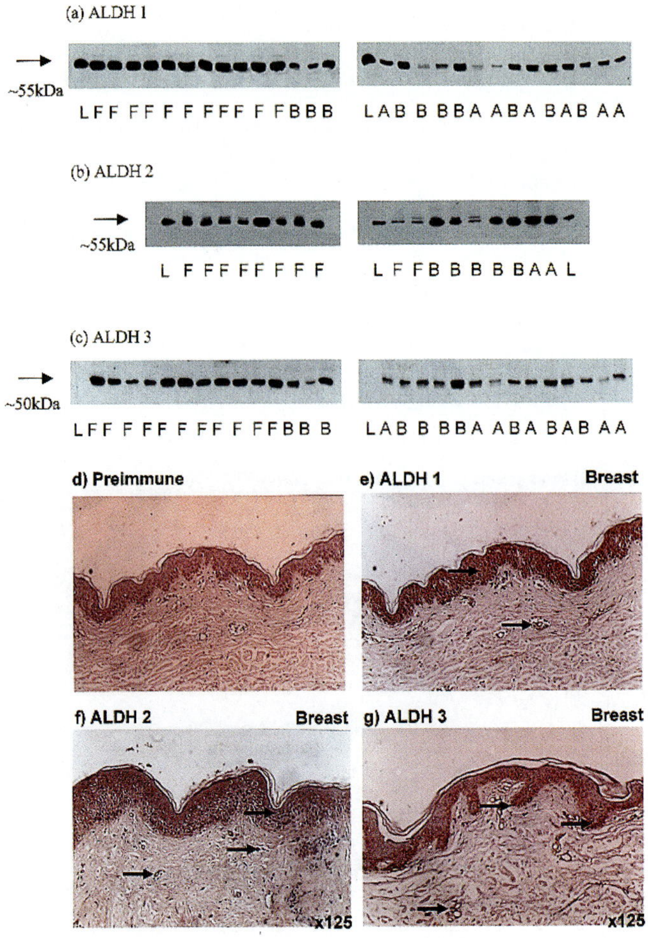

Figure 4.2: Expression and localisation of ALDH1 (a and e), ALDH2 (b and f) and ALDH3 (c and g) in human skin. Figures (a–c): Western blot analysis of ALDH enzymes in human skin cytosol and mitochondrial fractions. Nitrocellulose membranes were probed with antisera containing antibodies to: (a) ALDH 1 (diluted 1:3500); (b) ALDH 2 (diluted 1:7500); and (c) ALDH 3 (diluted 1:5000). Cytosol samples were loaded in (a) and (c), whereas, mitochondrial samples were loaded in (b). L = human liver sample (1 μg cytosolic and 1 μg mitochondrial protein loaded), F = foreskin sample (20 μg cytosolic protein loaded, age range 1 to 11 years with median age 5, n = 11; except for (b) 12 μg mitochondrial protein loaded, age range 1 to 11 years with median age 4, n = 10), B = breast skin sample (20 μg cytosolic protein loaded, age range 23 to 59 years with median age 35.5, n = 10; except for (b) 12 μg protein loaded, age range 28 to 45 years with median age 34, n = 5) and A = abdomen skin sample (20 μg cytosolic protein loaded, age range 30 to 78 years with median age 43, n = 7; except (B) 12 μg protein loaded, age range 39 to 64 years, n = 2). Figures (d–g): human skin sections (5 μm) were probed with antisera containing antibodies specific to different ALDH classes. Section (d) was incubated with pre-immune sera as a control. Sections were incubated with antisera to (e) ALDH 1 (diluted 1:250), (f) ALDH 2 (diluted 1:250) and (g) ALDH 3 (diluted 1:250). Sections (d) and (e) were taken from a 39-year breast skin sample. Section (f) was taken from a 27-year female breast skin sample. Section (g) was taken from a 24-year breast skin sample. All immunostaining was from diaminobenzidine (DAB) development (brown colour) and all sections were counterstained with Gill's haemtoxylin. Magnification ×125. Arrows on all sections indicate specific immunostaining. For experimental details relating to this work, please see Cheung *et al.*, 1999 and 2000b. (Original figure produced by Connie Cheung, Imperial College School of Medicine, London, UK.)

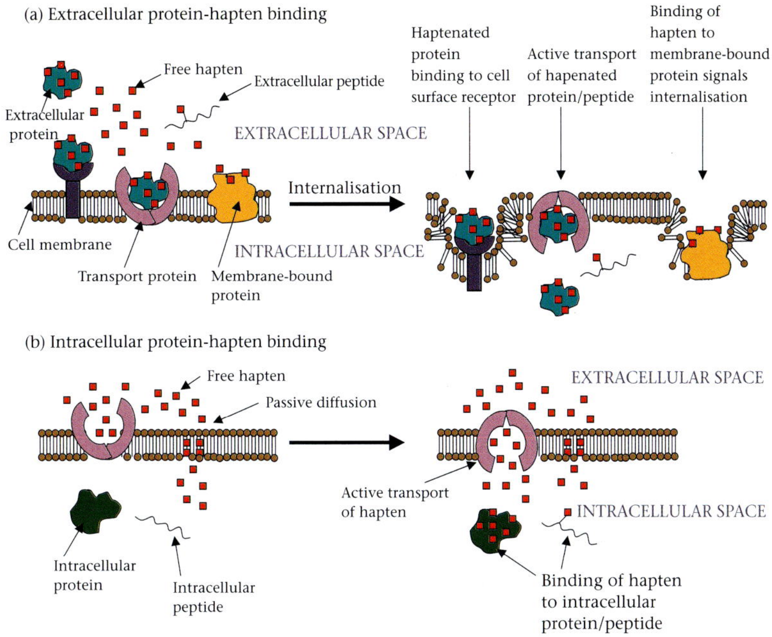

Figure 6.1: Possibilities for extracellular or intracellular protein-hapten binding. (a) Extracellular protein-hapten binding. A number of extracellular protein-hapten binding mechanisms could occur upon skin absorption of a xenobiotic: (i) the hapten may bind to extracellular proteins and the complexes generated could be recognised by cell surface molecules on APCs and internalised; (ii) the hapten may bind to extracellular proteins and the complexes generated could be actively transported into APCs by membrane-bound transport proteins; (iii) the hapten could bind to membrane-bound proteins on the surface of APCs and the binding of the hapten could signal the internalisation of the modified protein. The hapten could also bind to membrane-bound MHCs directly and not require internalisation.
(b) Intracellular protein-hapten binding. An alternative mechanism of protein-hapten binding is that the xenobiotic hapten enters the cell and binds to intracellular proteins. The hapten could either undergo: (i) active transport, or (ii) passive diffusion from the extracellular space, through the cell membrane and into the cytosol of APCs, with subsequent binding of the hapten to intracellular skin protein (or peptide). The protein (or peptide) is likely to be a 'self' molecule in both extracellular and intracellular scenarios. However, it is feasible that viral proteins or peptides, which could potentially invade the body and co-exist in a parasitic fashion without harmful effect to the individual, may be present to bind to hapten.

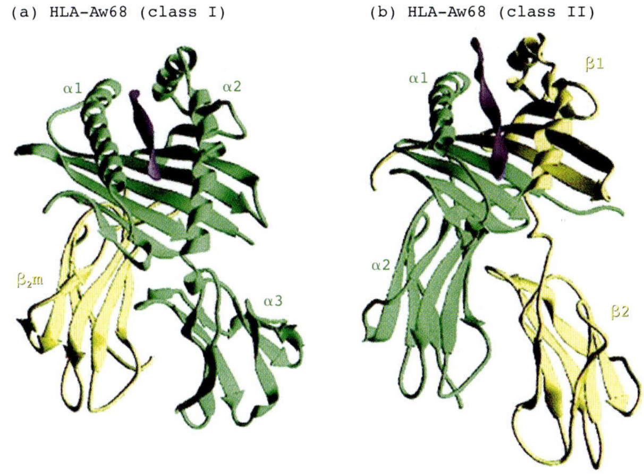

Figure 6.2: Ribbon diagrams of human leukocyte antigen (HLA) class I (Aw68 subtype) (a) and HLA class II (HLA-DR1 subtype) (b) molecules. In (a) the α1, α2 and α3 subunits are shown in green and the β_2m microglobulin domain is shown in yellow. In (b) the α1 and α2 subunits are shown in green and the β1 and β2 subunits are shown in yellow. In both (a) and (b) the peptide is shown as a dark purple ribbon residing between the two long α-helices of the peptide-binding groove. A β-sheet region (indicated by arrows) forms the base of this groove in both structures. (Reprinted from Structure 2(4) Stern and Wiley, 'Antigenic peptide binding by class I and class II histocompatibility proteins', 245–251. © 1994, with permission from Elsevier Science.)

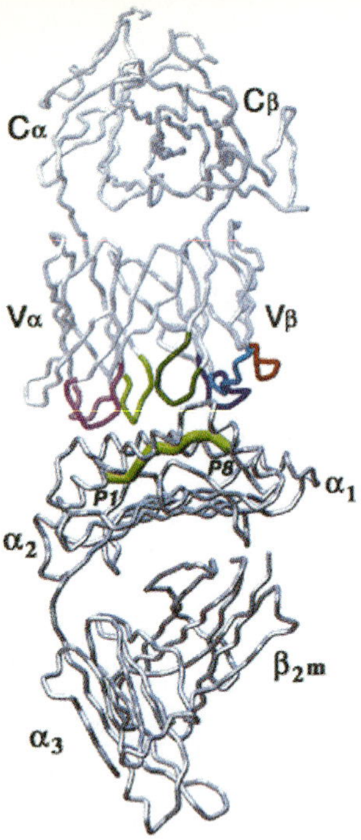

Figure 6.3: Structure of an MHC–peptide–T-cell receptor (TCR) complex. The Cα, Cβ, Vα and Vβ domains of the TCR are illustrated in light blue Cα-backbone worm format on the upper half of the diagram. The variable loops of the Vα and Vβ domains are multicoloured. The α1, α2, α3 and β_2m domains of the MHC molecule are shown in light blue worm format on the bottom half of the diagram. The bound peptide is shown in light green worm format and the positions of the P1 and P8 residues are labelled. (Reprinted with permission from Garcia *et al.* 'An alpha-β T cell receptor structure at 2-SA and its orientation in the TCR-MHC complex', Science, 274: 209–219. © 1996, American Association for the Advancement of Science.)

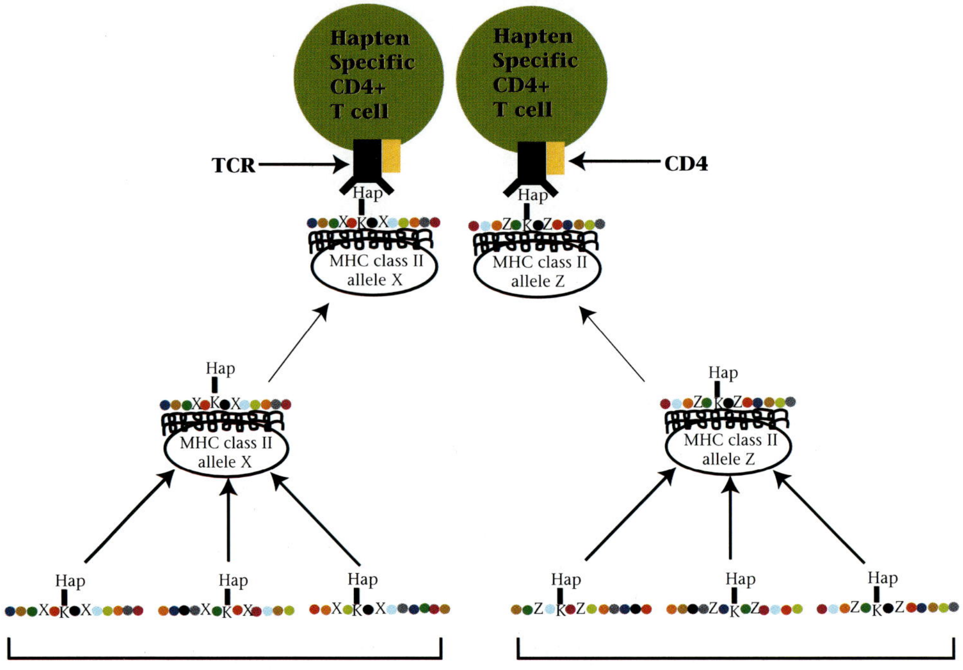

Figure 6.4: Hypothesis that hapten-specific T-cell clones could recognise different peptides, haptenated with the same xenobiotic but presented by different MHC alleles. Haptens can bind to a nucleophilic amino acid such as lysine (K) in peptides of varying sequence (different coloured dots represent different amino acid residues). In order to bind to MHC molecules, in this case class II molecules as the peptides are >10 amino acids, the peptides should contain MHC-binding motif residues (labelled X or Z). The motif residues are MHC allele specific and those that contain motif X could bind to allele X and those with the Z motif could bind to a different allele Z. However, these two different MHC-peptide-hapten antigens, could theoretically be recognised by the same lineage of hapten-specific T cells, if the only antigenic moiety was the hapten that the peptide carried.

post-affinity column eluent (Blacker *et al.*, 1991). The alpha form was only seen in intact human skin and the mu form was only seen in mouse and rat skin in these studies. Immunohistochemistry localised the pi and alpha forms in human skin to the hair follicles (Campbell *et al.*, 1991) and the pi and mu forms in the sebaceous glands and hair follicles in mouse skin (Raza *et al.*, 1991).

A putative sex difference in GST activity with some substrates has been reported to exist in both humans and rodents (Singhal *et al.*, 1992; Singhal *et al.*, 1993). Three GST isoforms, pi (pI = 4.8) and two alpha forms (pI 9.1 and 9.9, respectively), were affinity purified from both male and female human leg skin homogenates (Singhal *et al.*, 1993). The levels of GSH expression for these isoforms were all higher in females (F) than in males (M) (F/M ratios μg/mg total protein: 1.4 (pi), 1.7 (alpha 9.1) and 1.8 (alpha 9.9). Specific activities were also significantly higher for the pi and alpha 9.9 forms, in female skin: e.g. DNCB, male GST-pi, 30 400 ± 2320 nmol/min/mg; DNCB, female GST-pi, 43 900 ± 3210 nmol/min/mg; DNCB, male GST-alpha 9.9, 4260 ± 340 nmol/min/mg; DNCB, female GST-alpha 9.9, 5530 ± 316 nmol/min/mg. In contrast, in rodents GST activities were seen to be higher in males than in females (Singhal *et al.*, 1992).

Reactive electrophiles can also bind directly to GSH (to the —SH group of the cysteinyl group) without catalysis by GST. Depletion of GSH in rat skin (from 4.5 nmol/mg protein to 0.26 nmol/mg) has been shown following incubation of homogenates with DNCB for 90 min (Summer and Goggelmann, 1980). Hirai *et al.* (1997) also showed that on challenging both non-sensitised and sensitised mice with DNCB, there was an immediate drop in GSH levels in both sets of animals and normal levels were re-established within 24 hours.

4.2.1.2.6 Glycine conjugation

Very few studies have investigated glycine conjugation in skin. Nasseri-Sina *et al.* (1997) saw low level glycine conjugation of benzoic acid in human (2% conjugation) and rat (11% conjugation) keratinocyte cultures over 8 hours. Similarly, only low level glycine conjugation of benzoic acid has been observed after topical application on excised skin in flow-through diffusion apparatus: 2% recovery of glycine conjugate in rat skin and negligible recovery in human skin over 24 hours, and 7% recovery in hairless guinea-pig over 48 hours (Nathan *et al.*, 1990; Garnett, 1992).

4.2.1.3 Proteinases and peptidases

Proteolytic enzyme activity in the skin has been reviewed in detail by Hopsu-Havu *et al.* (1977) and, in particular, cutaneous exopeptidase activity has been reviewed by Steinstrasser and Merkle (1995). Peptides have become an important class of drugs and studies during the past two decades have begun to look at how peptides may potentially be metabolised and degraded by exopeptidases upon topical application (Sanderink *et al.*, 1988; Choi *et al.*, 1990; Shah and Borchardt, 1991).

Aminopeptidase, dipeptide hydrolase, dipeptidyl peptidase, carboxypeptidase and collagenase activities have all been demonstrated in human and rodent skin. Recently, confocal fluorescence microscopy, using rhodamine labelled peptide as an aminopeptidase probe, has been used to directly reveal the presence of aminopeptidase activity in human epidermis (Boderke *et al.*, 1997).

4.2.2 Relative activities of hepatic and cutaneous enzymes

Cutaneous enzymes are in general active at significantly lower constitutive levels than their hepatic counterparts (examples range from 0.1% to 28% for Phase I reactions and from 0.6% to 50% for phase II reactions) (see Table 4.2 and also review by Hotchkiss, 1998).[6] However, given the large surface area of the skin throughout which these enzymes are active, low basal level enzyme activities per gram of tissue become significant and it is clear that the skin is an efficient xenobiotic-metabolising organ.

Table 4.2 provides comparative cutaneous activities, for a range of enzymes and selected substrates, expressed as either % specific activity of hepatic counterparts or catalytic activity (moles of substrate converted/min/mg of tissue).

Three possible reasons may explain why cutaneous counterparts of hepatic enzymes have not been identified to date:

a the enzyme may not be expressed in skin;
b the level of constitutive (or inducible) enzyme expression may be too low to be detected by current methods; or
c the relevant experiments have not been performed.

In some cases, particularly when assaying for protein activity, it is difficult to distinguish whether (a) or (b) is the reason why an enzyme has not yet been observed in skin upon investigation. It is more appropriate to use more sensitive molecular biology techniques, such as RT-PCR, Northern blot analysis and *in situ*-hybridisation to look for the presence of low level enzymes. However, the detection of enzymes by these methods alone does not show that these enzymes are active.

4.2.3 Inducibility of cutaneous enzyme expression

Two difficulties arise when assessing the levels of induction of cutaneous enzymes by xenobiotics. Firstly, the levels of constitutive enzyme expression in skin are typically low and beyond the limit of detection of the analytical technique, and hence it is often difficult to compare induced expression levels with those of constitutive expression. Secondly, it has been shown that xenobiotic-metabolising enzyme expression can vary as a function of the stage of keratinocyte differentiation in the epidermis, which is linked to the level of intracellular Ca^{2+} ions (Reiners *et al.*, 1990; Sadek and Allen-Hoffmann, 1994). Also, induction of cutaneous enzymes often depends upon the route of application of the inducer, i.e. the most efficient induction is seen when the inducer is topically applied and induction in the skin is less likely if the inducer is administered systemically.

Human and rodent cutaneous CYP expression (in particular CYP1A1) has been shown to be inducible (in a similar fashion to hepatic enzymes) with classical inducers

TABLE 4.2

Cutaneous enzyme activities: specific activities and comparisons with hepatic activities

Substrate	Specific activity (% liver activity)	Catalytic activity (/mg of skin protein)	Reference
PHASE 1 ENZYMES			
CYTOCHROME P450			
aldrin (CYP2B/3A)	0.4–2.0	—	—
aminopyrene	1	—	—
aniline	6	—	—
benzo(a)pyrene (CYP1A1)	0.1–12.0	—	—
		62 fmol/min/mg	Bickers *et al.*, 1984
		240 fmol/min/mg	Storm *et al.*, 1990
benzo(a)pyrene-7,8-diol	9–11	—	—
7-benzoxyresorufin	6–9	—	—
butoxycoumarin	1	—	—
coumarin	<1	—	—
crysene	2–5	—	—
7,12-dimethylbenz(a) anthracene	3–7	—	—
diphenyloxazole	2–3	—	—
erythromycin (CYP3A)		1.1 nmol/min/mg	Jugert *et al.*, 1994
7-ethoxycoumarin (CYP1A/2B)	0.5–7	—	—
		0.36 pmol/min/mg	Bickers *et al.*, 1982
		24.3 pmol/min/mg	Moloney *et al.*, 1982
		0.11 pmol/min/mg	Cotovio *et al.*, 1996
7-ethoxyresorufin (CYP1A1)	0.1–15	3.6 pmol/min/mg	Pham *et al.*, 1989
		1.5 pmol/min/mg	Pham *et al.*, 1989
		18.0 pmol/min/mg	Moloney *et al.*, 1982
		20.6 pmol/min/mg	Jugert *et al.*, 1994
ethylmorphine	0.5	—	—
methoxycoumarin	1	—	—
p-nitroanisol	2–3	—	—
p-nitrophenol (CYP2E1)		0.04 nmol/min/mg	Jugert *et al.*, 1994
7-pentoxyresorufin	20–27	—	—
		3.7 pmol/min/mg	Pham *et al.*, 1989
		1.8 pmol/min/mg	Pham *et al.*, 1989
		1.7 pmol/min/mg	Jugert *et al.*, 1994
FLAVIN-CONTAINING MONOOXYGENASE			
Methimazole	10	—	Venkatesh *et al.*, 1992
Thiobenzamide	19	—	"
NAD(P)H:QUINONE REDUCTASE			
Dichlorophenol indo-phenol	118 (epidermis)	—	Khan *et al.*, 1987
	19 (dermis)		
	44 (whole skin)		
EPOXIDE HYDROLASE			
Benzo(a)pyrene-4,5-oxide	3–8	—	Pham *et al.*, 1989
Cis-stilbene oxide	9–11		
Trans-stilbene oxide	24–28		
Styrene oxide	6		

TABLE 4.2
Continued

Substrate	Specific activity (% liver activity)	Catalytic activity (/mg of skin protein)	Reference
PHASE 2 ENZYMES			
UDP-GLUCURONOSYLTRANSFERASE			
Benzo(a)pyrene-7,8-dihydrodiol	0.6–2	—	—
Bilirubin	3	—	—
3-hydroxybenzo(a)pyrene	0.6–5	—	—
1-naphthol	2–50	—	—
SULPHOTRANSFERASE			
5-hydroxymethyl chrysene	0.8–3	—	Okuda *et al.*, 1988
1-naphthol	10	—	Macpherson *et al.*, 1991
N-ACETYLTRANSFERASE			
2-acetylaminofluorene	6	—	—
p-aminobenzoic acid	18	—	—
2-aminofluorene	15	—	—
2-hydroxyamino-6-methyl dipyridoimidazole	18	—	—
GLUTATHIONE S-TRANSFERASE			
Benzo(a)pyrene-4,5-oxide	16	—	Mukhtar & Bickers, 1981
cis-stilbene oxide	49	—	Pham *et al.*, 1989
Styrene oxide	14	—	Mukhtar & Bickers, 1981
Butachlor	—	12 pmol/min/mg	Ademola *et al.*, 1993b

Data taken from Mukhtar & Khan, 1989 for specific CYP activities and Hotchkiss (1992) for specific UDP-GT and NAT activities.

such as PAHs, polychlorinated biphenyls, crude coal tar, TCDD, phenobarbitol and ethanol (Alvares *et al.*, 1972, 1973; Levin *et al.*, 1972; Wiebel *et al.*, 1975; Norred and Akin, 1976; Pohl *et al.*, 1976; Bickers *et al.*, 1982, 1986; Mukhtar and Bickers, 1982; Lawrence *et al.*, 1984; Asokan *et al.*, 1986; Das *et al.*, 1986; Lilienblum *et al.*, 1986; Finnen, 1987; Khan *et al.*, 1992; Raza *et al.*, 1992; Jugert *et al.*, 1994; Raffali *et al.*, 1994; Wolkenstein *et al.*, 1998). The levels of CYP1A1 induction can range from 1.5- to 162-fold higher than constitutive levels, depending upon the inducer and substrate analysed (see review by Hotchkiss, 1998).

Sutter *et al.* (1994) have also shown the induction of CYP1B1 mRNA in primary cultures of normal human keratinocytes, following incubation with 10 nM TCDD, which supports the hypothesis that this isoform activates chemical carcinogens. Also, topically applied dexamethasone (a steroid) induces a range of CYPs in mouse skin including CYP1A1, 2B1, 2E1 and 3A (Jugert *et al.*, 1994).

Other cutaneous enzymes are also induced by PAHs, including NAD(P)H:quinone reductase and GT (Lilienblum *et al.*, 1986; Khan *et al.*, 1987). In contrast to CYPs, induction of both of these latter enzymes could aid in detoxifying these chemical carcinogens.

4.3 INTER-SPECIES AND INTER-INDIVIDUAL VARIABILITY OF ENZYME EXPRESSION

Inter-species differences in enzyme expression may affect the accuracy and relevancy of extrapolating toxicity data from animal models to humans. Many of the studies described in section 4.2 and listed in Table 4.2 have shown that expression of xenobiotic-metabolising enzymes occurs across species, however, few *in vitro* studies have directly compared the levels of activity or expression for the same enzyme and substrate in skin from different species.

Mukhtar and Bresnick (1976) investigated glutathione-S-epoxide transferase (GSET) activity in adult mouse skin and human neonatal foreskin and found that activities for styrene oxide and 3-methylcholanthrene-11,12-oxide were 2-fold lower in the human samples. This finding may not be solely due to the difference in species however, but may also be influenced by developmental regulation.

Cheung *et al.* (1999, 2000b) have analysed species differences between alcohol dehydrogenase and aldehyde dehydrogenase enzymes in human and rodent skin. It was seen that ADH2 was absent in rat, mouse and guinea-pig skin but present in human skin, and that ALDH3 was absent in guinea-pig skin but present in human, rat and mouse skin. Their data suggest that genuine differences in ADH and ALDH protein expression exists between species.

Singhal *et al.* (1992, 1993) observed that for GST pi expression in humans, females had higher levels than males but the converse was true in rodents (see section 4.2.1.2.5).

Inter-individual and strain variabilities in cutaneous xenobiotic-metabolising enzyme expression has not been extensively investigated, although it is likely that predisposing genetic factors play major roles in determining whether an individual will be toxicologically susceptible to a xenobiotic. Some studies have begun to look at this phenomenon but due to difficulties in obtaining human skin and the labour-intensive methods used, sample sizes are relatively small.

Cheung *et al.* (1999) analysed skin samples from 28 human individuals for the presence of ADH and ALDH isoforms by semi-quantitative western blotting using densitometric analysis (see sections 4.2.1.1.3 and 4.2.1.1.4 above). These authors found that ADH and ALDH expression varied significantly with anatomical site (foreskin vs breast/abdomen skin) but did not vary significantly between individuals where tissue had been taken from the same site (e.g. breast or abdomen). However, observed site-specific differences in these studies may also be confounded by age-related and gender-related differences.

Oesch *et al.* (1980) evaluated epoxide hydratase and GST activities, with benzo(a)pyrene and DNCB as substrates respectively, in cultured fibroblasts from skin biopsies of different donors and from biopsies of the same donor. This study showed that differences in epoxide hydratase activity between individuals were negligibly small and varied 2.3-fold in 39 cultures from the same subject. GST activity varied equally in cultures from different donors (highest and lowest activities differed 2.3-fold) as in different cultures from the same donor. No significant differences were observed between males and females.

Dijkstra *et al.* (1986) have assayed fluorimetrically the levels of GSET in human hair follicles from smokers and non-smokers and found no differences. Mukhtar and Bresnick (1976) looked at styrene oxide and 3-methylcholanthrene-11,12-oxide metabolism by GSET in six strains of mice (C_3H, C_3Hf, $C_{57}Bl$, DBA/2^+, Balb/c^- and A^+) and found that, for both substrates, Balb/c-mice possessed ~1.5-fold higher activity than the rest.

In order to analyse definitively inter-individual variability in humans it is necessary to statistically analyse hundreds of individuals and at present, given the limitation of human skin sample availability, no such studies have been performed. With the advent of techniques to genotype individuals, this may be a way forward with respect to analysing interindividual differences. However, genotyping may confirm the presence or lack of a gene but does not yield information on the relative enzyme activities. Future advances in the fields of proteomics and metabonomics will hopefully aid in this respect.

4.4 SUMMARY

Although each cutaneous enzyme catalyses a specific biochemical reaction, these enzymes are promiscuous by having the capacity to bind to a range of different xenobiotic substrates, albeit limited by the size and chemical properties of their active sites. Likewise, the same xenobiotic can compete for a range of different enzymes, which would result in the formation of a variety of products. Hence, understanding the balance between detoxication and activation of xenobiotics by multiple metabolic pathways in the skin is crucial in assessing, monitoring or predicting local and systemic toxicity resulting from topical exposure to chemicals. Cutaneous metabolism provides beneficial contributions to the body's chemical defence mechanisms (by detoxifying toxicologically active chemicals to inactive metabolites) and in transdermal drug delivery (by activating inert pro-drugs). Alternatively, cutaneous metabolism may give adverse effects by activating inert compounds to toxicologically active species or by detoxifying an active drug to an inactive metabolite.

The following chapter focuses on how cutaneous metabolism may contribute to the observed levels of skin sensitisation seen for a range of small molecules *in vivo*. Many of the chemicals that come into contact with the skin could, on absorption, be substrates for the enzymes discussed above. For each family of chemicals, hypothetical mechanisms of activation (converting prohaptens to haptens) and detoxication (converting haptens to non-protein-reactive species) are presented and discussed.

NOTES

1 The other CYP families perform endogenous metabolism of, for example, steroids, cholesterol, fatty acids and vitamins.

2 Baron *et al.* (1998) has reported the detection of CYPs 1A1, 1B1, 2B1, 2B6, 2E1 and 3A in human keratinocytes by RT-PCR as confirmed by Northern blotting, immunoblot, immunostaining and catalytic assays. They also report constitutive expression of CYPs 1B1, 2B6 and 2E1 and inducible expression of CYPs 1A1 and 3A3/4 in skin-derived monocytes and macrophages, and constitutive expression of CYP1A1 in skin-derived T cells and endothelial cells. These authors suggest that the observed variations in CYP expression patterns in different skin-derived cells may be important

in the contribution of these cells in metabolising small molecules that may act as contact allergens. This work is currently under review by *J. Invest. Dermatol.*

3 It is also possible that the enzymes aldehyde oxidase and aldehyde reductase may convert aldehydes to acids and alcohols, respectively, but neither of these enzymes have been identified in skin.

4 Previous work by Dannan and Guengerich (1982) also showed the presence of FMO in pig skin by Western blot analysis.

5 These homogenates were prepared and fractionated after a 24 hour *in vitro* percutaneous absorption experiment using flow-through diffusion cells.

6 One notable exception exists, namely, NAD(P)H:quinone reductase, which shows higher specific activity in the epidermis than in the liver (see Table 4.2) (Khan *et al.*, 1987).

CHAPTER

5

Xenobiotics as Skin Sensitisers: Metabolic Activation and Detoxication, and Protein-binding Mechanisms

Contents

In order to act as a contact sensitiser, a small xenobiotic first has to penetrate the stratum corneum and be absorbed into the metabolically viable epidermis (see Chapter 1 (Figure 1.2) and Chapter 2 (Figures 2.1 and 2.3)). Once absorbed, the chemical must, hypothetically, bind to skin protein to form a macromolecular immunogen (see Chapters 1 and 6) or (if non-reactive) be metabolically activated into a protein-reactive metabolite by cutaneous enzymes (see Chapter 4). To go some way forward in understanding how protein-binding affinity and cutaneous xenobiotic-metabolism (both activating and detoxifying) may contribute to levels of observed sensitisation, a range of known skin sensitisers of varying potency are analysed. A compendium of (~200) low molecular weight compounds (<600 g/mol), grouped into chemical families based on functional group similarities and thus also on their potential to be enzyme substrate analogues, is provided. Within each family, the compounds are categorised (according to the classifications published in Cronin and Basketter (1994) and in reference to observed *in vivo* sensitisation data from LLNA and guinea-pig maximisation tests (see Appendix 1)) into sensitisers (strong, moderate and weak) and non-sensitisers.[1] Mechanistic hypotheses are discussed for each family, with respect to the protein-binding potential of the parent compounds and potential metabolism by cutaneous enzymes, in an attempt to rationalise observed levels of sensitisation in biochemical/molecular terms.

5.1 BINDING OF XENOBIOTICS TO BIOLOGICAL MACROMOLECULES

5.1.1 Binding of haptens to protein/peptide

As a hapten is too small to initiate or elicit an immune response (according to classical immunology theory), it has been hypothesised that a hapten must bind to protein or peptide and form an immunogen (see Chapters 1 and 6). This theory, originally postulated by Landsteiner and Jacobs (1936), remains to be proved in relation to skin sensitisation but has been widely accepted.

In order that the protein-binding potency of the parent xenobiotic and/or resulting metabolites can be assessed/predicted, an understanding of the reactions through which small molecules can bind to proteins is required. In general, small molecules that are sensitising haptens possess electrophilic ('electron-seeking') centres that react with peptide/protein nucleophilic (electron-rich) centres (typically on amino acid side chains) by a variety of mechanisms (Dupuis and Benezra, 1982; Roberts and Lepoittevin, 1998).

Roberts and Lepoittevin (1998) concluded from their analyses of a variety of skin sensitisers, that establishing the electrophilic characteristics of a molecule is a good predictor of whether a molecule will act as a sensitiser. This strategy can, however, lead to the occasional prediction of false positive and false negative conclusions (in terms of classifying molecules as sensitising or non-sensitising) as it does not take into account the potential role of skin metabolism, which may result in the activation or detoxication of the original molecule. The complex activation and detoxication of xenobiotics, in relation to observed sensitisation levels, will be discussed in more detail in section 5.3 below. First, for simplicity, we shall discuss the general mechanisms of hapten reactivity and protein-binding, prior to hypotheses of hapten formation and detoxication in skin.

5.1.1.1 Small molecule electrophiles

Figure 5.1 illustrates general examples of small molecule electrophiles. Haptens possessing polarised bonds include halogenated compounds, aldehydes, ketones and amides. Unsaturated (C=C double or triple bond) compounds require intramolecular activation by the inductive and/or mesomeric effects of 'electron-withdrawing' groups (e.g. α,β-unsaturated aldehydes, nitrobenzenes etc.). Table 5.1 shows substituents categorised in terms of their inductive effects. The importance of substituent effects on the reactivity of an electrophilic centre is discussed generally in section 5.1.1.3.2 and for more specific cases throughout section 5.3.

Ions may also be haptens. The most common positively charged species (cations) involved in ACD are Ni^{2+} and Cr^{3+}. The mechanisms through which these metal ions exert their allergic effects are expected to differ from those relating to organic xenobiotic ions (e.g. quaternary ammonium salts and metal salts, which may be subject to metabolism and also contain other electrophilic centres). Hence, nickel allergy will not be discussed in detail here but the reader is referred to the review by Maibach and Menné

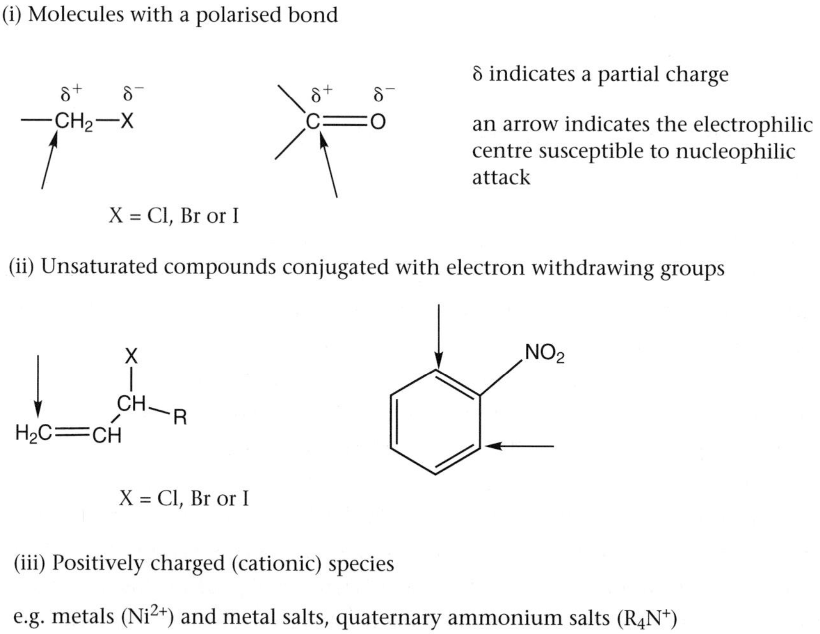

(i) Molecules with a polarised bond
δ+ δ−
CH2—X
δ+ δ−
C=O
δ indicates a partial charge
an arrow indicates the electrophilic centre susceptible to nucleophilic attack
X = Cl, Br or I
(ii) Unsaturated compounds conjugated with electron withdrawing groups
X
CH
R
H2C=CH
NO2
X = Cl, Br or I
(iii) Positively charged (cationic) species
e.g. metals (Ni2+) and metal salts, quaternary ammonium salts (R4N+)

Figure 5.1: Small molecule electrophiles.

TABLE 5.1
Inductive/mesomeric effects of substituents (Sub)

$\delta+$ >C ⟶ Sub Electron-withdrawing	$\delta-$ >C ⟵ Sub Electron-donating
HO — CH_3O — Cl > Br > I — NO_2 — C_2H_5 — $CH_5 = CH$ —	$CH_3 < CH_3CH_2 < CH_3CH_2CH_2-$ etc.

(1989). Metal ions associated with contact allergy often have the capacity to form co-ordination complexes where the bonds have some covalent character. It may be the case that Ni^{2+} and Cr^{3+} can bind in haem moieties *in vivo* replacing Fe or Co ions that are essential for haem activity. Hence, some enzymatic processes may be altered and as such normal metabolism may be affected, in addition to the allergic reactions seen with these metal ions.

5.1.1.2 Amino acid nucleophiles

Nucleophiles are either:

i atoms containing one or more unshared pairs of electrons; or
ii negatively charged ions (anions).

Free amino acids (Figure 5.2a) exist as zwitterions, which possess unusual reactivity. Amino acids are neither as strongly basic as amines nor as acidic as carboxylic acids due to the intramolecular interaction between the protonated amine and the negatively charged carboxylate group. Once incorporated into a polypeptide, an amino acid loses its zwitterionic properties (Figure 5.2b) and in terms of hapten binding to protein, only those amino acids that possess nucleophilic side chains are considered important. Figure 5.2c shows the major amino acid side chains that can act as nucleophiles.

Lysine (Lys) (ε-amino group), cysteine (Cys) (-SH group) and histidine (His) (imidazole group) are the strongest nucleophiles (Figure 5.2c). However, it should be noted that at physiological pH, a significant proportion of the Lys ε-amino group and His 'tele' nitrogens will be protonated and residues in this state will not be nucleophilic. Similarly, arginine (Arg) is a weaker nucleophile than either Lys or His and will be even more strongly protonated at physiological pH. It has been estimated that at pH 7.3, a mere 0.0006% of the arginine guanidino group exists in its unprotonated, nucleophilic form

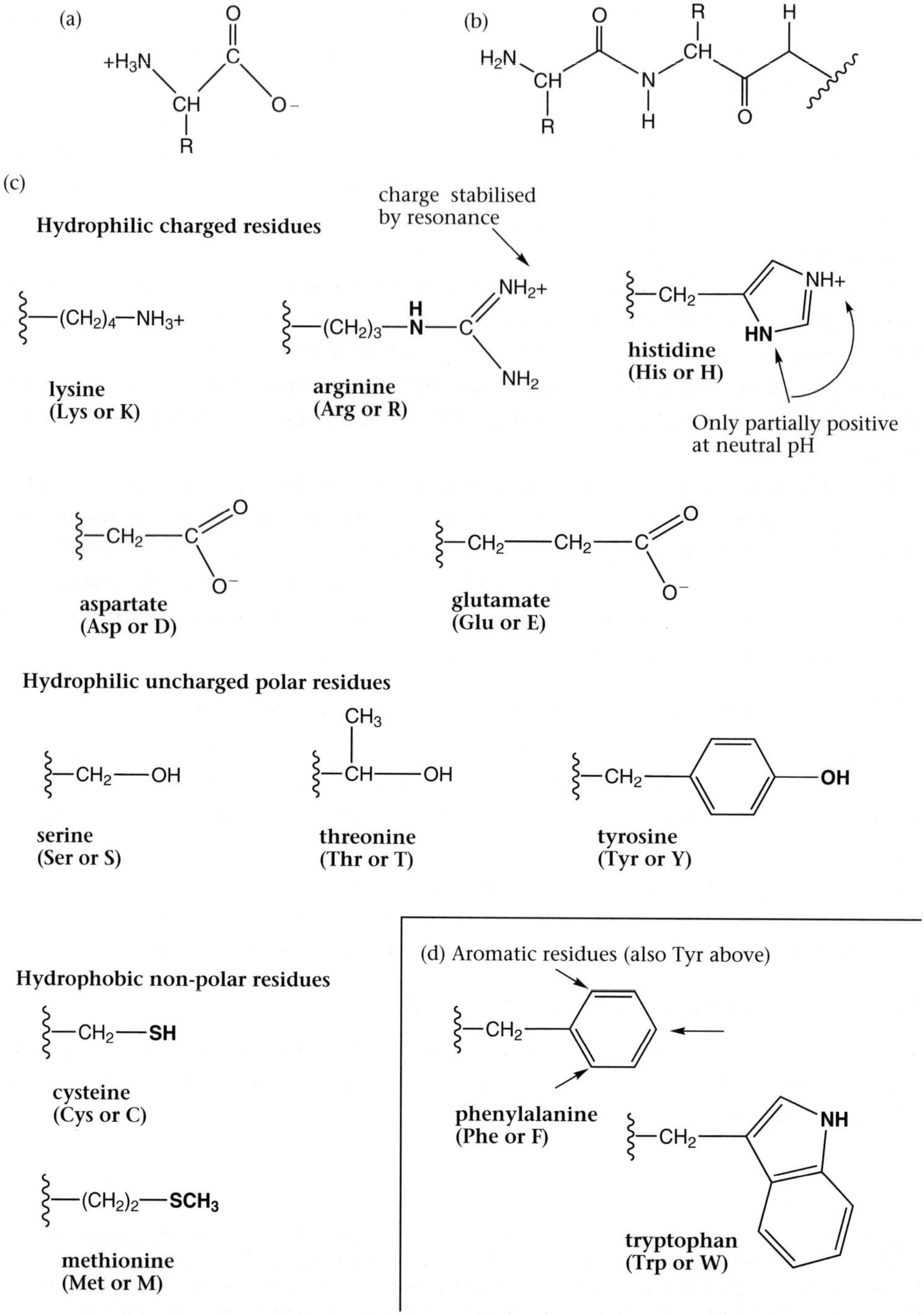
(a)
+H3N
CH
R
C
O
O-
(b)
H2N
CH
R
O
N
H
R
CH
O
H
(c)
Hydrophilic charged residues
charge stabilised
by resonance
(CH2)4—NH3+
lysine
(Lys or K)
(CH2)3—N—C
H
NH2+
NH2
arginine
(Arg or R)
CH2
NH+
HN
histidine
(His or H)
Only partially positive
at neutral pH
CH2—C
O
O–
aspartate
(Asp or D)
CH2—CH2—C
O
O–
glutamate
(Glu or E)
Hydrophilic uncharged polar residues
CH2—OH
serine
(Ser or S)
CH3
CH—OH
threonine
(Thr or T)
CH2
OH
tyrosine
(Tyr or Y)
Hydrophobic non-polar residues
CH2—SH
cysteine
(Cys or C)
(CH2)2—SCH3
methionine
(Met or M)
(d) Aromatic residues (also Tyr above)
CH2
phenylalanine
(Phe or F)
CH2
NH
tryptophan
(Trp or W)

(Greenstein and Winitz, 1961).[2] In contrast, the pKa of Cys has been calculated to be ~6.0, therefore it should be substantially ionised to the thiolate anion at physiological pH. Cys residues are typically involved in disulphide bridges in proteins however, and there are few free Cys residues available for hapten binding, unless the protein is in a reducing environment.

The —OH group of serine (Ser), threonine (Thr) and tyrosine (Tyr) residues may act as a weak nucleophile, but only in cases where the electrophilic xenobiotic contains a good leaving group, e.g. a halogen. Ser may act as a good nucleophile when the environment is tailored, as in the case of the histidine-activated serine in the reactive catalytic triad of serine proteases such as trypsin and chymotrypsin.

Aspartate (Asp) and glutamate (Glu) residues possess negatively charged side chains and can potentially form ionic bonds to xenobiotic cations, e.g. quaternary ammonium salts (see section 5.1.1.4.9) or their CO^{2-} groups can act as nucleophiles.

Aromatic amino acids, such as phenylalanine (Phe), tryptophan (Trp) and tyrosine (Tyr), can act as one-electron acceptors i.e. react with free radicals (see section 5.1.1.3.8 below).

It is also possible that the free amine group at the N-terminus (pKa = 7.1) of a protein/peptide is able to bind to xenobiotics and this amine will be less protonated than other side chain amine groups at physiological pH.

The specific nucleophilic protein/peptide residues at which particular compounds can covalently bond will have relevance to the specific types of peptide antigens that they can form and this is discussed in more detail in Chapter 6.

5.1.1.3 Molecular properties affecting electrophile/nucleophile reactivity

Simple chemicals can be classified in many ways including acidity/basicity, their position on the hard–soft scale and by the extent to which they are sterically hindered. If quantitative parameters could be theoretically determined to predict the electrophilic or nucleophilic character of an unknown chemical (based on prior empirically determined and rule-based values for a large selection of chemicals of known sensitisation) this may contribute to future models that could predict sensitisation potential. Some chemical studies have been performed in an attempt to empirically determine values for reactivity parameters.

5.1.1.3.1 Measurement of nucleophile reactivity

Swain and Scott (1953) developed the following equation for measuring nucleophilicity of a compound that reacts by an S_N2 reaction (see section 5.1.1.4.1 below) relative to a reference standard:

Figure 5.2: Protein residues that may react with xenobiotics. The structures of: (a) a general amino acid; and (b) the general protein backbone, are shown, where variation in the R group determines the residue type. R groups that are potential nucleophiles are shown in (c) — the groups are drawn in their protonated states as they are likely to exist at physiological pH — and (d) shows the aromatic side chains that may act as one-electron acceptors.

$$\log(k/k_s) = s(n - n_s)$$

where s = electrophile susceptibility, n = nucleophilicity of the unknown, n_s = nucleophilicity of the reference nucleophile, k = rate constant for reaction of the nucleophile with a reference electrophile, k_s = rate constant for reaction with reference standard. The reference electrophile used in their study was methyl bromide and the reference standard nucleophile was water. The n value can be determined for a given nucleophile by defining the s value of the reference electrophile as unity and the n_s value of water as zero. Log of the ratio of the measured rate constant for methyl bromide reaction with a nucleophile (k) and the rate constant for hydrolysis in water ($k_s = k_w$) gives the value n for that nucleophile. Conversely, once n values have been calculated, s can be determined for a variety of electrophiles. Rate constants for the reaction of the electrophile with nucleophiles of known n value (k) and for its reaction with water ($k_s = k_w$) are determined. The slope of the plot of log (k/k_w) vs n yields s.

It should be noted, however, that such calculations are not absolute and may not be directly applicable in predicting chemical reactivity in biological systems. However, an *in vitro* correlation with sensitisation potency might exist that could be used in predictive modelling for xenobiotics.

5.1.1.3.2 Measurements of electrophile reactivity — 'reactivity parameter'

As the substituents on a molecule affect the reactivity of the electrophile, models have been derived using linear free energy relationships (i.e. Hammett (σ^-) and Taft (σ^*) constants for the substituents), which have successfully predicted whether a compound is electronegative enough to perform a haptenation reaction via an S_N mechanism (see section 5.1.1.4) (Roberts, 1995). The general model has been termed the reactivity parameter (RP) but different models are required for different types of compound. For example, the RP as derived by Roberts (1995) for dinitrohalobenzenes is calculated as follows:

$$\text{RP} = \Sigma\sigma^-(o, m, p) + 0.45\sigma^*(i)$$

where o, m and p represent the ortho, meta and para positions on the aromatic groups relative to the group displaced and $\sigma^*(i)$ is the Taft constant, a measure of the inductive properties, for the group displaced. In this study it was shown that if a substituted nitrophenol molecule had an RP of greater than 3.80 it was a positive sensitiser and if it was less than 3.65 it was a non-sensitiser. In general, calculated RPs can replace the $a \log k$ term in the RAI model (described in section 5.4.1).

5.1.1.3.3 Hard and soft theory

The classical hard and soft theory of acids and bases can also be applied to electrophiles and nucleophiles (Fessenden and Fessenden, 1990; Roberts and Lepoittevin, 1998). Hard electrophiles preferentially react through their low-energy vacant orbitals with the occupied orbitals of hard nucleophiles, and are of low polarisability (Roberts and Lepoittevin,

1998). Similarly, soft electrophiles preferentially react with soft nucleophiles through higher energy orbitals and are of higher polarisability. Examples of hard nucleophiles are water, hydroxide ions, carboxylate anions, alcohols and alkoxides. Primary amines can also be considered as hard to intermediate nucleophiles. Thiols, thiolate anions and sulphides are examples of soft nucleophiles.

Therefore, based on this theory, soft xenobiotic electrophiles are more likely to react with soft thiol groups or thiolate anions in Cys residues than to any other protein nucleophile.[3] Similarly, hard xenobiotic electrophiles are more likely to react with hard nucleophiles such as Lys, Thr and Ser in proteins than with Cys. Hence, hardness and softness of the xenobiotic electrophile may also be a factor in predicting its type of reaction with protein.

5.1.1.3.4 Steric effects

It may be the case that a molecule contains an electrophilic centre but it is sterically hindered by neighbouring substituents. Hence, steric effects can contribute to the reactivity of a molecule and for some compounds, a measurement of steric hindrance could be incorporated into an RP calculation (see section 5.1.1.3.2 above) although the effects may be too subtle to quantify reliably. A look at the energy minimised 3D structure of a xenobiotic using molecular graphics would confirm that this needs consideration.[4]

5.1.2.4 Mechanisms of protein-binding

Some examples of two-electron (nucleophilic substitution, addition-elimination and nucleophilic addition) and one-electron (radical) reactions are generically shown below for a range of small molecule electrophiles (Schemes 5.1–5.8). These reactions result in covalent bonding between molecules. Scheme 5.9 shows how xenobiotics may also bind to proteins via ionic bonding.

5.1.2.4.1 Nucleophilic substitution (S_N)

No evidence exists to suggest that S_N1 (unimolecular nucleophilic substitution) reactions are involved in sensitisation. Similarly, no naturally occurring skin sensitising haptens have had their allergenicity proved as a result of their ability to react with protein via an S_N2 (bimolecular) reaction (Scheme 5.1), although several synthetic primary halide S_N2 electrophiles are sensitising (Roberts and Lepoittevin, 1998). In S_N2 reactions, the nucleophile acts as the attacking group and the group (in Figure 5.1a the halogen, X) bonded to the electrophilic centre acts as the leaving group. It should be noted that although S_N2 reactions lead to an inversion of molecular configuration for attack at tertiary carbon atoms, only primary halides are reactive enough under physiological conditions to react with proteins by an S_N2 mechanism and hence inversion does not arise.

In the case of aromatic halides, the nucleophilic substitution mechanism is called an S_NAr reaction. This reaction will only occur on aromatic molecules that are activated by electron-withdrawing substituents (e.g. NO_2, CN, etc.). Such is the case for the classical strong sensitiser dinitrochlorobenzene (DNCB) (Figure 5.16a).

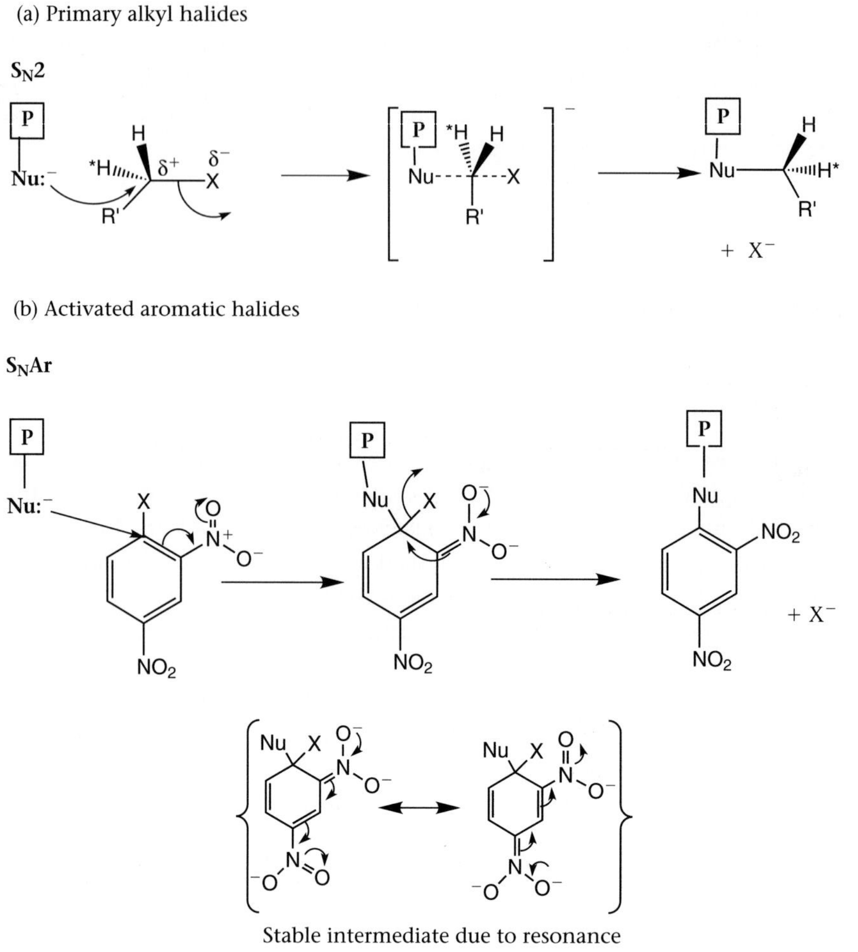

Scheme 5.1: Nucleophilic substitution of halogenated compounds.

5.1.2.4.2 Addition-elimination of aldehydes and ketones; Schiff base formation

The net effect of addition-elimination at an unsaturated centre is nucleophilic substitution (also termed S_NAr), via the replacement of a functional group in the xenobiotic with the nucleophilic group of the protein residue, thus forming a covalent bond to the protein. The rate-determining step of this reaction is the attack of the nucleophile. When the protein nucleophile is a primary —NH_2 group, as in the case of the ε-amino group of lysine, the resulting product formed is a Schiff base (an imine) (Scheme 5.2). If the nucleophile is an —OH group, as in serine residues, the product formed would be a hemiacetal.

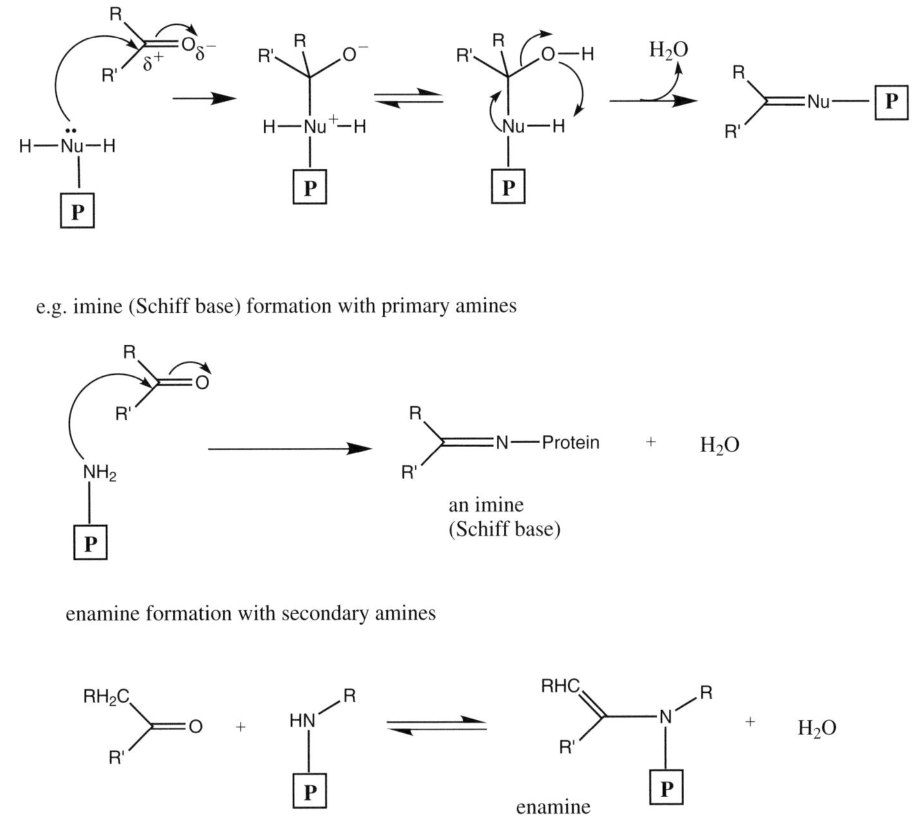

Scheme 5.2: Addition-elimination of aldehydes and ketones; Schiff base formation.

5.1.2.4.3 Addition-elimination of acids, esters and amides

A typical addition-elimination reaction for acids, esters and amides is shown in Scheme 5.3. These kinds of reactions are different from addition-elimination of aldehydes and ketones, in that expulsion of the leaving group and not the attack of the nucleophile is the rate-determining step. For example, in xenobiotic esters an MeO- leaving group is not as good a leaving group as an ArO- group as the conjugate acid is less stable for the former. ArO- groups in the presence of electron withdrawing substituents are even better leaving groups. It is often the case that the acyl or amide group requires activation by another neighbouring carbonyl or amide group within the molecule in order to be reactive enough for addition-elimination to occur. The reactive acyl or amide group is a hard electrophile and typically reacts with hard nucleophiles such as Lys and His.

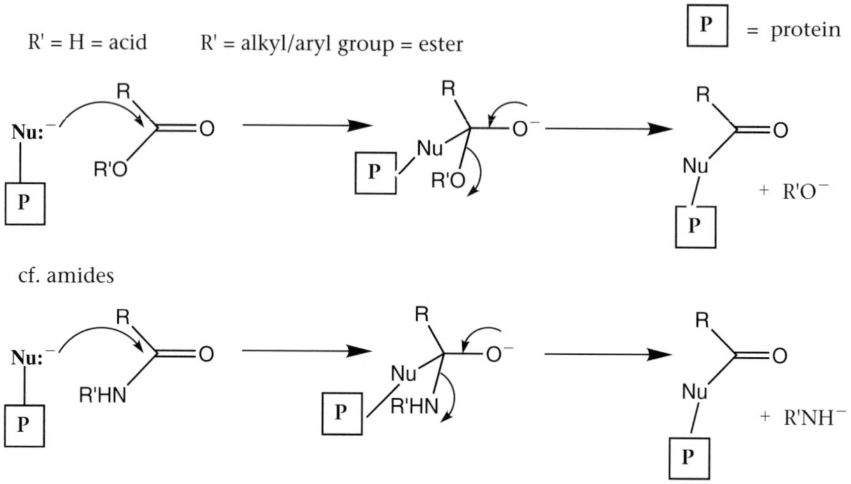

Scheme 5.3: Addition-elimination of acids, esters and amides.

5.1.2.4.4 Nucleophilic addition of aldehydes and ketones

Many nucleophilic addition reactions, especially those involving weak nucleophiles, are acid-catalysed and result in the formation of a saturated compound, due to there being no leaving group (Scheme 5.4). There is no evidence as to whether nucleophilic addition of aldehydes and ketones can occur *in vivo*, but the skin is typically acidic and hence such reactions may be possible. Although it should also be noted that in order for a ketone to be a reactive enough electrophile to sensitise, electron-withdrawing substituents (Table 5.1) are required in neighbouring positions to the carbonyl group.

5.1.2.4.5 Michael addition of α,β-unsaturated compounds

α,β-Unsaturated compounds possessing a double (or a triple) bond (soft electrophile) activated by an electron-withdrawing group, such as a carbonyl, have the capacity to act as Michael acceptors (Scheme 5.5). One naturally occurring sensitiser that reacts via this

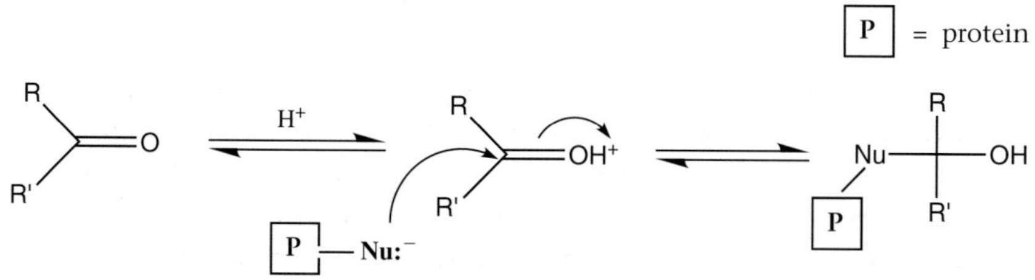

Scheme 5.4: Nucleophilic addition of aldehydes and ketones.

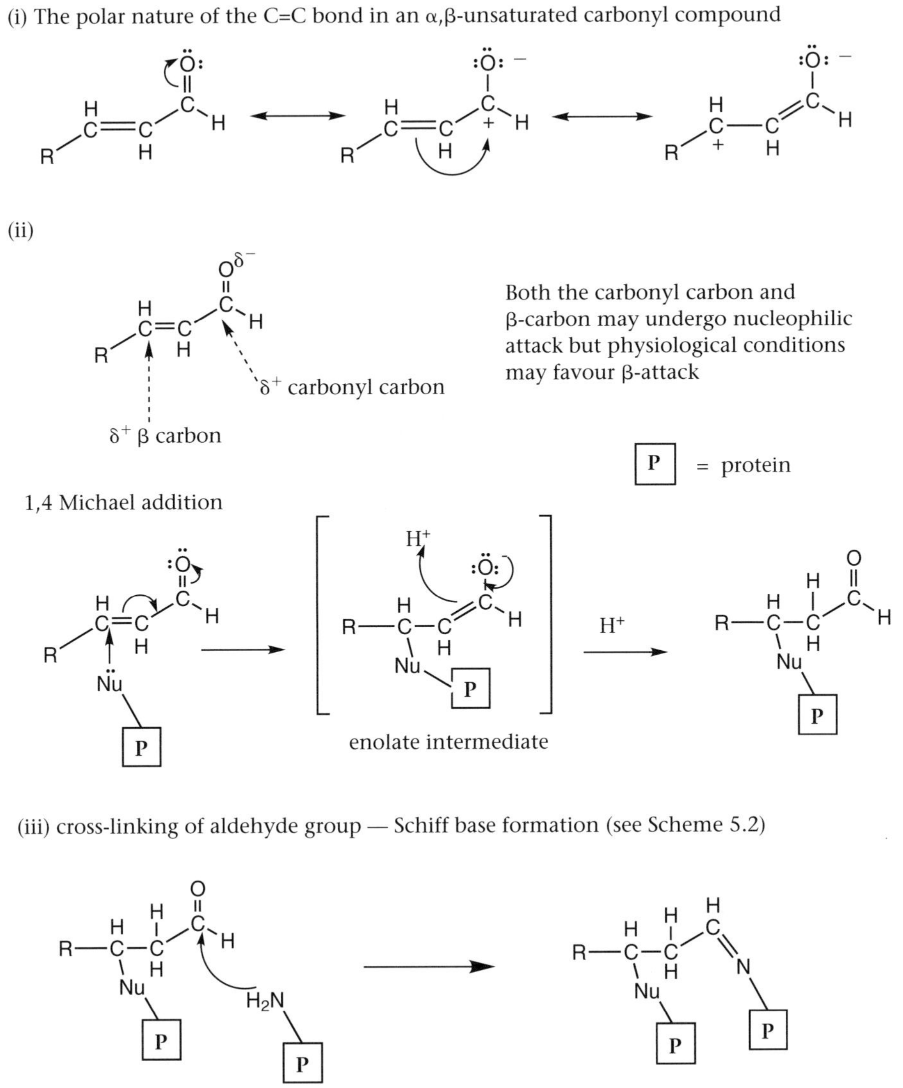

Scheme 5.5: Michael addition of α,β-unsaturated compounds and the potential cross-linking of proteins.

mechanism is tulipalin A, the allergen of tulip bulbs (Slob, 1973). Examples of synthetic chemicals that can act as Michael acceptors are acrylates and methacrylate esters. Scheme 5.5 shows a typical 1,4-Michael addition reaction between a general α,β-unsaturated compound and a soft protein nucleophile such as Cys.

α,β-Unsaturated aldehydes (such as cinnamaldehyde) are unusual in that they possess dual functionality with respect to protein-binding. Both 1,4-Michael addition across the double bond as well as Schiff base formation with protein primary amines (Scheme 5.2) can occur. This may well allow for the existence of cross-linking between two proteins/peptides. However, it is anticipated that Michael addition should occur before Schiff base formation, as without the aldehyde group activating the β-carbon of the double bond, the reactivity of the latter will be nullified. This is a theory that remains to be proven.

5.1.2.4.6 Nucleophilic addition by ring-cleavage of epoxides

Nucleophilic addition to epoxides can be acid-catalysed or non-catalysed to yield the same product (Scheme 5.6). In Scheme 5.6, the first step of the reaction is an S_N2 reaction.

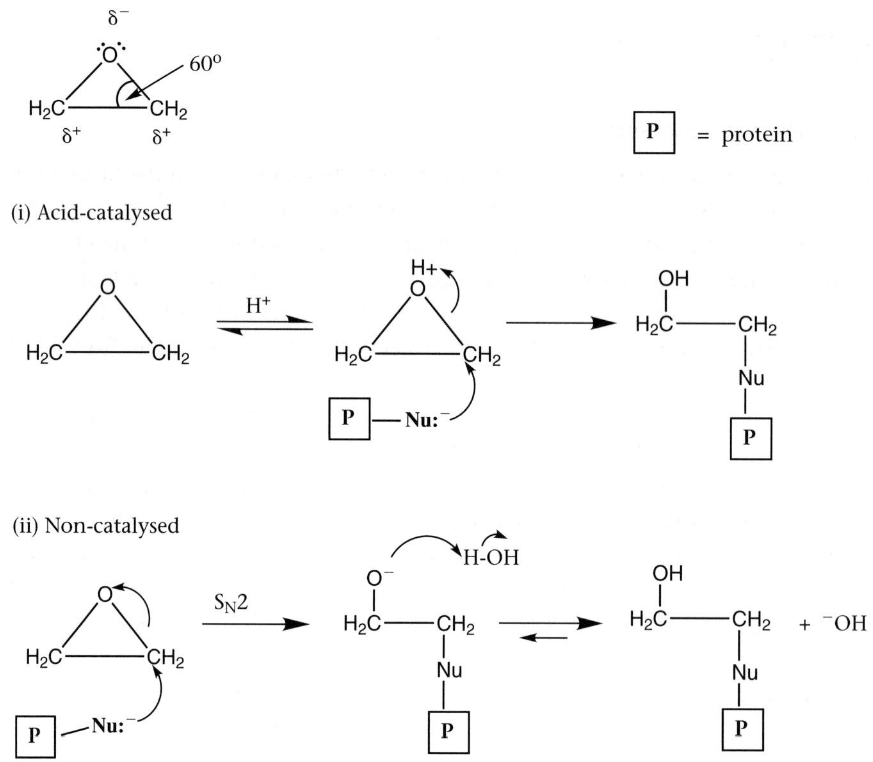

Scheme 5.6: Addition by ring-cleavage of epoxides.

5.1.2.4.7 Electrophilic substitution of diazonium salts

A general electrophilic substitution reaction between diazonium salts and aromatic protein side chains is illustrated in Scheme 5.7.

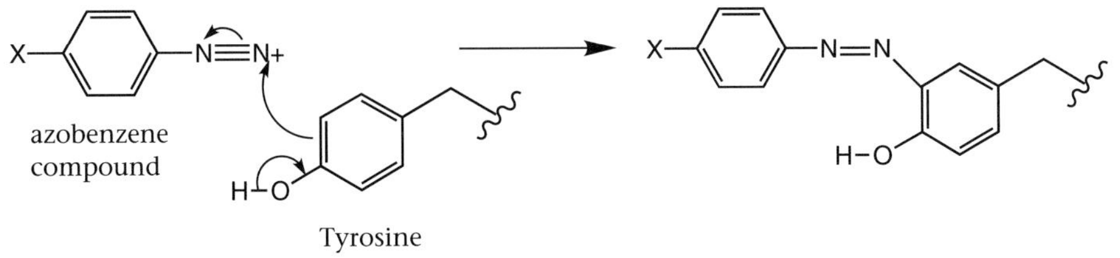

Scheme 5.7: Electrophilic substitution of diazonium salts.

5.1.2.4.8 Radical reactions

Free-radicals are produced as by-products of normal metabolism and the body possesses a variety of effective mechanisms for their elimination. However, during oxidative stress, exerted by metabolic disorders or exposure to environmental challenges, such as ultraviolet irradiation or xenobiotics, radicals may be overproduced. Endogenous free-radicals that may cause modification of protein side-chains include: hydroxyl radical (•OH), superoxide anion radical ($O_2^{\bullet}$-), thiyl radical (RS•) and nitric oxide (•NO) (Wallace, 1997).[5]

All protein residues are susceptible to attack by hydroxyl radicals but in particular, the aromatic ring of residues Tyr, Phe and Trp and the imidazole of His are the major one-electron acceptors (Figure 5.2). Substituents on an aromatic ring have an electron-directing effect in terms of the position of radical-binding. In tyrosine, the —OH group directs the radical to bind at the position α to it (see Scheme 5.8). In phenylalanine, the *ortho* and *para* positions are favoured due to lower electron density at these positions (Wheland and Pauling, 1935). Tryptophan also directs radicals to its α position.

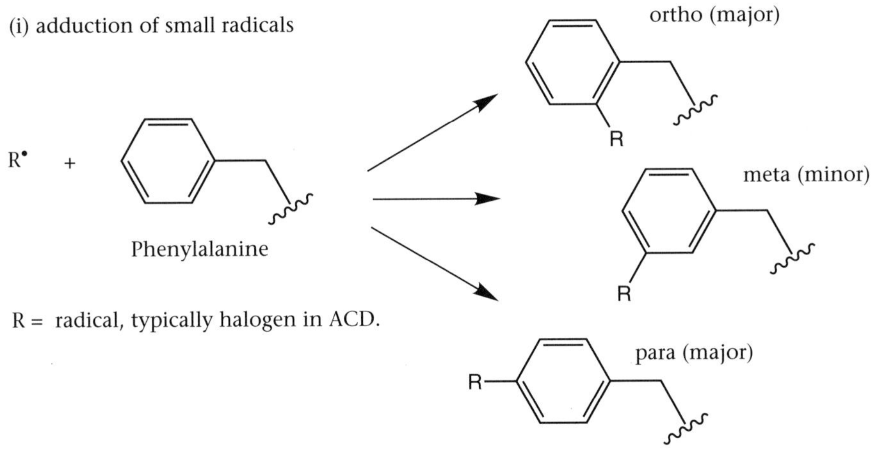

(ii) adduction of larger radicals

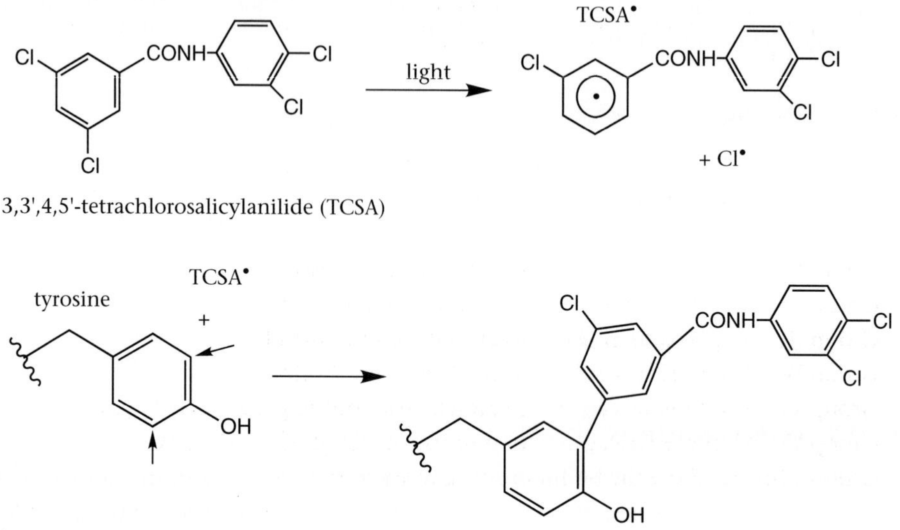

Scheme 5.8: Radical adducts to proteins.

5.1.2.4.9 Ionic bonding

Charged xenobiotics, such as quaternary ammonium ions and metal ions (e.g. nickel and chromium) may bind to charged amino acids via ionic bonding (Scheme 5.9). It is not expected that ionic bonding contributes to sensitisation of ammonium ions, however (see section 5.3.18).

(i) ionic bonds

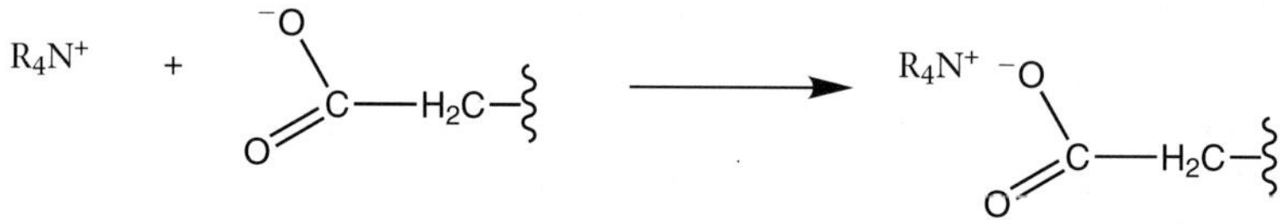

(ii) hydrogen bonds

e.g.

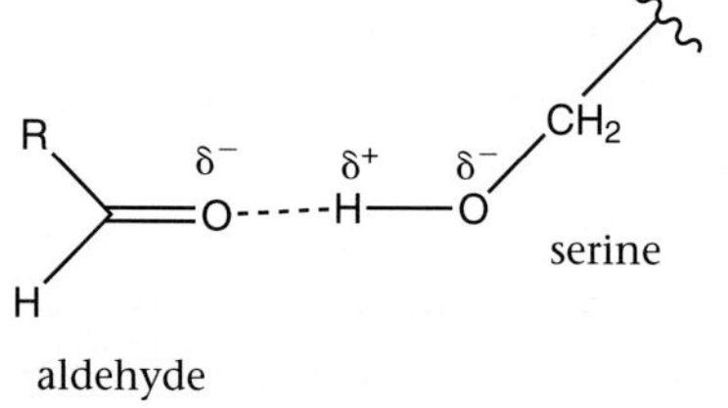

Scheme 5.9: Electrostatic interactions.

Another example of charge bonding is hydrogen bonding, although such bonds are characteristically weak and are not expected to be important in antigen formation. However, intramolecular hydrogen bonding may affect the reactivity and availability of an electrophilic centre.

5.1.2.5 Classification of haptens

Throughout this chapter, haptens will be classified (according to the groups defined initially by Dupuis and Benezra (1982) and based on the reactions above) as follows:

Group I: Haptens susceptible to nucleophilic substitution (S_N)
Group II: Haptens susceptible to addition-elimination
Group III: Haptens susceptible to electrophilic substitution
Group IV: Haptens susceptible to nucleophilic addition
Group V: Haptens susceptible to radical reactions (e.g. loss of halogen)
Group VI: Haptens susceptible to multiple nucleophilic reactions
Group VII: Metallic salts with chelating properties

In all of the figures in section 5.3, the electron deficient site of nucleophilic attack in a hapten is marked with an arrow.

5.2 CONCEPTS OF PROHAPTEN ACTIVATION AND HAPTEN DETOXICATION

To reiterate, an early event in the sensitisation phase required to generate the xenobiotic-specific immune response that causes ACD (see Chapter 1) is, hypothetically, binding of the parent xenobiotic and/or its metabolites to skin macromolecules (Landsteiner and Jacobs, 1936; Dupuis and Benezra, 1982; Roberts and Lepoittevin, 1998). For covalent binding to occur, it is likely that the small molecule contains an electrophilic (electron-deficient) centre that will react with protein nucleophiles (electron-rich) (Dupuis and Benezra, 1982; see also section 5.1 above for mechanisms). Such a protein-reactive small molecule, that when bound to a polypeptide forms an antigen, is called a 'hapten'. All haptenic groups in the figures relating to section 5.3 are emboldened.

In evaluating whether a molecule has the capacity to act as a hapten, a number of considerations other than its electrophilic character also need to be made. Some potential haptens may not penetrate the stratum corneum (see Chapter 2), therefore lipophilic properties (such as log $P_{o/w}$) and solubility in aqueous solutions (molar refractivity (MR) values) need to be analysed. Some haptens may bind to skin proteins directly upon absorption and go on to cause sensitisation, but the affinity of protein binding may be a factor with regards to potency. Alternatively, some potential haptens may penetrate the skin but show little effect as they are detoxified by metabolism (although to date, evidence for this in relation to sensitisation is not available in the literature).

Conversely, some skin sensitisers do not appear to be protein-reactive molecules at all or at least have a very weak electrophilic character. It has therefore been hypothesised that such sensitising compounds undergo cutaneous activation to become haptens (Dupuis and Benezra, 1982). In this scenario, the parent molecule is termed a 'prohapten' and the activated compound acts as the true sensitising hapten.

5.2.1 Prohapten activation and hapten detoxication by skin metabolising enzymes

It is hypothesised that skin enzymes (predominantly located in the epidermis as described in Chapter 4) can metabolise absorbed xenobiotics via reactions analogous to those determined in the liver (as described in Chapter 3).[6] Xenobiotic metabolism (both phase I and phase II) could therefore result in:

a activation of an initially unreactive compound into a protein-reactive hapten;
b detoxication of a (protein-reactive) compound, by modification of chemical group functionalities or increasing solubility; or
c performing no net effect and the chemical remains effectively unchanged.

5.2.2 Non-enzymatic xenobiotic oxidoreduction

Xenobiotics can also be activated by non-enzymatic autoxidation and reduction mechanisms. Such mechanisms should also be considered, alongside metabolic mechanisms, when attempting to assess the potential biotransformation of small molecules in skin.

5.2.2.1 Autoxidation

On exposure to air, for example whilst on the skin surface, some chemicals can undergo autoxidation (Karlberg *et al.*, 1999). Therefore, when attempting to determine the haptenic species of a known allergen, especially when the parent compound is a prohapten, it is important to consider whether any products of air oxidation may be haptenic as well as the potential metabolic products of the parent compound. A classical example of this is the sensitising hydroperoxide formed in air-oxidised turpentine (see section 5.3.6). Another example is the air oxidation of the ethoxylated surfactant $C_{12}H_{25}(OCH_2CH_2)_5OH$ (Bergh *et al.*, 1998). It has been shown that upon exposure to air a range of aldehyde products can be formed with the general formula $C_{12}H_{25}(OCH_2CH_2)nOCH_2CHO$ (n = 0–4). The major aldehyde, dodecyltetraoxy-ethyleneoxyacetaldehyde (n = 4), was shown to be as sensitising in guinea-pigs as formaldehyde. This illustrates that impurities in a chemical preparation may account for allergenicity and not the major parent compound in the preparation.

Within tissues, autoxidation mechanisms involve the transfer of an electron from a chemical to O_2 and are often associated with trace amounts of metals e.g. Fe and Cu. For example the reduced metals Cu(I) and Fe(II) when bound to cell components can mediate the production of free radicals e.g. $^{\bullet}OH$ radical generation from $O_2^{\bullet-}$ and H_2O_2.

The parent chemical can often be regenerated by the action of reducing agents (see section 5.2.2.2 below) and effectively non-enzymatic redox cycling occurs.

5.2.2.2 Non-enzymatic reductants

Throughout cells, radicals can be generated by the reaction of xenobiotics with endogenous reductants. For example, nitroso compounds are reduced non-enzymatically to radical species by NAD(P)H, GSH, ascorbate, cysteine or (in erythrocytes) haemoglobin. Also, arene diazonium compounds can be chemically reduced by NADH and ascorbate to aryl radical species. Cellular reductants can also generate radicals from metals including Ni(II) and Cr(III).

It is noteworthy that such non-enzymatic chemical modification of xenobiotics can occur within the skin, however the extent to which these mechanisms are involved in allergenicity is unknown.

5.3 HYPOTHETICAL BIOTRANSFORMATIONS OF SMALL MOLECULES IN SKIN

Although the following chemicals are grouped into families, it is important to emphasise that when attempting to predict whether a compound will be sensitising or not, the properties of each individual compound should perhaps be taken into consideration rather than the sole use of generic rules. As will be shown, within each chemical family, there are compounds with the same chemical group functionalities but very different sensitisation properties. This is mainly due, perhaps, to the variation in reactivity of the functional group, which is affected by the rest of the substituents of the molecule. Variations in log $P_{o/w}$, molecular weight, solubility etc. must be taken into account for each compound. However, it remains useful to classify sensitisers (weak, moderate and strong) and non-sensitisers into chemical families as a base from which to begin understanding the relationships between chemical reactivity and sensitisation potential.

5.3.1 Alcohols

Alcohols are often used as industrial solvents (e.g. methanol, ethanol etc.) and as components of mixtures (e.g. ethanol, cinnamic alcohol, eugenol, isoeugenol etc.) in the fragrance and flavourings industries[7] and are therefore commonly encountered xenobiotics, both in the workplace and at home (Suit and Estes, 1990; Johansen *et al.*, 1996). The majority of alcohols are non-sensitising but some of the substituted benzyl alcohols and phenols (e.g. cinnamic alcohol, eugenol, isoeugenol, catechols etc.) are moderate or strong sensitisers (Johnson *et al.*, 1972; Epstein *et al.*, 1974; Basketter, 1992; Roberts and Benezra, 1993; Bertrand *et al.*, 1997; see Appendix 1) (Figures 5.4a–c). Sensitising alcohols are prohaptens (when no other protein-reactive functionalities are present in the molecule). A discussion of alcohol structure, potential metabolism and sensitisation levels follows.

5.3.1.1 Aliphatic alcohols

All aliphatic alcohols tested to date are either non-sensitisers or weak sensitisers with respect to ACD (Figure 5.3a) (e.g. Jedrychowski *et al.*, 1990; Kobayashi *et al.*, 1999; see Appendix 1). Small aliphatic alcohols are water-soluble and once penetrated may be excreted easily. Alcohols with long aliphatic chains, such as octanol and decanol, are

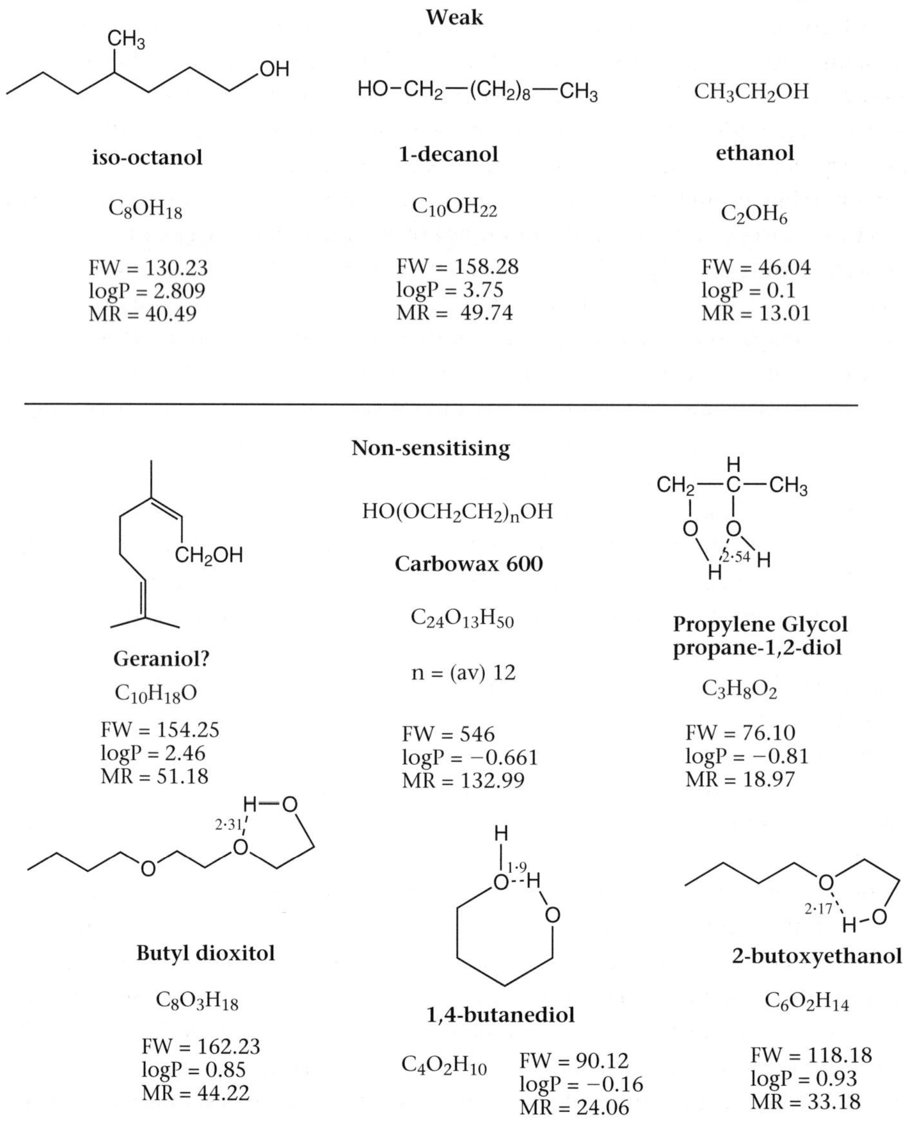

Figure 5.3a: Aliphatic alcohols.

less water-soluble (typical log $P_{o/w}$ values 2.5–4.0) and therefore may reside in the hydrophobic compartments of the skin for a longer time than smaller chain alcohols. The stratum corneum may also be more penetrable for longer chain alcohols possessing moderate levels of hydrophobicity.

The alcohol group is chemically unreactive with respect to protein-binding and hence if a low level of sensitisation is produced by an alcohol (for example, with ethanol) it is a prohapten that hypothetically requires metabolic activation. Mammalian systems are known to have the capacity to metabolically activate aliphatic alcohols, by classes of alcohol dehydrogenases (ADHs) (Wilkin and Stewart, 1987; see sections 3.3.1.2.1 and 4.2.1.1.3), or CYPs (Lieber, C.S., 1999; see sections 3.3.1.1.2 and 4.2.1.1.1) to protein-reactive aldehydes, which react via Schiff base formation (Scheme 5.2). The presence and localisation of cutaneous human ADH enzymes has been shown by Cheung *et al.* (1999) (see Figures 4.1 and 4.2) and the presence of CYPs in human keratinocytes has been shown by Western blotting (Baron *et al.*, 1998).

One notable example within the family of small aliphatic alcohols is ethanol, which can act as a weak sensitiser (positive in 6 out of 93 individuals) when encountered as a xenobiotic (Stotts and Ely, 1977). Ethanol, an endogenous alcohol, is a major substrate for both class 1 ADH and CYP2E1 enzymes. These enzymes perform oxidation of ethanol (prohapten) to acetaldehyde (hapten), a compound known to cause injury to a variety of organs through the formation of acetaldehyde adducts with proteins (Tuma *et al.*, 1987; Lieber, 1988; Nicholls *et al.*, 1992; Conduah Birt *et al.*, 1998). It is likely that the formation of acetaldehyde-polypeptide adducts may be responsible for observed skin reactions to ethanol. A more in-depth discussion of acetaldehyde protein adducts is provided in section 5.3.2.1 below, concerning aliphatic aldehydes. Under normal circumstances, the production of acetaldehyde during endogenous metabolism will be tightly controlled. However, if the body is exposed to high concentrations of ethanol, it may be the case that the system becomes overloaded with acetaldehyde and the detoxifying enzymes become saturated, hence toxic levels of acetaldehyde are produced. Such a scenario would imply that the kinetics of acetaldehyde formation are faster than acetaldehyde detoxication.

The preferred substrates for class 3 ADH are long chain aliphatic alcohols and phenols (Li and Bosron, 1981). 1-Decanol and iso-octanol have both been seen to be weak sensitisers in the LLNA, which may be the result of their oxidation by ADH class 3 to their respective aldehydes.[8]

It seems, however, that the xenobiotic aliphatic alcohols classified as non-sensitisers by *in vivo* tests (Figure 5.3a) may not be sufficiently activated to toxic levels of aldehydes in the skin or else their levels of sensitisation would, in principle, be higher than observed. These alcohols may not be suitable substrates for any of the potentially activating enzymes. One chemical observation that is common for all of the non-sensitising aliphatic alcohols (except geraniol) and may contribute to reactivity and enzyme substrate suitability, is that they all have the capacity to form intramolecular hydrogen bonds (Figures 5.3b), which may confer additional structural stability on these molecules.[9]

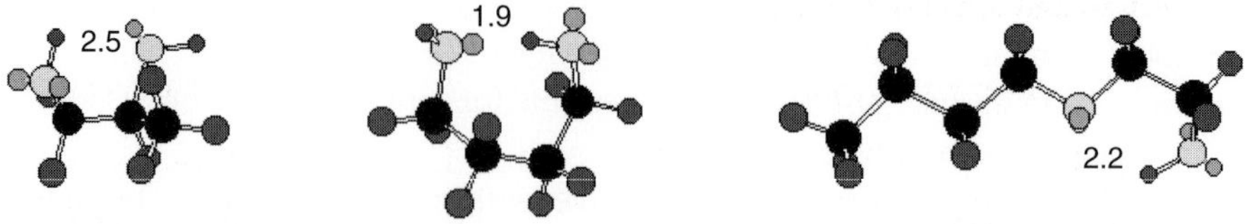

Figure 5.3b: Ball-and-stick representations of propane-1,2-diol, butane-1,4-diol and butoxyethanol. The potential intra-molecular hydrogen-bonding distances between neighbouring oxygen atom (large light grey circle) and hydrogen atom (small black circle) in each molecule are given in angstroms.

Alternatively, for non-sensitisers, the levels of aldehyde production may be effectively controlled by detoxication mechanisms (e.g. by aldehyde dehydrogenase). ADH (as well as potentially activating alcohols and aldehydes) has also been observed to act as an aldehyde dismutase (Svensson *et al.*, 1996) and it may be the case that alcohol to aldehyde to acid conversion (see Figure 3.9a) is effected concomitantly by the same enzyme and no free aldehyde becomes present in the system.[10]

It is arguable as to whether the classification of geraniol and propylene glycol (1,2-propanediol) (by *in vivo* rodent methods) as non-sensitisers is true;[11] these chemicals have both been postulated to cause contact allergy in humans (Cardullo *et al.*, 1989; Catanzaro and Smith, 1991). It may be that in humans but not in rodents, geraniol is metabolised to geranial (possibly by ADH class 2 that is absent in rodent skin (Cheung *et al.*, 2000b) and similarly that 1,2-propanediol is metabolised to 1,2-propanedione and these are the sensitising haptens?

5.3.1.2 Phenols and benzylic alcohols

Within the family of phenolic compounds, a range of sensitisation potentials exists depending upon the substitution of the aromatic ring.

5.3.1.2.1 Catechols and the urushiol mechanism

It is hypothesised that any phenolic compound that contains vicinal (1,2-) hydroxyl functions may be oxidised enzymatically (probably via a CYP) to an orthoquinone (Group IV hapten) that will go on to covalently bind to proteins via nucleophilic Michael-type addition (Scheme 5.10a) (Dupuis, 1979; Roberts and Benezra, 1993). This is the case for the prohapten urushiol (pentadecylcatechol component of poison ivy) (Figure 5.4a), which has been known to be a strong sensitiser for many years (Johnson *et al.*, 1972; Dupuis, 1979). Sensitisation to 4-methylcatechol and 2-methoxy-4-methyl phenol (Figure 5.4a) may occur through analogous formation of quinones.

Methylation of both vicinal hydroxyls in pentadecylveratrole, produces a non-sensitiser (Baer *et al.*, 1970). In contrast, 2-methoxy-4-methyl phenol is a strong sensitiser. Therefore, it is apparent that one demethylation reaction (probably effected by a CYP, see Figure 3.5) may occur to produce the required hydroxy substituent for orthoquinone

Catechols and urushiol (Prohaptens)

Strong/moderate

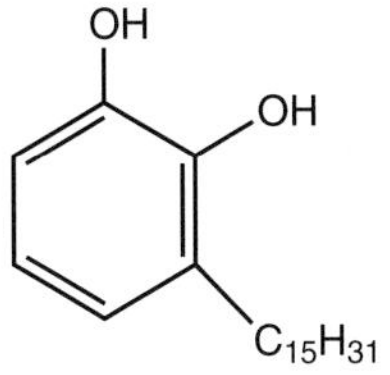

Urushiol (pentyldecylcatechol)

$C_{21}H_{36}O_2$

FW = 320.91
logP = 7.89
MR = 98.9

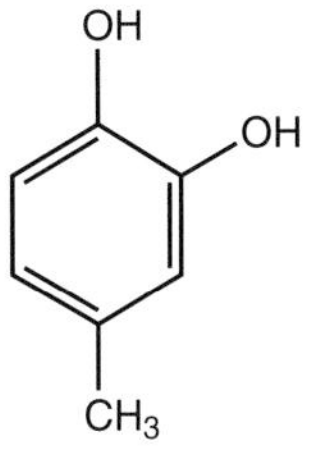

$C_7H_8O_2$

4-methylcatechol

FW = 124.05
logP = 1.50
MR = 34.49

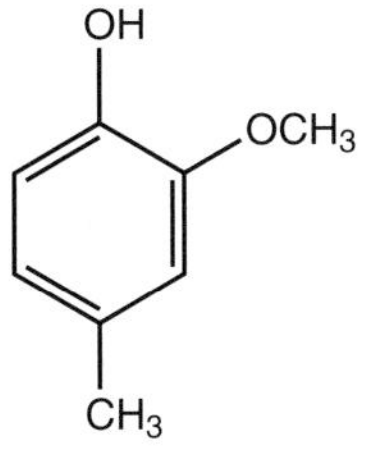

$C_8H_{10}O_2$

2-methoxy-4-methyl phenol

FW = 138.17
logP = 2.02
MR = 39.26

Weak/Non-sensitising

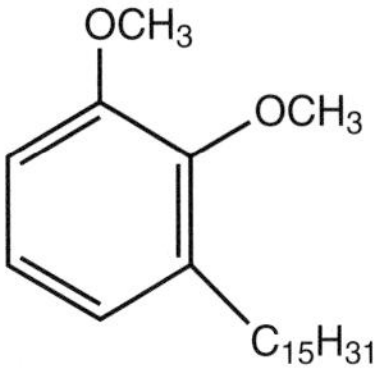

pentyldecylveratrole

Figure 5.4a: Phenolic compounds — catechols and urushiol.

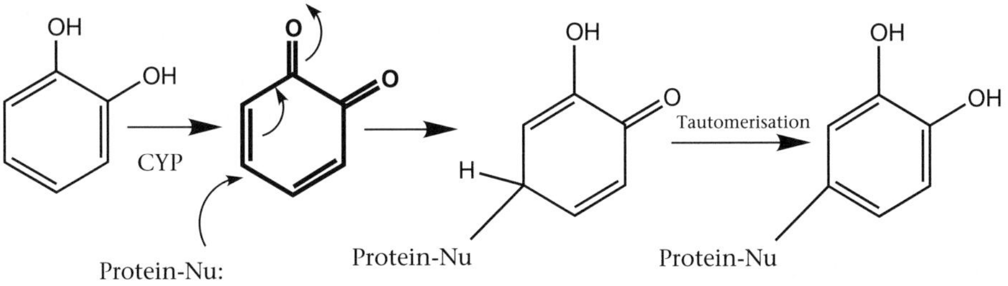

Scheme 5.10a: Nucleophilic addition (Michael addition) to catechol-derived orthoquinones.

formation, but two demethylation reactions do not occur to a sufficient extent to lead to quinone formation and hence cause sensitisation.

Lepoittevin and Benezra (1986) analysed the cross-reactivities between the unsaturated urushiol and saturated urushiol derivatives (*trans,trans*- and *cis,trans*-3-alkyl-1,2-cyclohexanediols). Cyclohexanediols with an alkyl substituent of C10 or greater were seen to be sensitising in guinea-pigs. In animals sensitised against cyclohexanediols, cross-reactivity was seen upon challenge with urushiol. Conversely, animals sensitised against urushiol were not cross-reactive to cyclohexanediols upon challenge. Cross-reactivity was also not observed between *trans, trans* and *cis, trans* cyclohexanediol sensitisers suggesting that there is not a common metabolite.

It is also interesting to consider the possibility of ring opening of catechols as a mechanism of activation. Bacterial catechol-4,5-dioxygenases are known to exist (e.g. LigAB; Sugimoto *et al.*, 1999) and the reaction performed is shown in Scheme 5.10b.[12] It is postulated that if a mammalian form of such an enzyme exists, or even if a CYP can perform a similar reaction (as the requirements are a ferrous ion and dioxygen), then resulting aldehydes could also act as haptens for prohaptenic catechols.

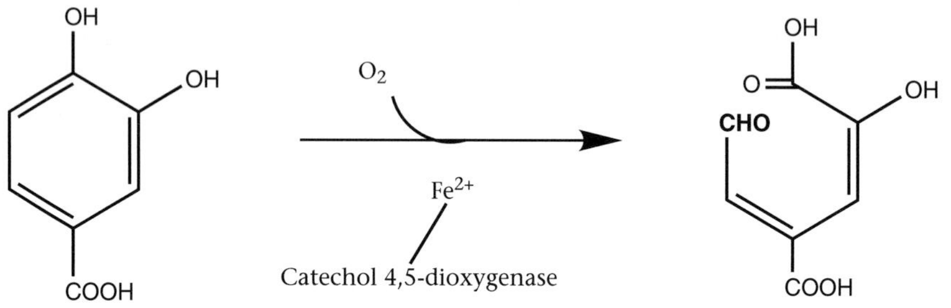

Scheme 5.10b: Ring opening of catechols performed by bacteria.

5.3.1.2.2 Eugenol and isoeugenol relatives

In recent years, some of the most extensively studied phenolic compounds, with respect to QSAR and contact sensitisation, have been eugenol (4-hydroxy-3-methoxy-allylbenzene) and isoeugenol (4-hydroxy-3-methoxy-propenylbenzene), and their structural relatives (Figure 5.4b). Eugenol and isoeugenol are both prohaptens that require biotransformation to a protein-reactive hapten to become sensitising. Although they are close structural isomers, isoeugenol and eugenol show markedly different levels of sensitisation and are only weakly cross-reactive in *in vivo* tests: isoeugenol is a strong sensitiser and eugenol is moderate (Barratt and Basketter, 1992).

Barratt and Basketter (1992) suggested that isoeugenol and eugenol do not share a common mechanism of sensitisation. This is supported by the fact that only limited cross-reactivity exists between these two compounds in humans. A complex picture for the difference between isoeugenol and eugenol sensitisation may be postulated by also

Eugenol/Isoeugenol relatives (Prohaptens)

Strong

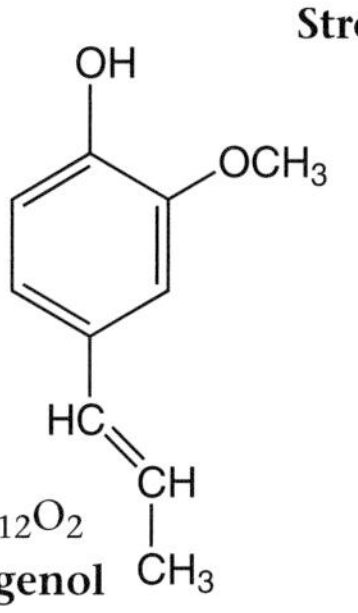

$C_{10}H_{12}O_2$

Isoeugenol

FW = 164.2
logP = 2.49
MR = 49.58

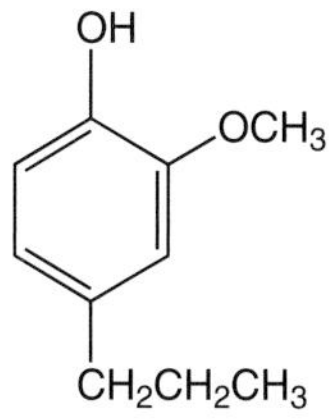

$C_{10}H_{14}O_2$

Dihydroeugenol

FW = 166.22
logP = 2.94
MR = 48.46

Moderate

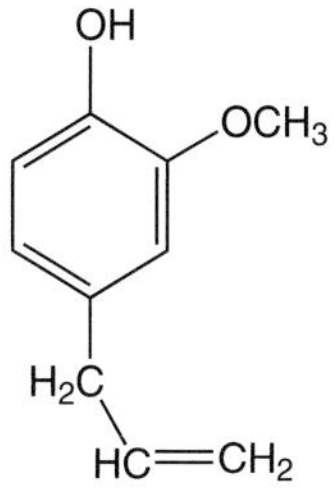

Eugenol

$C_{10}H_{12}O_2$

FW = 164.2
logP = 2.69
MR = 48.5

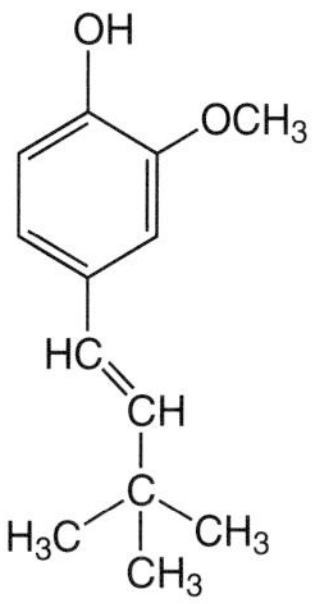

9,9,9-trimethylisoeugenol

$C_{13}H_{18}O_2$

FW = 206.28
logP = 3.95
MR = 63.2

Weak

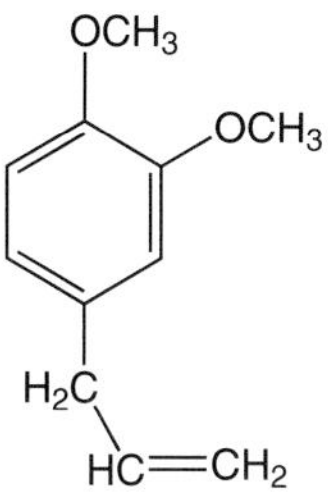

Methyleugenol

$C_{11}H_{14}O_2$

FW = 178.23
logP = 3.21
MR = 53.27

Non-sensitising

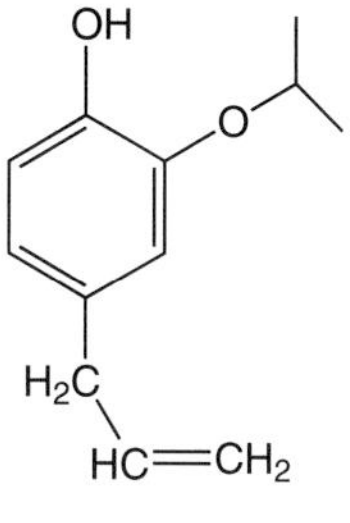

2-Isopropyleugenol

$C_{12}H_{16}O_2$

FW = 192.25
logP = 3.23
MR = 57.67

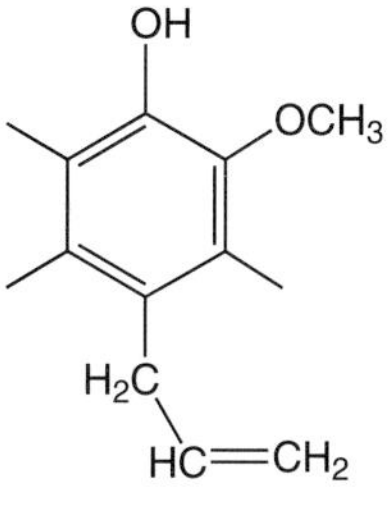

3,5,6-trimethyleugenol

$C_{13}H_{18}O_2$

FW = 206.28
logP = 3.94
MR = 63.63

Figure 5.4b: Phenolic compounds — eugenol/isoeugenol relatives.

considering the metabolism studies of Fischer *et al.* (1990) and Thompson *et al.* (1991), along with QSAR analysis by Bertrand *et al.* (1997) (Scheme 5.11). Such a combined theory from a variety of data acts as a good example to illustrate the many considerations that need to be taken into account for substituted aromatic compounds when trying to predict their sensitisation potential and metabolism.

Both eugenol and isoeugenol have the potential to be converted to quinone methide (QM) and/or orthoquinone (OQ) species. It is unknown as to which endogenous epidermal enzymes may perform the initial oxidation to QM/OQ but in the liver, peroxidase and CYP1A1 have been suggested for QM formation (Thompson *et al.*, 1991) and CYP is proposed to convert catechols to OQ. QM is a Michael acceptor and may either bind covalently to protein (via soft nucleophiles) or alkylate protein (Bolton, Turnipseed and Thompson, 1997) or bind to and deplete intracellular GSH (Scheme 5.11). Similarly, OQ is also susceptible to Michael addition (Scheme 5.10). QM formation occurs by oxidation via a semiquinone radical and it may be the case that this undergoes redox cycling (Scheme 3.22), generating damaging superoxide and hydroxyl radical species.

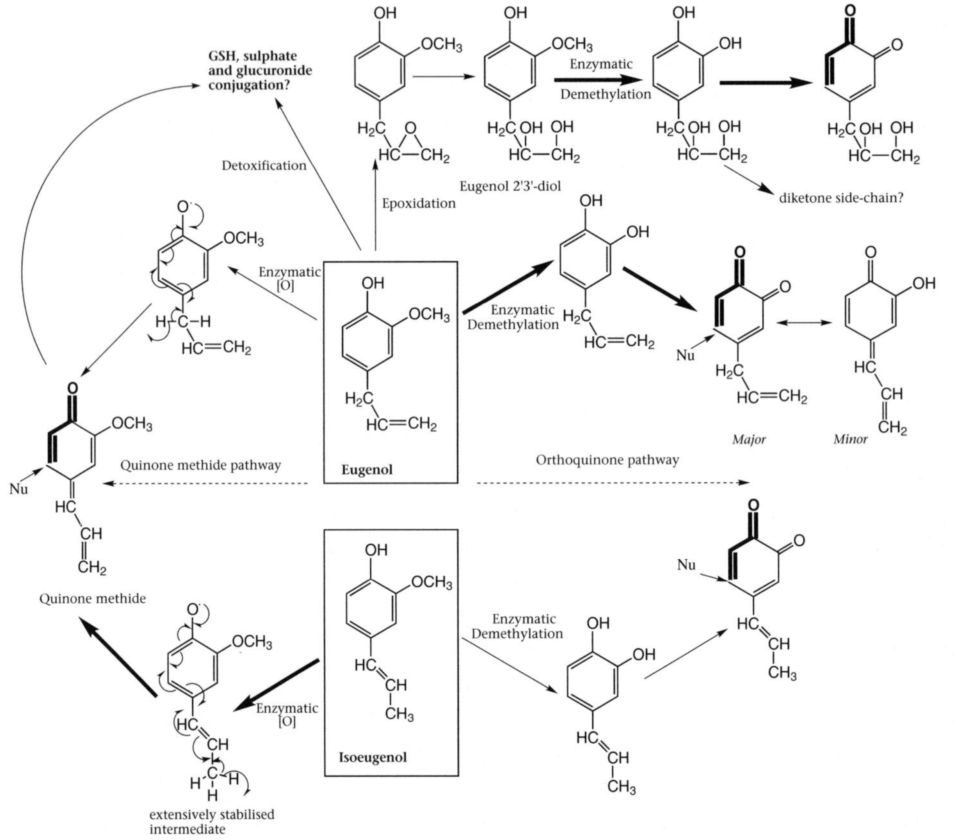

Scheme 5.11: Potential metabolism of eugenol and isoeugenol.

By selectively methylating a variety of positions on isoeugenol and eugenol and performing LLNA for the compounds generated,[13] Bertrand *et al.* (1997) suggested that isoeugenol is preferentially metabolised to a QM. A substantially decreased level of T-cell proliferation in the LLNA was seen with the isoeugenol analogue 9,9,9-trimethylisoeugenol (Figure 5.4b), which is a derivative that cannot be directly oxidised to QM but can be converted to orthoquinone. However, the levels still remained slightly above those for eugenol suggesting that other mechanisms could also play a role for this analogue.

Eugenol also has the capacity to be converted to QM (Scheme 5.11). However, it is considered that this is not an important mechanism of activation for this molecule for two reasons. First, the complete loss of T-cell proliferation in the LLNA when the 2-methoxy group in eugenol was substituted for an isopropoxy group (Figure 5.4b) suggests that an O-demethylation reaction, which leads to the ultimate production of a protein-reactive OQ is the preferred (if not the only) mechanism of sensitisation for eugenol. However, OQ derived from eugenol can also spontaneously tautomerise to the more electrophilic QM (Bolton *et al.*, 1994) but if the nature of the allyl substituent in eugenol derivatives is changed this may not be possible. Secondly, the QM intermediate semiquinone radical cannot be resonance stabilised by the eugenol side chain as extensively as is the case for isoeugenol (Scheme 5.11).

In a similar way as with eugenol, the methoxy group was substituted for isopropoxy in isoeugenol and in contrast to eugenol, this made virtually no difference to the LLNA result, suggesting that in isoeugenol O-demethylation was not involved in producing sensitisation.

It has also been postulated that eugenol may undergo epoxidation across its non-conjugated allylic double bond leading to the formation of the non-protein-reactive eugenol 2′3′-diol (Delaforge *et al.*, 1980; Fischer *et al.*, 1990). However, this may still lead to a pathway of activation as the diol can be converted to an α,β-diketone, which can potentially react with protein (see Scheme 5.15).

In the case of methyleugenol (Figure 5.4b), which is a much weaker sensitiser than eugenol, two O-demethylation reactions would be necessary to produce OQ and enzymatically this may not be as achievable as a single O-demethylation reaction; the skin enzyme that performs the O-demethylation reaction is at present unknown but is believed to be a CYP. 4-Allylphenols and catechols are known to be substrates for the oxidative enzyme tyrosinase (Krol and Bolton, 1997) but at present this enzyme has not been detected in skin. In this study in rat liver, eugenol was not converted to either OQ or QM by tyrosinase, however, in contrast methyleugenol did undergo tyrosinase-catalysed QM formation. These contradictory results with respect to the contact sensitisation of eugenol and methyleugenol suggest that tyrosinase is not the oxidative enzyme in skin.

A complete loss of sensitisation potential is observed with 3,5,6-trimethyleugenol (Figure 5.4b), which could be attributed to steric hindrance on the demethylase action or be the result of the decrease in electrophilicity of the ring system by the electron-donating inductive effects of the additional methyl groups.

The detoxication mechanisms of eugenol and isoeugenol remain unknown. However, it is expected that these molecules can undergo glutathione, glucuronide and sulphate conjugation.

5.3.1.2.3 Low-molecular weight phenols and alkyl phenols

A range of low molecular weight phenols (Figure 5.4c) are contact sensitisers (Hagdrup *et al.*, 1994; Bruze and Zimerson, 1997) and are prohaptens, and Bruze and Zimerson have identified significant cross-reactivity in humans.

Those that cross react share a common structural motif (highlighted as the blue pro-

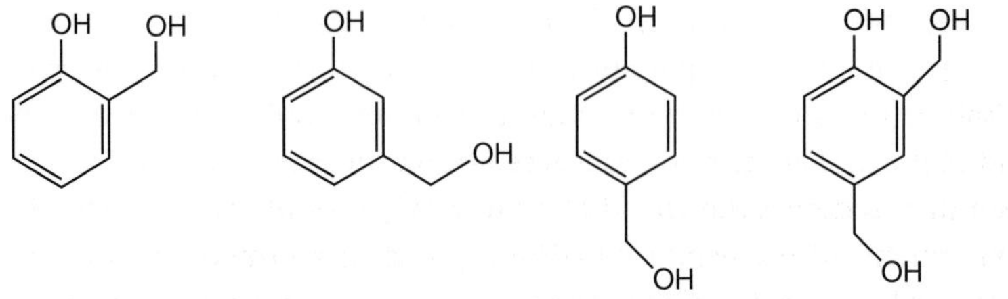

2-MP **3-MP** **4-MP** **2,4-MP**

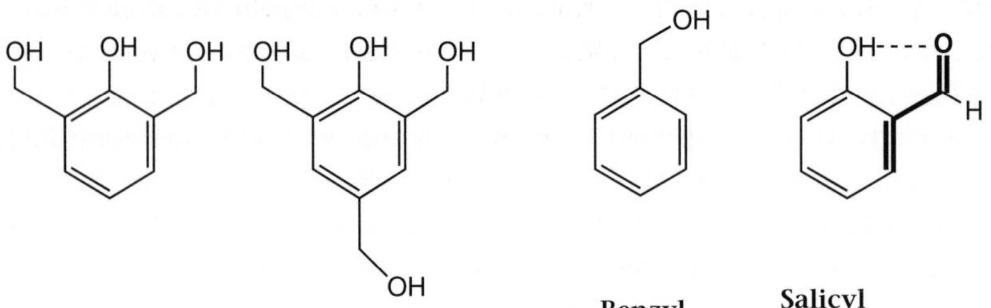

2,6-MP **2,4,6-MP** **Benzyl alcohol** **Salicyl aldehyde** c.f. benzaldehyde, which is non-sensitising?

	Patient no.									
Compound	1	2	3	4	5	6	7	8	9	10
2-MP	+	+	+	-	-	+	+	+	+	+
3-MP	-	-	-	-	+	-	-	-	-	-
4-MP	+	-	-	-	+	+	+	-	-	-
2,4-MP	+	+	+	+	+	+	+	-	-	+
2,4,6-MP	-	+	+	+	+	+	+	-	-	+
Benzyl alcohol	-	-	-	-	-	-	-	-	-	-
Benzaldehyde	-	-	-	-	-	-	-	-	-	-
Salicyl aldehyde	+	+	NT	-	-	-	NT	+	-	+

(Adapted from Bruze & Zimerson, 1997)

Figure 5.4c: Cross-reactivities of the methylol phenols and related chemicals. (Adapted from Bruze & Zimerson, 1997.)

hapten in Figure 5.4c). The hydroxyl group on the 2 position on the aromatic ring appears to be a requirement for sensitisation as the close relative benzyl alcohol is seen to be non-sensitising in this study (and is classified as such in *in vivo* animal tests). (However, some studies postulate that benzyl alcohol is sensitising in humans (Corazza *et al.*, 1996; Verecken *et al.*, 1998; Podda *et al.*, 1999). This is intriguing as benzyl alcohol is non-electrophilic and the likely metabolic product, benzaldehyde (Figure 5.6b), is also seen to be a non-sensitiser by Bruze and Zimerson and in *in vivo* animal tests.) Salicyl aldehyde, however, which is a benzylic aldehyde, is a sensitiser and it is hypothesised that the positioning of a phenolic group adjacent to the aldehyde group on the aromatic ring allows tautomerisation to take place. Such tautomerisation would lead to the formation of a compound that could act as a Michael acceptor on the aromatic ring. This could also be a mechanism that underlies the sensitisation to 2-MP, 2,4-MP and 2,4,6-MP. However, in an acidic environment, if the benzylic hydroxyl group in methylol phenols becomes protonated, this would allow the OH_2^+ group to act as a good leaving group and through rearrangement, a quinone methide electrophile could be formed. Alternatively, the OH_2^+ could leave the molecule and result in the formation of a benzylic carbonium ion.

Hydroquinone (quinol) (Figure 5.4d) is a 1,4 aromatic diol that shows strong/moderate sensitisation potential in the LLNA (Kimber *et al.*, 1998b) and it is presumed that some of the compound may be oxidatively metabolised to 1,4-benzoquinone (Group IV hapten), which is itself a strong sensitiser, and some may be excreted. The benzoquinone formed would bind covalently to protein by nucleophilic Michael-type addition in a similar fashion to orthoquinones derived from catechols (Scheme 5.10).

Resorcinol, the related 1,3-aromatic diol, has been classified as a non-sensitiser as determined by mouse, guinea-pig and human predictive tests: oxidation to a 1,3-quinone cannot occur i.e. it is impossible to draw a structure for this that satisfies all atomic valencies. However, Barbaud *et al.* (1996) have identified a systemic allergic reaction as a result of topical application of resorcinol but the mechanism through which this may occur has not been identified.

5.3.1.2.4 Others

Cinnamic alcohol (Figure 5.4d) is a moderate sensitiser but is not a protein reactive compound, due to the absence of intramolecular double bond activation by a carbonyl group (c.f. cinnamaldehyde), and is therefore a prohapten. It has been hypothesised that cinnamic alcohol can be oxidised by ADH/CYP to cinnamaldehyde (Scheme 5.14) (Basketter, 1992), a stronger sensitiser, the metabolism of which is discussed in section 5.3.2.2.3. However, in 24 h human skin absorption and metabolism experiments with cinnamic alcohol, no cinnamaldehyde was seen to penetrate or remain free within the skin, although low levels of alcohol-derived cinnamaldehyde evaporated and remained on the surface of the skin at the end of the experiment (Smith *et al.*, 1999, 2000a). Also, cinnamic acid was seen to penetrate and reside within the skin, that was presumably formed via a cinnamaldehyde intermediate (Scheme 5.14). Human skin metabolism data for cinnamic alcohol is presented and discussed in more detail, together with cinnamaldehyde metabolism data, in section 5.3.2.2.3.

Moderate

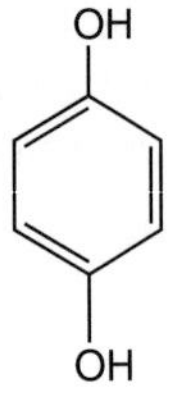

Quinol (1,4-hydroquinone)

FW = 110.11 $C_6H_6O_2$
logP = 1.09
MR = 29.45
cf. benzoquinone - strong

Non-sensitising

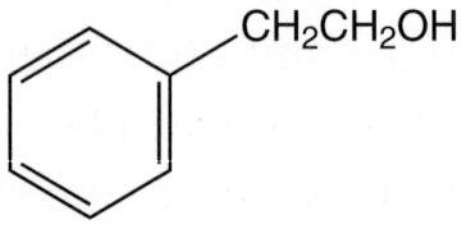

Phenylethyl alcohol

FW = 122.17 $C_8H_{10}O$
logP = 1.57
MR = 37.63

Weak

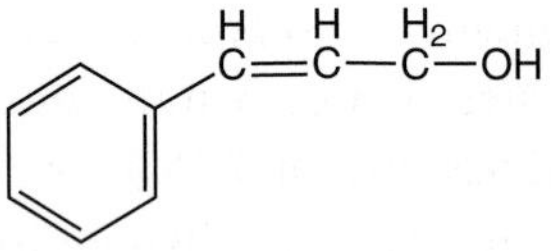

Cinnamic alcohol

FW = 134.18 $C_9H_{10}O$
logP = 1.58
MR = 43.19

Very weak/Non-sensitising

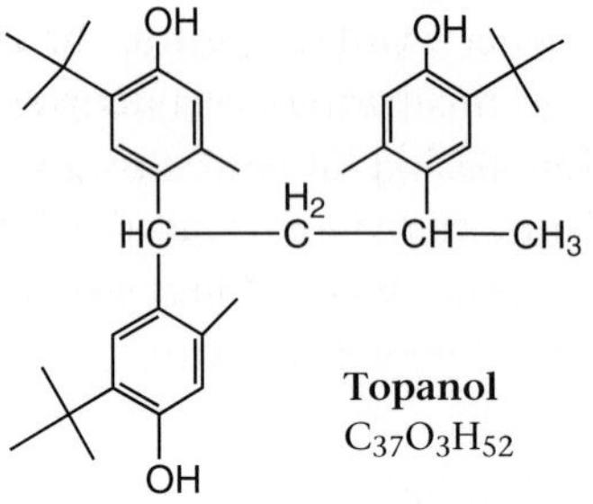

Topanol
$C_{37}O_3H_{52}$

FW = 544.39
logP = 12.22
MR = 170.39

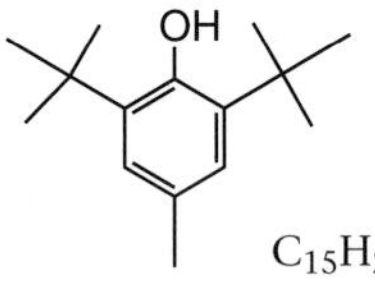

$C_{15}H_{24}O$

Butylated hydroxytoluene

FW = 220.36
logP = 5.64
MR = 70.13

Figure 5.4d: Quinol and other benzyl alcohols.

Topanol and butylated hydroxytoluene (BHT) (Figure 5.4d) are not skin sensitisers. However, toxic metabolites (quinone methide and hydroperoxide analogues) of BHT produced by CYP oxidation have been observed in hepatic and pulmonary microsomes and implicated in pulmonary tumours (Bolton and Thompson, 1991). These compounds may be non-sensitising due to a lack of such activating metabolism in skin. Both topanol and BHT are highly substituted molecules and steric hindrance may also play a role in their lack of sensitisation.

5.3.2 Aldehydes

Aldehydes are used commonly in industry and in consumer products (at low constituent levels) as fragrance and flavouring agents. Aldehydes are highly reactive molecules, many of which are strong sensitisers.

5.3.2.1 Aliphatic aldehydes

All aliphatic aldehydes have the capacity to act as Group II haptens by binding to protein nucleophiles via a Schiff base mechanism to either the ε-amino group of Lys or the α-amino N-terminal amine group (Scheme 5.2). The aldehydes illustrated in Figure 5.5 are strong sensitisers and their direct conjugation to hard protein nucleophiles (Lys or N-terminal amine) is thought to be responsible for this.

A recent study looking at the nature of acetaldehyde binding to peptides *in vitro* may have relevance in general with respect to the binding of aldehydes to protein (Conduah Birt *et al.*, 1998). On incubating acetaldehyde with a 21-mer peptide, which contained one of each amino acid (plus an extra glycine), at pH 6.5 and at 37°C, the major acetaldehyde adduct was seen to be at the N-terminus (Val) i.e. to the free N-terminal NH_2 group.[14] Also, the ultimate adduct was not an imine (i.e. a Schiff base) but a more

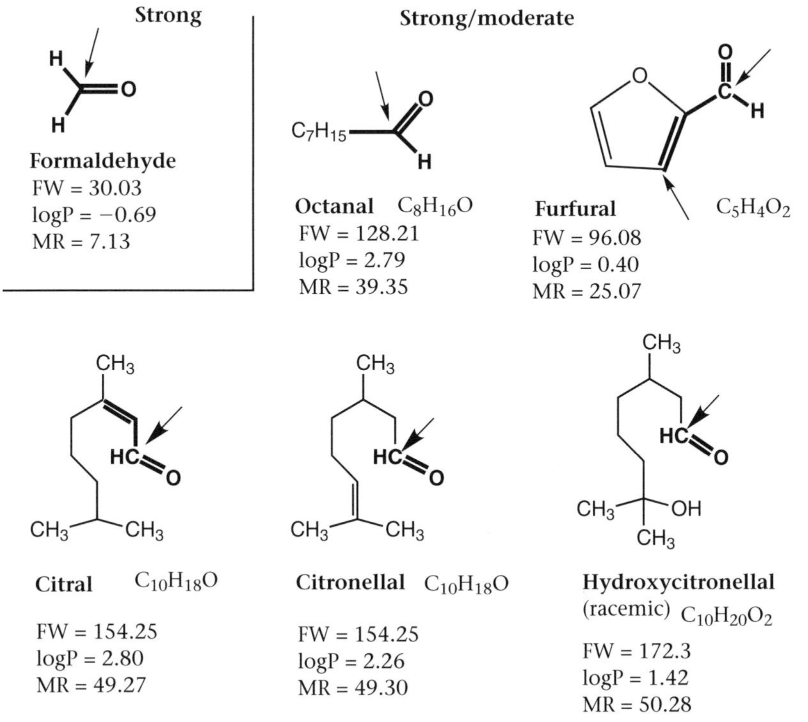

Figure 5.5: Aliphatic aldehydes.

stable imidazolidinone, a heterocyclic adduct that is believed to spontaneously form from a Schiff base (Scheme 5.12). This chemistry can only occur at the N-terminal amine. If this is the only major form of adduction between aldehydes and protein, this will have consequences for the immune recognition of the aldehyde-protein adduct (see Chapter 6).

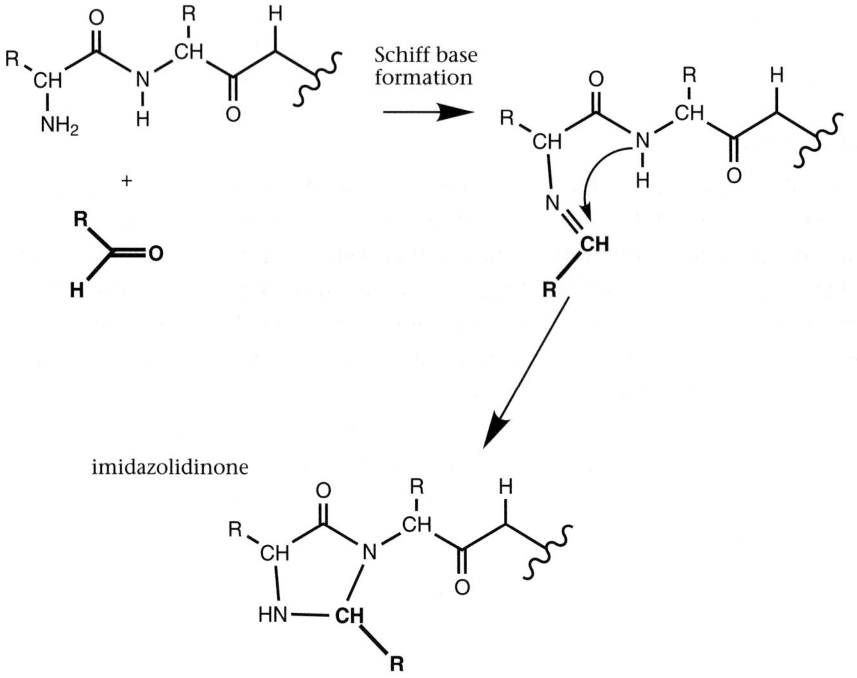

Scheme 5.12: Hypothesis of aldehyde binding to the N-terminus of proteins/peptides based on structural analyses of acetaldehyde binding to peptides *in vitro*.

Why then are such toxic xenobiotic aldehydes not totally detoxified within the skin by the cutaneous enzymes that have been shown to be present (e.g. alcohol and aldehyde dehydrogenases) (see Figures 4.1–4.2 adapted from Cheung *et al.*, 1999, 2000b)? One hypothesis is that there is a concentration dependence and that the low levels of detoxifying enzymes cannot cope with the levels of xenobiotic aldehyde exposure. Another hypothesis is that these strongly sensitising xenobiotic aldehydes are not substrates for any of the aldehyde metabolising enzymes.

5.3.2.1.1 Formaldehyde

The oxidation product of methanol (via ADH, catalase or a CYP), i.e. formaldehyde (Figure 5.5), is not only a strong sensitiser (Epstein and Maibach, 1966; Lee *et al.*, 1984; Andersen *et al.*, 1985; Krecisz and Kiec-Swierczynska, 1998; Agner *et al.*, 1999; Bergh and

Karlberg, 1999) but is also a highly cytotoxic molecule. Formaldehyde will easily form protein adducts via reactions with hard protein nucleophiles.

Formaldehyde can be detoxified by forming a spontaneous adduct with glutathione (S-hydroxymethyl-glutathione) (Yang, Bosron and Hurley, 1997). Class 3 alcohol dehydrogenase acts as a glutathione-dependent formaldehyde dehydrogenase (FDH), whose action is depleted by a single Asp57Leu mutation (in the human enzyme) indicating that a negative charge is required at this position for FDH activity (Estonius *et al.*, 1994). It appears from site-directed mutagenesis studies that the FDH action is mutually exclusive to alcohol dehydrogenase action on primary and secondary alcohols.

5.3.2.1.2 Others

The naturally occurring aldehydes, citronellal and hydroxycitronellal (HC) (Figure 5.5) are known sensitisers (Johansen *et al.*, 1996) and again it is believed that the Schiff base mechanism (Scheme 5.2) is responsible for this (Dupuis and Benezra, 1982). Detoxication of these aldehydes is most likely to take place enzymatically: the oxidation to their corresponding acids is most probably mediated by aldehyde dehydrogenase or aldehyde oxidase; the reduction to their corresponding alcohols is likely to be mediated by alcohol dehydrogenase (class 3) or aldehyde reductase. To date, however, neither aldehyde oxidase or aldehyde reductase have been detected in skin, although three ADH and three ALDH classes have been shown to be present in human skin (Cheung *et al.*, 1999, 2000b). Hydroxycitronellol and hydroxycitronellic acid metabolites of HC were first detected in urine (Ishida *et al.*, 1989) but have subsequently been detected in skin homogenates and in receptor fluid after absorption of hydroxycitronellal through full-thickness human skin using a validated flow-through diffusion cell skin absorption model (Tonge, 1995).

Citral and furfural (Figure 5.5) are also common sensitisers (Steltenkamp *et al.*, 1980) and are α,β-unsaturated carbonyl compounds (similar to cinnamaldehyde), which may undergo 1,4 Michael addition across the C=C bond (Scheme 5.5).[15] However, Schiff base formation, similar to that for citronellal and hydroxycitronellal, is also a possibility.

5.3.2.2 Aralkyl (semi-aromatic) and aromatic aldehydes

In discussing aldehydes that contain an aromatic ring, it is important to differentiate between those that are truly aromatic (where electronic conjugation and resonance stabilised — canonical — structures can be drawn across the whole molecule) and those that are semi-aromatic (i.e. where there is an aromatic ring but there is no resonance stabilisation between this and the aldehyde group). The aromaticity of a compound can significantly affect its reactivity, as discussed below.

5.3.2.2.1 Aralkyl (semi-aromatic) aldehydes

All of the aralkyl (semi-aromatic) aldehydes (Group II haptens) shown in Figure 5.6a are strong sensitisers (Fregert, 1970; Steltenkamp, 1980) and all possess hard electrophilic carbonyl groups that can form a Schiff base as illustrated in Scheme 5.2. The aldehydic

Strong

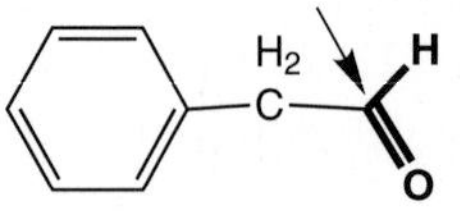

Phenyl acetic aldehyde

C_8H_8O FW = 120.15
logP = 1.53
MR = 36.44

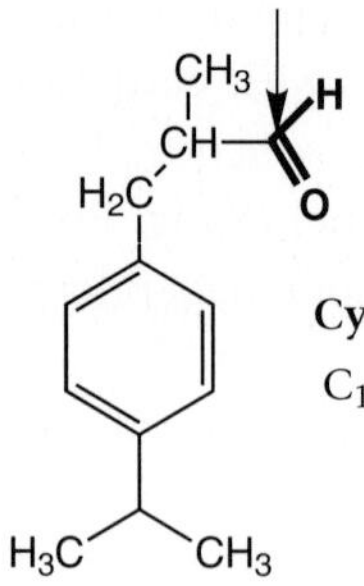

Cyclamen aldehyde

$C_{13}H_{18}O$ FW = 190.29
logP = 3.26
MR = 59.81

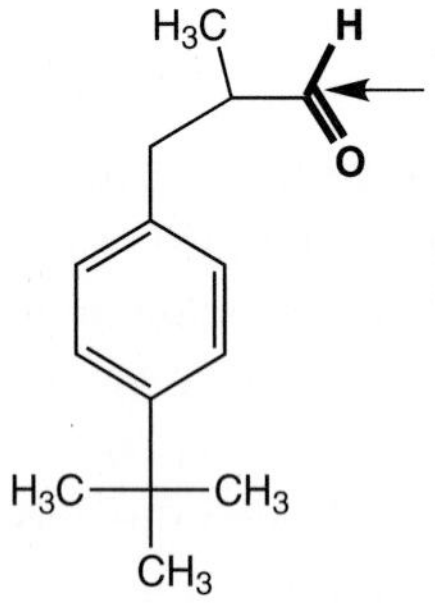

Lillial P FW = 204.31
$C_{14}H_{20}O$ logP = 4.06
MR = 64.28

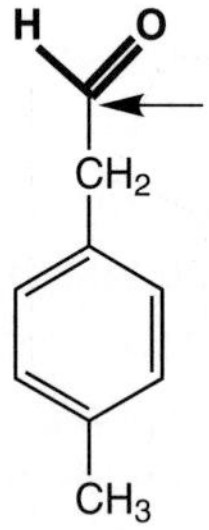

Syringa aldehyde

$C_9H_{10}O$ FW = 134.18
logP = 1.94
MR = 41.48

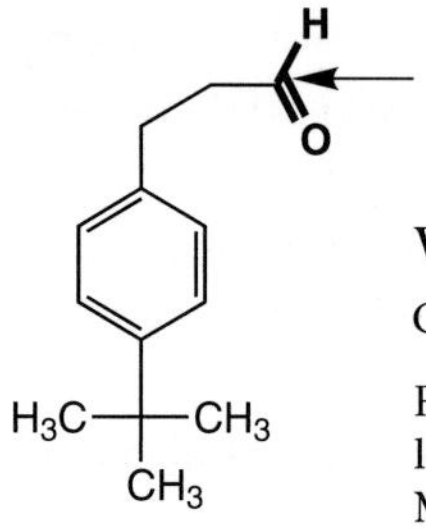

V. strong

$C_{13}H_{18}O$

FW = 190.28
logP = 3.86
MR = 59.71

Bourgeonal
p-t-butyl dihydro
cinnamic aldehyde

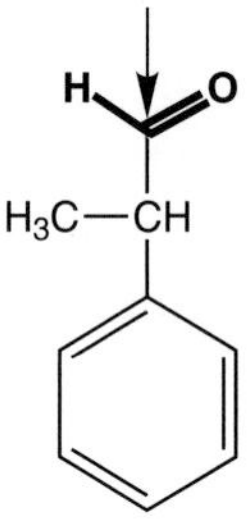

Phenyl propionaldehyde

$C_9H_{10}O$ FW = 134.18
logP = 1.73
MR = 41.01

Figure 5.6a: Aralkyl (semi-aromatic) aldehydes.

carbonyl is strongly electrophilic in these molecules, due to the electron withdrawing effects of the benzyl group, and nucleophilic attack would occur easily.

5.3.2.2.2 Aromatic aldehydes

In contrast to the semi-aromatic aldehydes, the aromatic aldehydes in Figure 5.6b are weak sensitisers (vanillin (Robinson *et al.*, 1990), heliotropin) or non-sensitising (benzaldehyde and anisic aldehyde) (see Figure 5.6d). The carbonyl group in these molecules is directly conjugated to the aromatic ring and the distribution of the δ^+ charge across the whole molecule (Scheme 5.13) reduces the reactivity of the aldehydic group

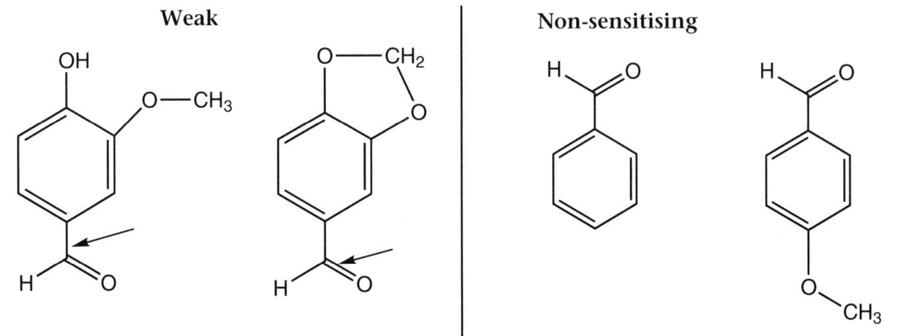

Weak		Non-sensitising	
Vanillin	**Heliotropin**	**Benzaldehyde**	**Anisic aldehyde**
$C_8H_8O_3$	$C_8H_6O_3$	C_7H_6O	$C_8H_8O_2$
FW = 152.15	FW = 150.13	FW = 106.12	FW = 136.15
logP = 1.09	logP = 0.58	logP = 1.34	logP = 1.47
MR = 40.81	MR = 38.42	MR = 32.65	MR = 39.11

cf. catechols and urushiol — strong

Figure 5.6b: Aralkyl (semi-aromatic) aldehydes (cont.).

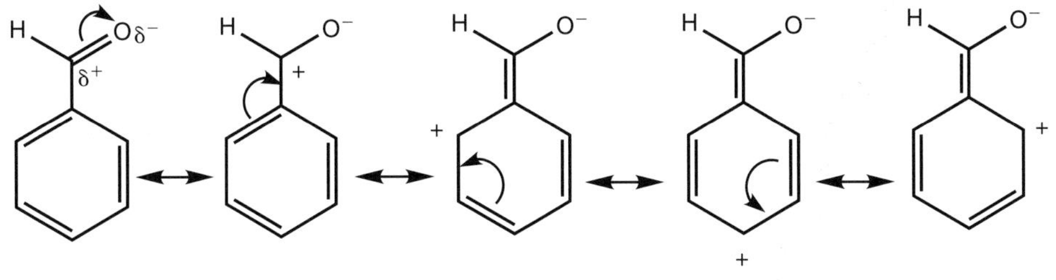

Scheme 5.13: Resonance stabilisation of benzaldehyde. (Applies to all of the structures in Fig. 5.6b.)

sufficiently enough, presumably, to make the molecule non-susceptible to nucleophilic attack. In the event of a nucleophilic reaction with the aldehyde group, the conjugation between the ring system and the carbonyl group would be lost in the resulting intermediate and hence the activation energy barrier that needs to be overcome for a reaction to occur at all would be high. The urushiol mechanism described in section 5.3.1.2 (Scheme 5.10) could act as an alternative for vanillin and heliotropin (prohaptens) allowing some sensitisation potential to exist with these molecules, via metabolic activation.

5.3.2.2.3 Cinnamaldehyde

Cinnamaldehyde, a known sensitiser that is commonly used in the fragrance and flavouring industries and is a major component of the European standard fragrance mix, is an α,β-unsaturated carbonyl compound that contains two potential protein-binding sites (Group IV hapten) (Figure 5.6a) (Goh and Ng, 1988; Weibel and Hansen., 1989a, b; Meding, 1993; Johansen and Menne, 1995; Johansen *et al.*, 1996; Katsarou *et al.*, 1999). Preliminary immunochemical studies, using specific anti-RSA-cinnamaldehyde sera[16], have shown that cinnamaldehyde can form adducts with many, as yet unidentified, skin proteins (Elahi *et al.*, 2000). Contradictory observations have led to confusion over the exact mode of protein-cinnamaldehyde binding. Under physiological conditions, where *in vivo* hard bases are characteristically weak, it is known that for α,β-unsaturated carbonyl compounds 1,4 Michael addition between the activated double bond (a soft electrophile) and Cys residues (soft nucleophiles) should be favoured over the Schiff base mechanism at amine groups (hard nucleophiles) (Schauenstein *et al.*, 1977; Fessenden and Fessenden, 1990). Weibel and Hansen (1989b) have provided evidence that cinnamaldehyde binds to protein primarily at thiol groups, although some conjugation to the ε-amino groups of Lys residues was not ruled out. Majeti and Suskind (1977) on the other hand have argued that Schiff base formation between the hard aldehydic electrophile and hard nucleophilic free primary amine groups is the preferred mode of action. Further molecular characterisation studies are required to prove whether Schiff base formation, Michael addition or both can occur *in vivo*.

Cinnamaldehyde may also be metabolically detoxified by ADH/CYP and ALDH enzymes to cinnamic alcohol and cinnamic acid, respectively (Scheme 5.14).[17] Cinnamic alcohol (Scheme 5.14) can also be activated to cinnamaldehyde. Hence, the interconversion between cinnamaldehyde and cinnamic alcohol and the rates of activation/detoxication may also contribute to observed sensitisation levels for these compounds. It has been hypothesised that cinnamaldehyde acts as the true hapten in cinnamic alcohol sensitisation (Basketter, 1992), as these molecules are cross-reactive *in vivo* (Weibel *et al.*, 1989).

In studies by Weibel and Hansen (1989a and 1989b), cinnamaldehyde was seen to be converted to cinnamic alcohol and cinnamic acid in human skin, *in vitro* over 150 h taking samples every 24 h. However, in their study, no activating metabolism of cinnamic alcohol to cinnamaldehyde (as hypothesised) or cinnamic acid was observed. Recently, however, it has been shown that cinnamaldehyde and cinnamic alcohol are both metabolised in fresh skin during 24 h (Smith *et al.*, 2000a). Total recovery data

Strong

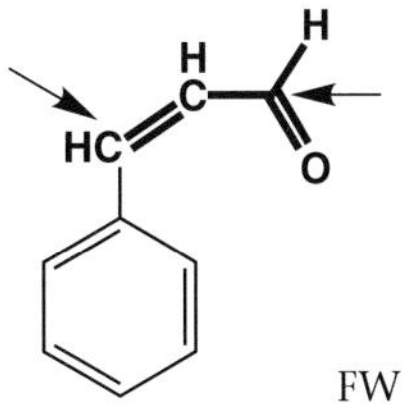

FW = 132.16
logP = 2.08
C_9H_8O MR = 42.13

Cinnamaldehyde

Weak

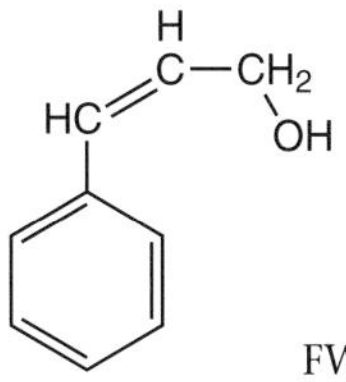

FW = 134.18
logP = 1.58
$C_9H_{10}O$ MR = 43.19

Cinnamic alcohol

Non-sensitising

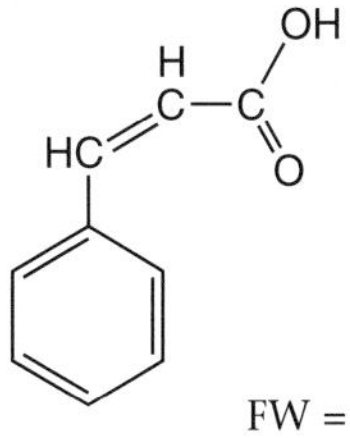

FW = 148.16
logP = 1.96
$C_9H_8O_2$ MR = 43.06

Cinnamic acid

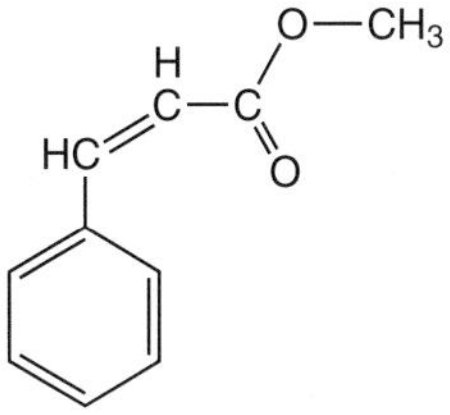

Methyl cinnamate FW = 162.19
$C_{10}H_{10}O_2$ logP = 2.43
MR = 47.83

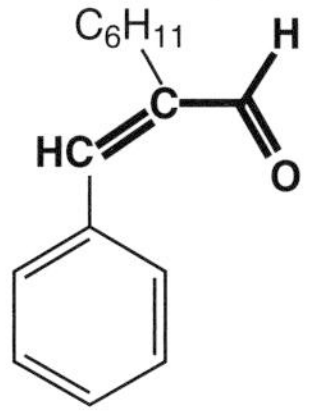

FW = 216.32
logP = 4.35
$C_{15}H_{20}O$ MR = 69.50

Hexylcinnamaldehyde

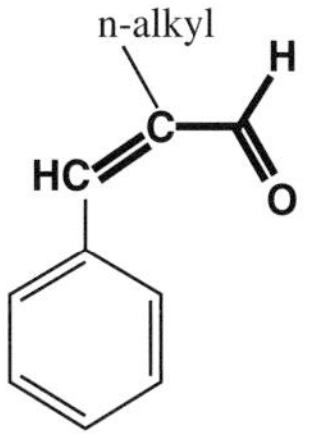

n-alkyl = methyl, butyl, amyl

a-alkyl substituted cinnamaldehyde

Figure 5.6c: Cinnamic compounds.

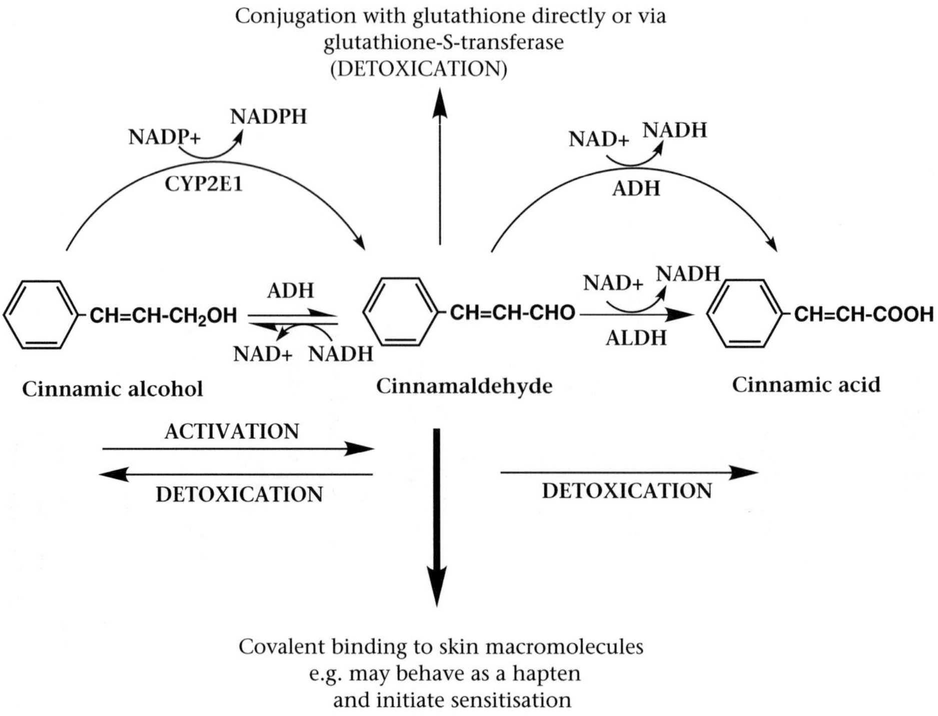

Scheme 5.14: Potential metabolism of cinnamaldehyde and cinnamic alcohol.

from this 24 h *in vitro* fresh human skin absorption and metabolism study, following 78 μmoles (10 μl neat) cinnamaldehyde or cinnamic alcohol application are presented in Figure 5.6d.

Cinnamic alcohol was seen to be converted to cinnamaldehyde in this study, but only on the surface of the skin (possibly as a result of skin microflora conversion of cinnamic alcohol or back diffusion of cinnamaldehyde generated by metabolism from within the skin). Cinnamic alcohol-derived cinnamic acid (presumably formed via a cinnamaldehyde intermediate) had penetrated and remained within the skin. It is expected that any low-level cinnamaldehyde generated within the skin had bound to skin protein or glutathione.

In an attempt to investigate the effects on sensitisation of α-substitution of cinnamaldehyde (i.e. α-methyl-, α-butyl-, α-amyl- and α-hexyl-cinnamaldehyde), local lymph node assays (*in vivo* mouse sensitisation tests (Kimber *et al.*, 1986)) were run on this series of chemicals (see Appendix 1 and Patlewicz *et al.*, 2001). All of the α-substituted cinnamic compounds exhibited markedly reduced sensitisation levels in comparison to cinnamaldehyde;[18] benzaldehyde was used as a non-sensitising negative control (see Appendix 1). A previous GPMT study (which is arguably a less definitive/quantitative assay) indicated that there was a tendency for a QSAR to exist with increasing

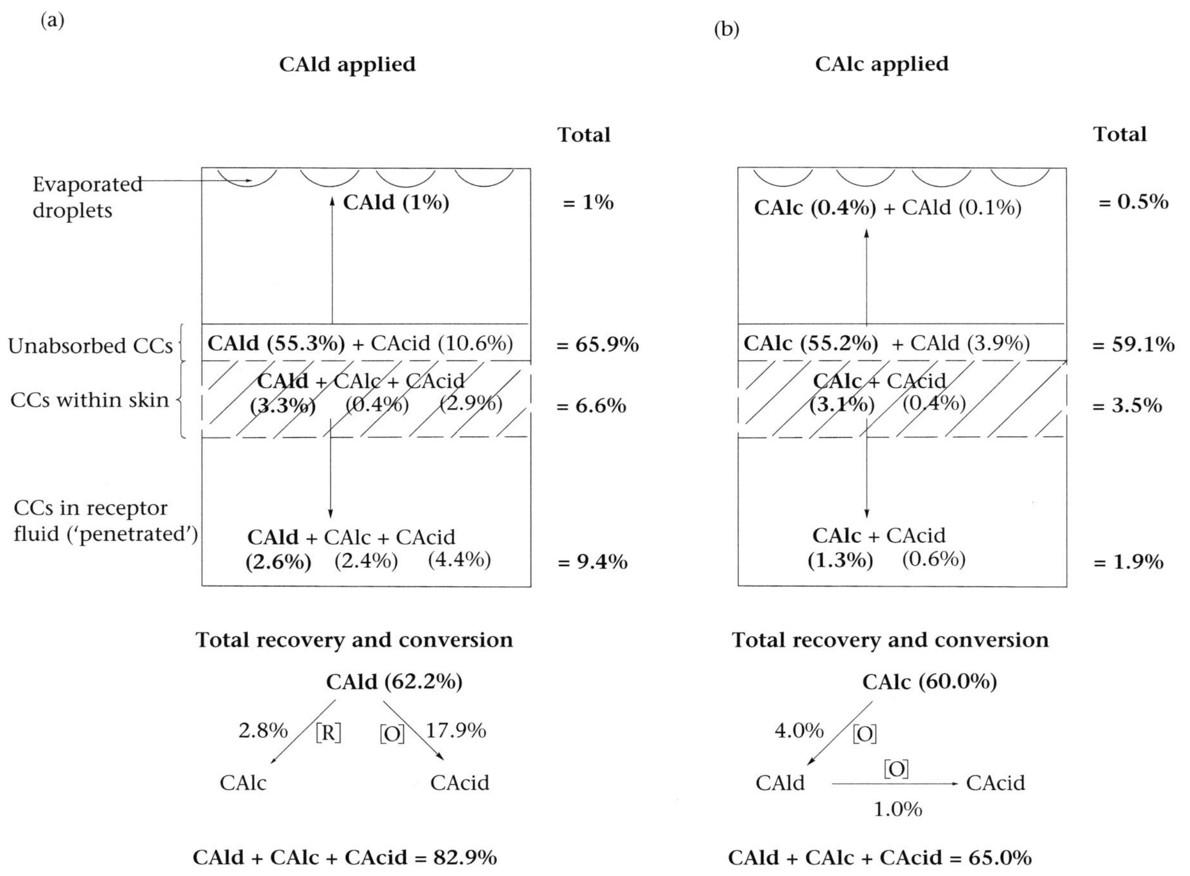

Figure 5.6d: Recovery of cinnamic compounds from 24 h human skin absorption studies. This schematic shows the total recoveries, partitioning and conversion of cinnamic compounds in human skin following application of: (a) cinnamaldehyde, or (b) cinnamic alcohol in the *in vitro* skin absorption model system. Data are shown as % of initial applied dose (78 μmoles) for the levels of cinnamic compounds (CCs) that had evaporated from the skin surface, remained unabsorbed on the skin surface, were extracted from within the skin and penetrated the skin into receptor fluid, after 24 h. [R] = reduction, [O] = oxidation. (Reproduced from Smith *et al.*, 2000a.)

α-substituent alkyl chain length (Senma *et al.*, 1978) and this was corroborated by the LLNA results. It is unknown as to whether these observed differences in sensitisation are due to differences in relative absorption, metabolism (detoxication) or protein-binding potential. Differences in absorption and metabolism are being investigated currently for this series of compounds. It is anticipated that the electropositivity of the β-carbon (see Scheme 5.5) would be most seriously affected by the presence of an electron-donating α-substituent, rather than the reactivity of the more strongly polarised aldehydic carbon. It may be the case that α-substitution completely diminishes the protein-reactivity or sterically hinders these substituted cinnamaldehydes and possibly enzymatic dealkylation (perhaps by CYP) is required before they can bind to protein residues. Hence, if this occurs, cinnamaldehyde would be the common hapten for all members of this series and the additional metabolism required by α-substituted compounds may increase the dose-dependency. There is at present no information on the cross-reactivities of cinnamaldehyde and α-substituted compounds in humans to support this common hapten hypothesis.

As in the case of eugenol/isoeugenol detailed above, there is a complex balance for cinnamaldehyde and cinnamic alcohol between the varied reactivities of the molecules and their propensity to be metabolised that contributes to their overall sensitisation potential.

5.3.3 Ketones

Due to the electron donating properties of alkyl groups, ketones are less protein-reactive and in general less sensitising than aldehydes. When carbonyl groups in ketones are activated by neighbouring electron-withdrawing groups however, they can be sufficiently protein-reactive to be sensitising. As the carbonyl group is a hard electrophile, it is expected that protein-binding should occur with hard protein nucleophiles such as free primary amines. Such may be the case for the aromatic ketones and diketones (which are used in sunblock), that are shown in Figure 5.7a.

In α,β-dicarbonyl compounds (Group IV haptens) such as the sensitisers glyoxal (Krecisz and Kiec-Swierczynska, 1998; Schnuch *et al.*, 1998a), diacetyl, 1-phenylpropane-1,2-dione and the more complex steroid derivatives 21-dehydro-17-deoxy-hydrocortisone and 21-dehydro-hydrocortisone (Figure 5.7b), two carbonyl groups are juxtaposed. These compounds have the ability to react with the guanidino group of arginine residues in proteins,[19] by forming heterocyclic adducts (Scheme 5.15) (Bundgaard, 1980; Roberts *et al.*, 1999). As with other diketones, the nature of the substituents will affect the reactivity of the carbonyl groups and one carbonyl group may preferentially react with the arginine residue first. The reactivity of each carbonyl group can be calculated using the RP (see section 5.1.1.3.2). For example, in a study of α,β-diketones by Roberts *et al.* (1999), the two carbonyl groups in 1-phenylpropane-1,2-dione (Figure 5.7b) were seen to have different RPs. The carbonyl attached to the phenyl group has an RP of 2.56 and the carbonyl attached to the methyl group has an RP of 2.20, indicating that the phenyl-linked carbonyl is the more electron deficient and is more likely to react preferentially with an amino group of arginine first.

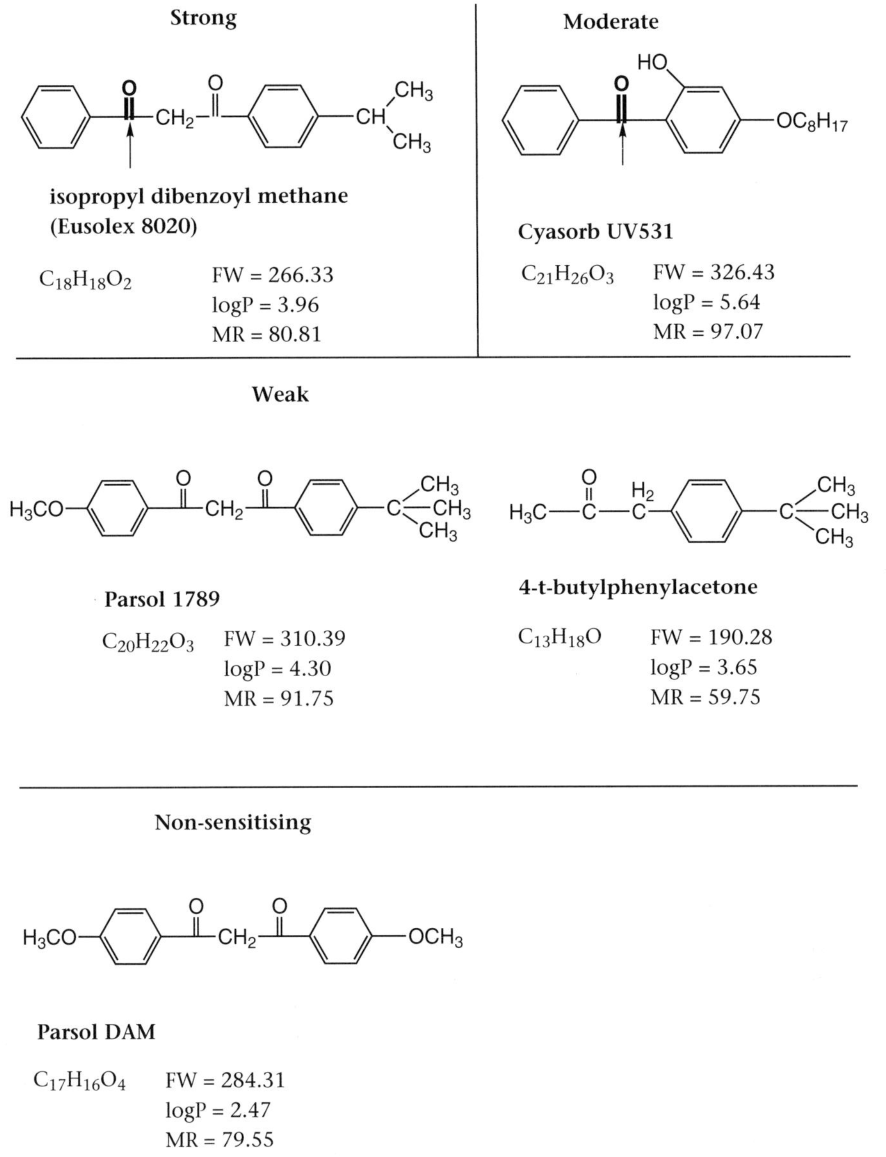

Figure 5.7a: Ketones and diketones.

Roberts *et al.* (1999) also showed that a high correlation ($r^2 = 0.958$) exists between the RAI of a selection of α,β-diketones and log (T/C) ratios from LLNA results, where varying doses were applied. RP, logP and log (T/C) values for the chemicals analysed (furil (non-sensitising), camphorquinone (Malanin, 1993) and butane-2,3-dione (moderate) and 1-phenylpropanedione (strong) (Figure 5.7b)) are given in Table 5.2.

Strong

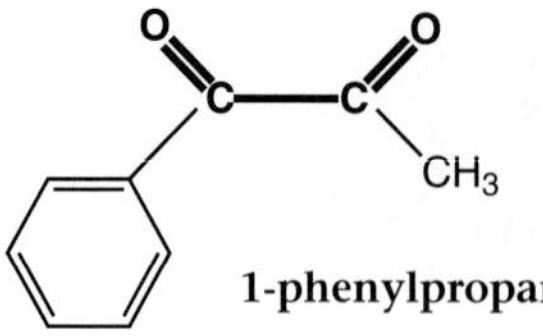

1-phenylpropane-1,2-dione

FW = 148.16
logP = 0.63
MR = 41.92

Moderate

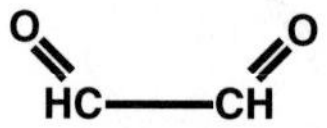

Glyoxal

FW = 58.04
logP = −0.61
MR = 12.56

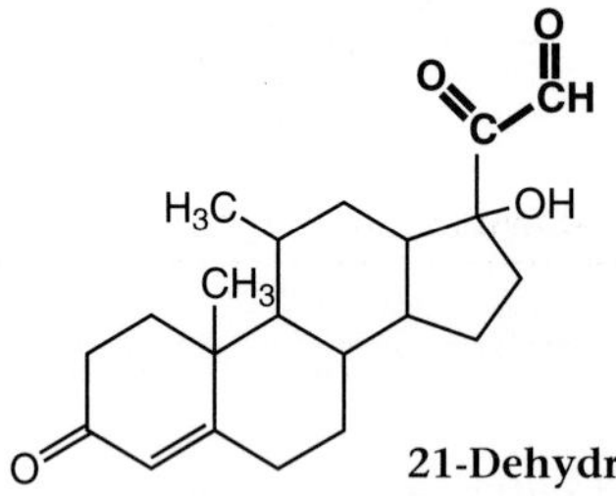

21-Dehydrocortisone

FW = 344.44
logP = 2.01
MR = 95.34

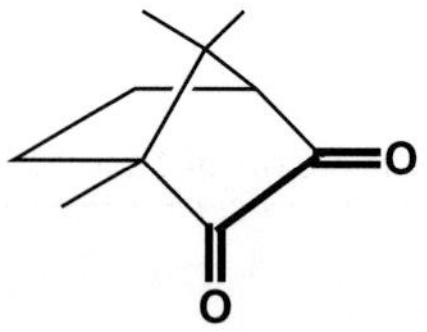

Camphorquine

FW = 166.22
logP = 1.7
MR = 45.49

Weak

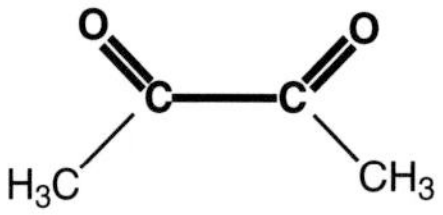

Butane-2,3-dione

FW = 86.09
logP = −0.66
MR = 21.77

Non-sensitising

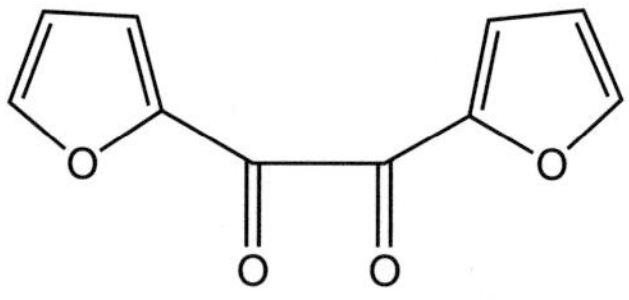

Furil

FW = 190.15
logP = 0.01
MR = 46.92

Figure 5.7b: α,β-diketones.

5.3.4 Carboxylic acids

Carboxylic acids are not protein reactive and are unlikely to be actively metabolised into protein-reactive species and hence all such compounds, in the absence of any other functionality, have been found to be non-sensitising in *in vivo* tests. Carboxylic acids are also the products of aldehyde detoxication, formed via an irreversible reaction performed by the enzyme aldehyde dehydrogenase (Scheme 3.9a).

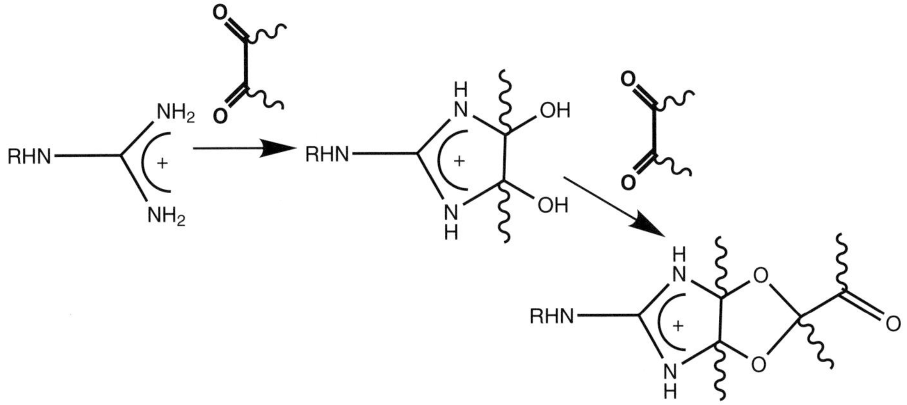

Scheme 5.15: Formation of heterocyclic adducts between α,β-diketones and arginine.

TABLE 5.2

LLNA results and chemical properties of four α,β-diketones

Compound	Dose (%)	T/C ratio	Classification	RP	logP	M. pt.
Furil	5	1.2	Non	0.50	1.42	164°C
	10	1.7	Non			
	25	2.2	Non			
Camphorquinone	5	2.8	Weak	1.62	0.69	200°C
	10	3.0	Moderate			
	25†	1.7	Non			
Butane-2,3-dione	5	1.4	Non	1.81	−1.22	<20°C
	10	2.8	Weak			
	25	5.2	Strong			
1-Phenylpropane-1,2-dione	5	12.8	Strong	2.56	1.02	84°C
	10	17.7	Strong			
	25*	20.1	Strong			

Data taken from Roberts *et al.* (1999). Structures for the listed chemicals are given in Figure 5.7b.
Classification is based on the formal regulatory classification that a T/C > 3.0 designates the molecule as sensitising.
† This dose of camphorquine does not correlate well and it is hypothesised that due to a relatively high melting point it may precipitate out of solution during passage through the stratum corneum.
* This dose of 1-phenylpropane-1,2-dione generates a lower T/C value than expected from extrapolation, probably due to overload effects.

In some studies it has been shown that some carboxylic acids can inhibit delayed-type hypersensitivity responses. For example, cis-1-methyl-4-isohexylcyclohexane carboxylic acid (IG-10) has been seen to inhibit contact dermatitis to *p*-phenylenediamine when administered orally at 100 mg/kg post-challenge in guinea pigs (Koda *et al.*, 1985; Nakatomi *et al.*, 1987). It is suggested by the authors of these studies, that inhibition is

Non-sensitising

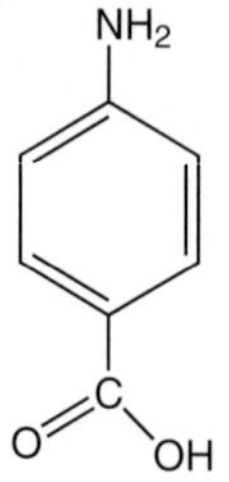

4-aminobenzoic acid

$C_7H_7NO_2$ FW = 137.14
logP = 0.41
MR = 37.52

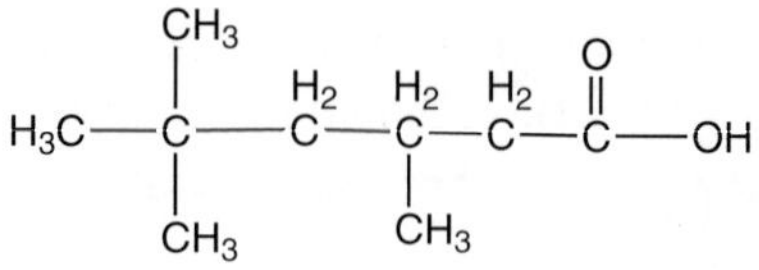

3,5,5 trimethyl hexanoic acid

$C_9H_{18}O_2$ FW = 158.24
logP = 2.97
MR = 44.65

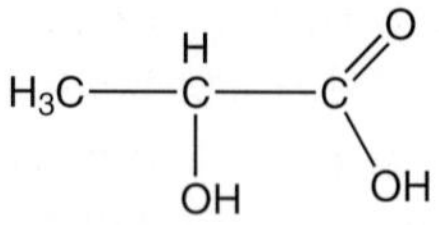

Lactic acid

$C_3H_6O_3$ FW = 90.08
logP = −0.97
MR = 18.84

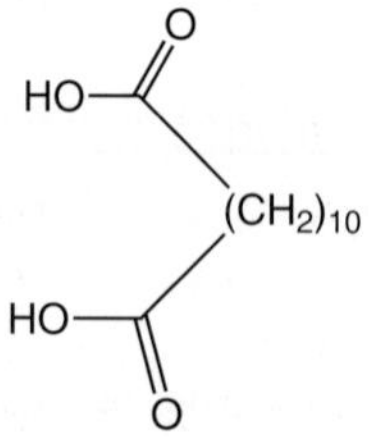

Dodecanedioic acid

$C_{12}H_{22}O_4$ FW = 230.30
logP = 3.17
MR = 60.35

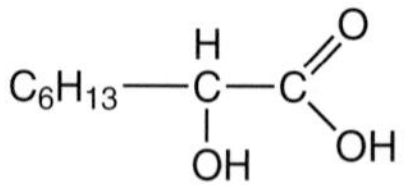

alpha-hydroxycaprylic acid

$C_8H_{16}O_3$ FW = 160.21
logP = 1.31
MR = 41.77

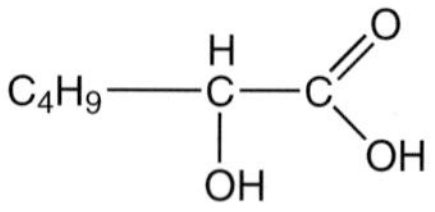

alpha-hydroxycaproic acid

$C_4H_{12}O_3$ FW = 132.16
logP = 0.40
MR = 32.57

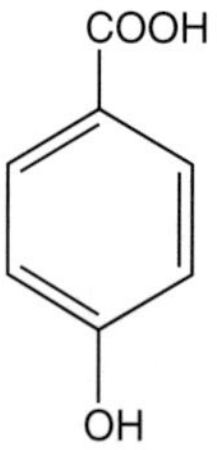

p-hydroxybenzoic acid

$C_7H_6O_3$

FW = 138.12
logP = 0.83
MR = 34.51

Figure 5.8: Carboxylic acids.

effected through the drug's action on chemokines (such as monocyte chemoattractant protein-1 (MCP-1) and macrophage migration inhibition factor (MIF)) and lymphokines (such as skin reactive factor (SRF)) during the elicitation phase of ACD. However, the exact mechanism of action remains unknown.

5.3.5 Esters

5.3.5.1 Aliphatic esters

A range of aliphatic esters are shown in Figures 5.9a and b. In general, although some esters are strong sensitisers, the ester group in aliphatic esters is not a hapten. However, the presence of an ester group adjacent to a weak electrophilic centre (e.g. C=C) can activate the latter, for example in acrylates (used in the paint industry), and render the compound sensitising (Katsuno *et al.*, 1996; Kanerva *et al.*, 1997a; Borelli and Nestle, 1998; Rustemeyer *et al.*, 1998).

The two strong sensitisers 2-hydroxyethyl acrylate and triethyl aconitate (TEA) are Group IV haptens as they possess an activated C=C bond that can bind to protein by acting as a Michael acceptor at the position shown (see Scheme 5.5). The carbonyl group in acrylates and methacrylates is thought to be insufficiently electrophilic to react with protein nucleophiles. This is clear from comparison with the close relative of TEA, triethyl citrate, which lacks the double bond (or any electrophilic centre) and is non-sensitising.

The moderate sensitisers, ethylidene heptanoate acetate (EHA) and methacrolein diacetate (MADA) are prohaptens but are activated esters and can act as acetyl (-$COCH_3$) transfer agents. Also, these compounds can be readily hydrolysed to aldehydes. It is suspected that acetaldehyde or 2-methyl-1,2-propen-3-al are the true haptens leading to sensitisation with these compounds.

Methyl stearate was classified as a weak sensitiser (Cronin and Basketter, 1994) and yet there are no obvious mechanisms via which this can act as a hapten or be metabolised into a hapten. Triethyl citrate (Figure 5.9a) and the esters in Figure 5.9b are all non-sensitisers as all of them are non-electrophilic in character and presumably there are no known mechanisms of metabolic activation.

Of interest, is the comparison between acrylates e.g. 2-hydroxyethyl acrylate (HEA) (Figure 5.9a) and methacrylates, e.g 2-hydroxypropylmethacrylate (HPMA) (Figure 5.9b). Both of these chemicals have been seen to be sensitising in guinea-pig and humans (Katsuno *et al.*, 1996; Kanerva *et al.*, 1997a; Borelli and Nestle, 1998; Rustemeyer *et al.*, 1998). However, comparisons of sensitisation potency between these chemicals does not appear to have been reported. A study in guinea-pigs has suggested that HPMA is only sensitising at high dose in petrolatum (Clemmensen, 1985). It is expected that a similar situation as described for the β-carbon in cinnamaldehyde and α-alkylated cinnamaldehydes would occur for acrylates and methacrylates (see section 5.3.2.2.3) (Figure 5.6d).[20] In CAld and HEA (both strongly sensitising haptens) the soft activated β-carbon electrophile can act as a Michael acceptor by bonding with soft nucleophilic Cys residues. When an alkyl group (methyl or larger) is substituted at the α-carbon in relation to the carbonyl group, it may reduce the sensitisation potential of alkylacrylates in comparison

Strong

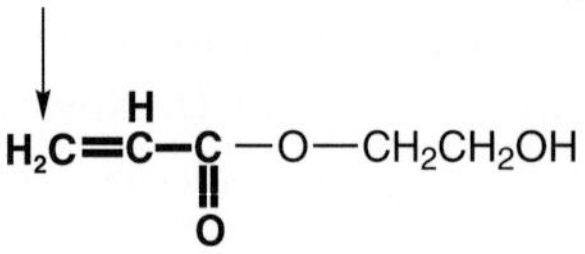

2-Hydroxyethyl acrylate

$C_5H_8O_3$ FW = 116.12
logP = 0.28
MR = 28.35

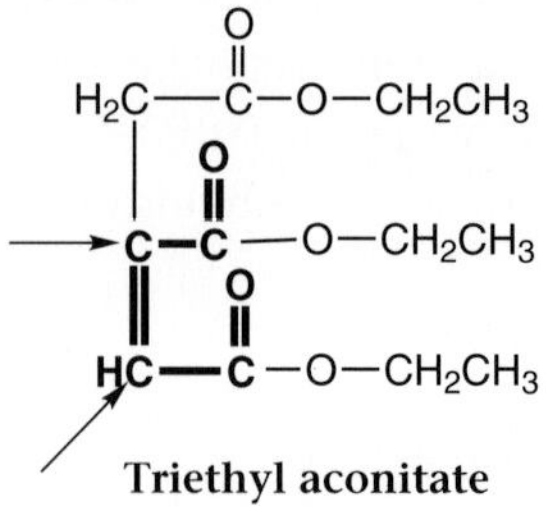

Triethyl aconitate

FW = 258.27 $C_{12}H_{18}O_6$
logP = 0.81
MR = 63.78

Moderate

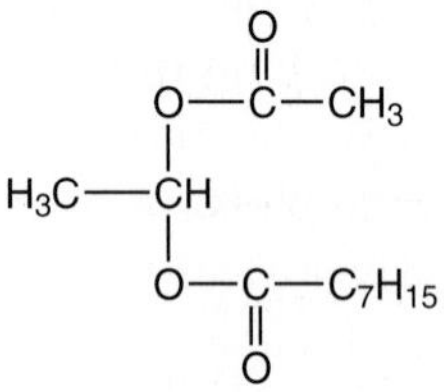

Ethylidene heptanoate acetate

$C_{12}H_{22}O_4$

FW = 230.30
logP = 2.93
MR = 60.14

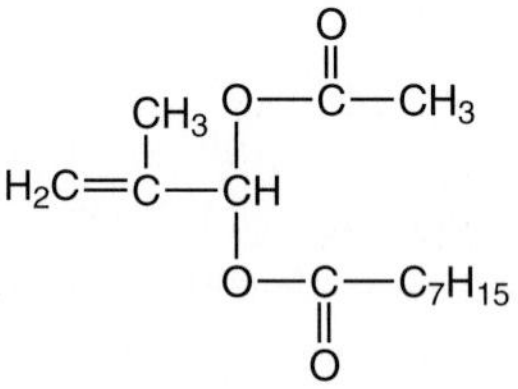

Methacrolein diacetate

$C_{14}H_{24}O_4$

FW = 256.34
logP = 3.72
MR = 68.67

Weak

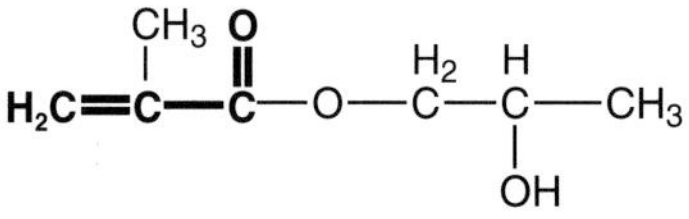

2-hydroxypropylmethacrylate

$C_7H_{12}O_3$ FW = 144.17
logP = 0.560
MR = 38.16

Non-sensitising

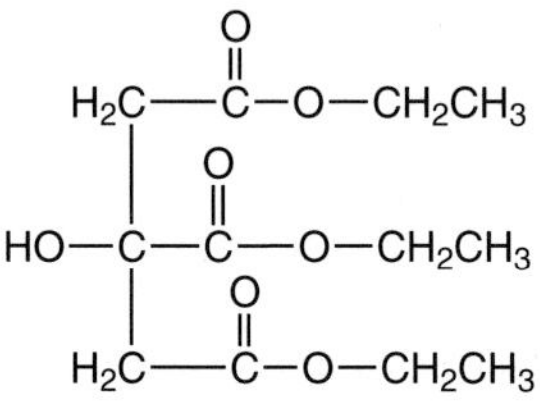

Triethyl citrate

$C_{12}H_{20}O_7$

FW = 276.28
logP = 0.12
MR = 64.18

c.f. triethylaconitate
strong sensitiser!

Figure 5.9a: Aliphatic esters.

Non-sensitising

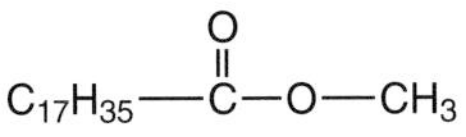

Methyl stearate

$C_{19}H_{38}O_2$

FW = 298.50
logP = 7.70
MR = 91.05

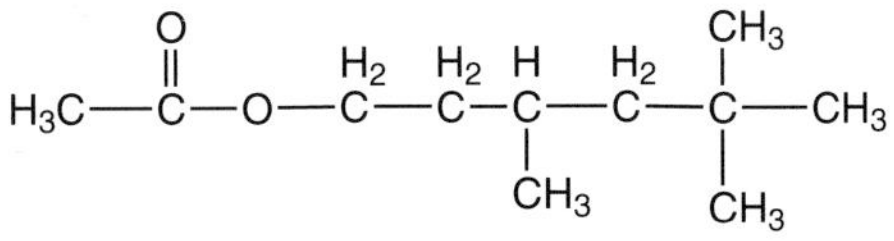

inonyl acetate
3,5,5-trimethylhexylacetate

$C_{11}H_{22}O_2$

FW = 186.29
logP = 3.72
MR = 54.06

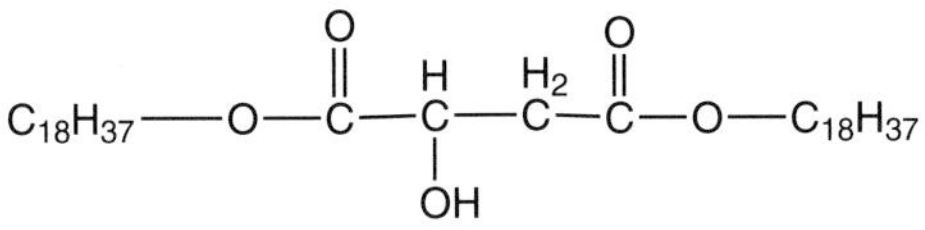

Cosmol

$C_{40}H_{78}O_5$

FW = 638.04
logP = 17.478
MR = 192.60

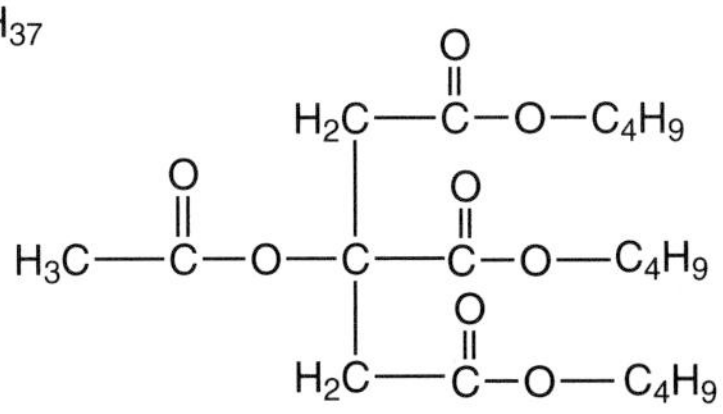

Acetyl tributyl citrate

$C_{20}H_{34}O_8$

FW = 402.29
logP = 4.781
MR = 102.09

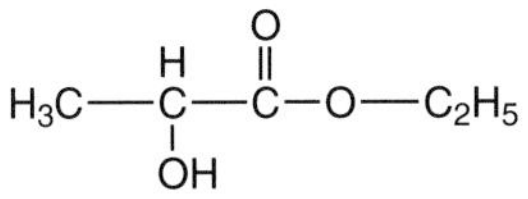

Ethyl lactate

$C_5H_{10}O_3$

FW = 118.13
logP = 0.31
MR = 28.38

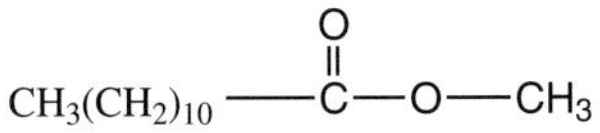

Methyl laurate

$C_{13}H_{26}O_2$

FW = 214.34
logP = 4.96
MR = 63.45

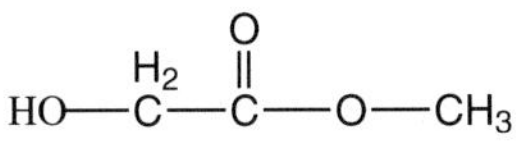

Methyl glycolate

$C_3H_6O_3$

FW = 90.08
logP = −0.530
MR = 1.911

Figure 5.9b: Aliphatic esters (cont.).

to acrylates due to the electron-donating inductive properties of the alkyl group. Such electron-donating induction would reduce the electrophilicity of the β-carbon and hence reduce the capacity for protein-binding.

Esterases, which are active in the skin, can metabolise ester groups to alcohol and acid (Scheme 3.20) and ester hydrolysis can be detoxifying (see sections 3.3.1.5.1 and 4.2.1.1.18). However, molecules that possess a conjugated —C=C—C=O system (e.g. HEA and TEA) may not be suitable substrates for cutaneous esterases and may therefore not be metabolically detoxified in the skin.

5.3.5.2 Aromatic esters

Aromatic esters are commonly used in sunscreens and incidences of sunscreen contact allergies have been reported (Ricci *et al.*, 1997). All of the activated benzoate esters in Figure 5.10a are strong sensitisers and are all Group I haptens. They can undergo nucleophilic substitution at the position indicated and all of the respective leaving groups form reasonably acidic conjugate acids.

Benzocaine (Figure 5.10b) and other 'caine' esters are used as local anaesthetics and can cause allergic reactions in humans, though true immune reactions are rare (Eggleston and Lush, 1996). Benzocaine is moderately sensitising and is a prohapten. It is postulated that metabolic activation (probably by a CYP-mediated oxidative radical reaction), which results in the conversion of NH_2 to NO_2 that is activated by the p-CO_2Et group, is responsible for hapten formation.

Ethylidene benzoate acetate (Figure 5.10b) is only weakly sensitising. However, it possesses a good leaving group for nucleophilic attack at the position shown and is also an acetaldehyde precursor, hence it is surprising that this chemical does not exhibit higher observed sensitisation levels in the LLNA.

Parsol (Figure 5.10b) is sensitising (Ricci *et al.*, 1997) but only appears to be a weak sensitiser. It has the capacity to act as a Michael acceptor at its double bond but its log P is relatively high and hence skin absorption may be a limiting factor. Anther and aspartame (Figure 5.10b) acting as sensitisers are difficult to explain in chemical terms. Neither of these chemicals possess sufficiently reactive electrophilic centres. It is possible that sulphation of aromatic esters can activate the ester group (see section 5.3.14).

It may also be possible that ester hydrolysis by esterases (see Scheme 3.20) leads to the formation of acid and alcohol derivatives (e.g. benzoic acid and benzyl alcohol from benzyl benzoate or 1-pheylethanoic acid and isobutanol from anther). However, neither of these chemical species would be protein-reactive nor would further metabolism of the generated benzyl alcohol by ADH/CYP lead to a sensitising aldehyde, as benzaldehyde is known to be non-sensitising from *in vivo* animal tests. Formation of ADH-derived isobutanal from anther may account for weak sensitisation observed for this molecule.

Methyl cinnamate, gardocyclene and dimethyl isophthalate are all regarded as non-sensitisers. The two latter compounds do not possess electrophilic centres. Methyl cinnamate, however, possesses a potential Michael acceptor but the reactivity of the β-carbon, in comparison to the strongly sensitising cinnamaldehyde (Figure 5.6c), will be substantially lower due to the presence of the strongly electron withdrawing

Strong

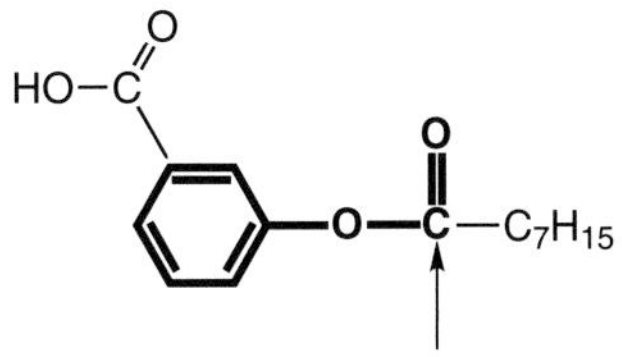

3-carboxyphenyl heptanoate

$C_{15}H_{20}O_4$ FW = 264.32
logP = 3.92
MR = 71.58

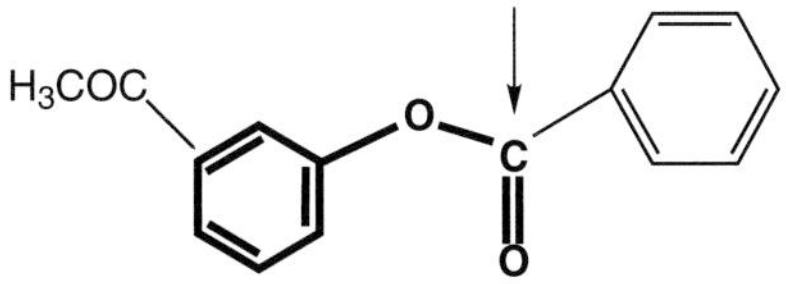

3-acetyl phenyl benzoate

$C_{15}H_{12}O_3$ FW = 226.27
logP = 2.83
MR = 67.77

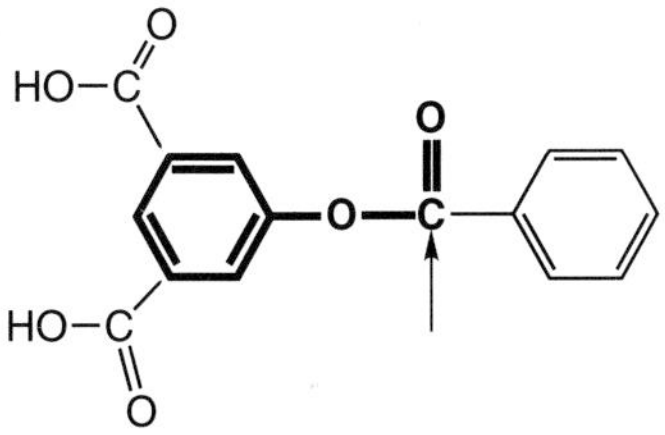

Benzoyloxy-3,5-benzene dicarboxylic acid

$C_{15}H_{10}O_6$ FW = 286.24
logP = 2.63
MR = 70.88

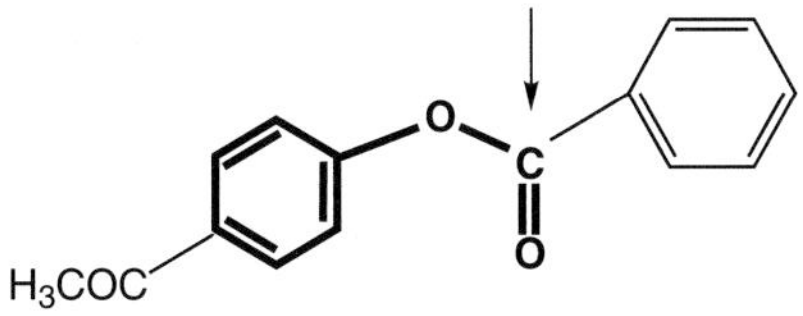

4-acetyl phenyl benzoate

$C_{15}H_{12}O_3$ FW = 226.27
logP = 2.83
MR = 67.77

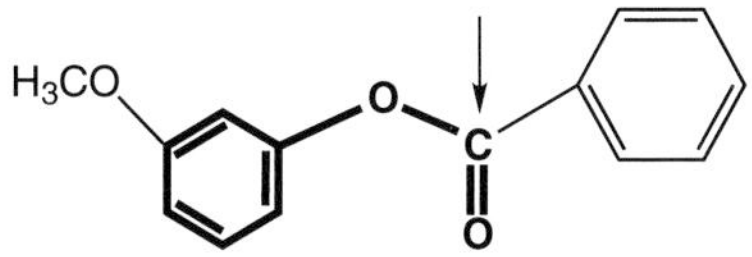

3-methoxy phenyl benzoate

$C_{14}H_{12}O_3$ FW = 228.24
logP = 3.02
MR = 63.85

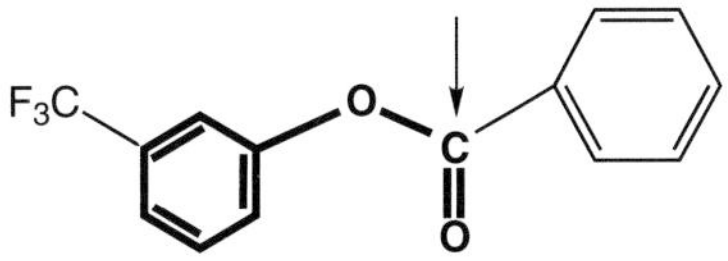

3-trifluoromethyl phenyl benzoate

$C_{14}H_9F_3O_2$ FW = 266.22
logP = 4.44
MR = 63.34

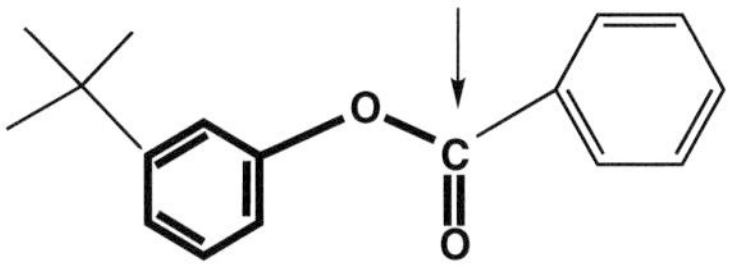

3-tert-butyl phenyl benzoate

$C_{15}H_{14}O_2$ FW = 254.32
logP = 4.77
MR = 76.03

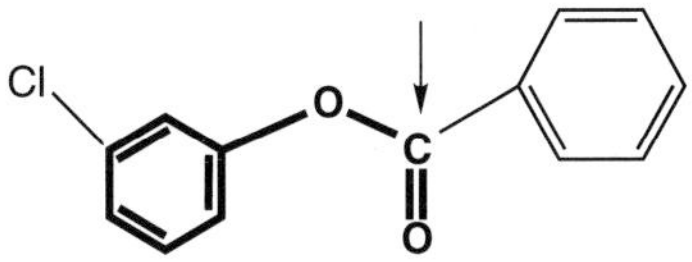

3-chloro phenyl benzoate

$C_{13}H_9ClO_2$

FW = 232.66
logP = 3.51
MR = 62.17

Figure 5.10a: Aromatic esters.

Moderate

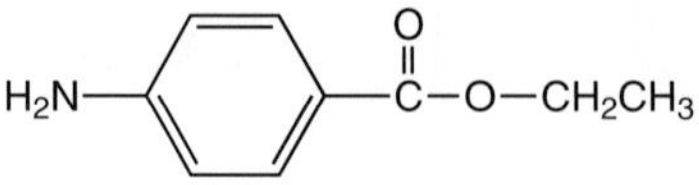

Benzocaine

FW = 165.19 $C_9H_{11}NO_2$
logP = 1.17
MR = 47.03

Weak

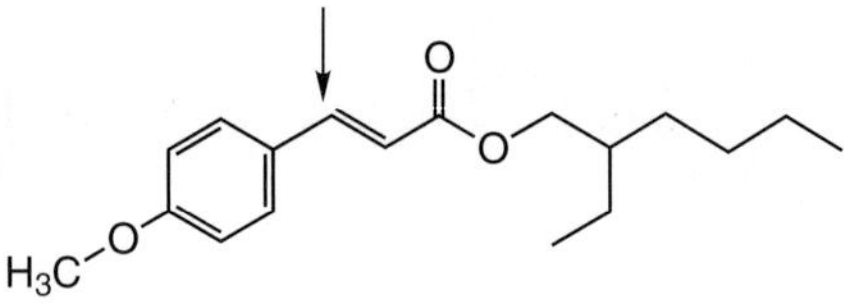

Parsol MCX

$C_{18}H_{26}O_3$ FW = 290.4
logP = 6.057
MR = 8.875

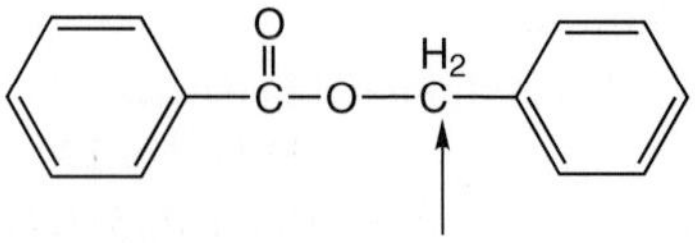

Benzyl benzoate

$C_{14}H_{12}O_2$

FW = 212.24
logP = 3.00
MR = 62.20

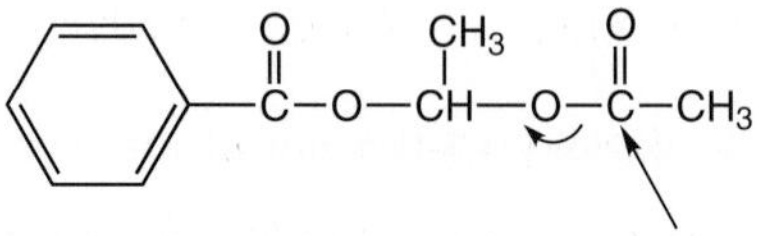

Ethylidene benzoate acetate

$C_{11}H_{12}O_4$

FW = 208.21
logP = 2.09
MR = 52.68

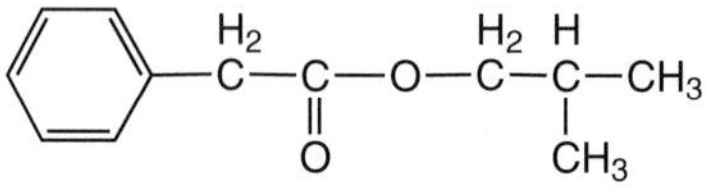

Anther

$C_{12}H_{16}O_2$ FW = 192.25
logP = 2.83
MR = 55.88

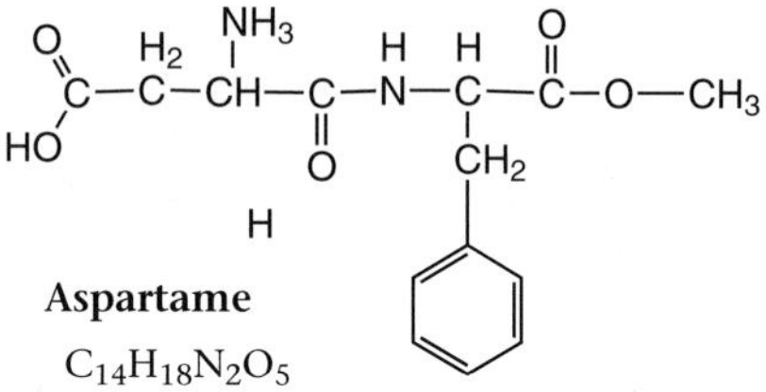

Aspartame

$C_{14}H_{18}N_2O_5$

FW = 294.30
logP = −0.39
MR = 73.22

Figure 5.10b: Aromatic esters (cont.).

Non-sensitising

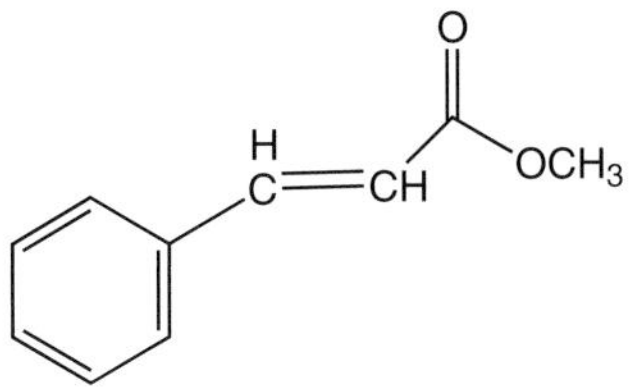

Methyl cinnamate

$C_{10}H_{10}O_2$

FW = 162.19
logP = 2.43
MR = 47.83

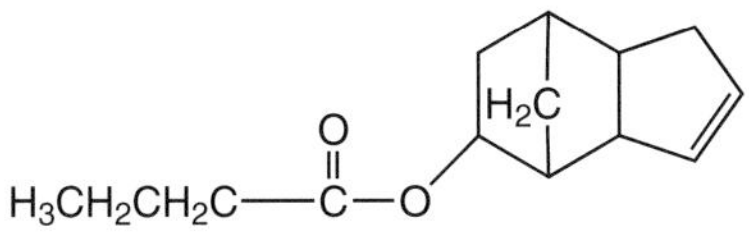

Gardocyclene

$C_{14}H_{20}O_2$

FW = 220.31
logP = 2.65
MR = 63.28

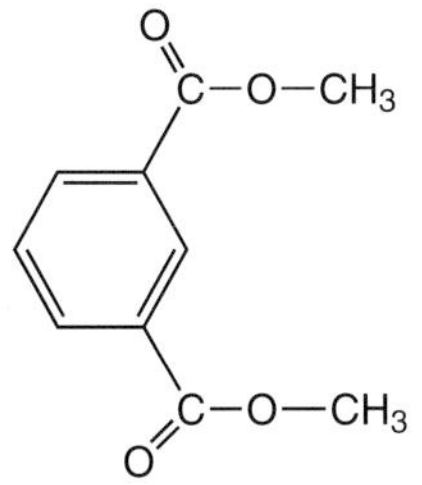

Dimethyl isophthalate

$C_{10}H_{10}O_4$

FW = 194.18
logP = 1.67
MR = 49.11

Figure 5.10c: Aromatic esters (cont.).

methoxy group of the ester. It is therefore hypothesised that methyl cinnamate is non-sensitising due to insufficient reactivity of the β-carbon.

5.3.5.3 Epoxy esters

The epoxy esters, ethyl phenyl glycidate and ethyl methyl phenyl glycidate (Figure 5.11) are both strong sensitisers (Group IV haptens). They can undergo direct nucleophilic attack as shown in Scheme 5.16.

It is feasible that epoxide hydrolase could detoxify the epoxy group by conversion to a diol via hydrolysis (see Figure 3.25). Also, the action of esterases may lead to the generation of ethanol, which could then be reduced by ADH/CYP to protein-reactive acetaldehyde (Scheme 5.17).

Strong

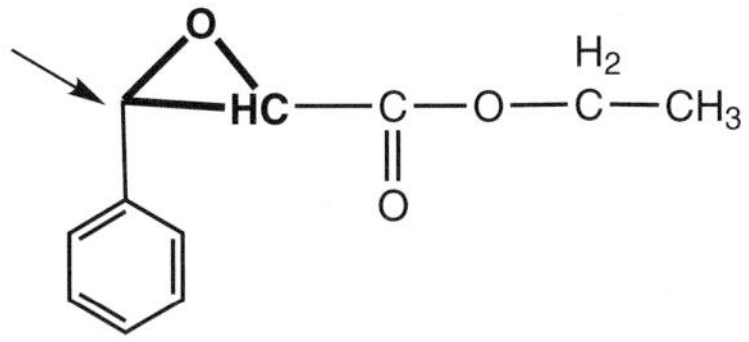

Ethyl phenyl glycidate

$C_{11}H_{12}O_3$

FW = 192.21
logP = 1.58
MR = 50.67

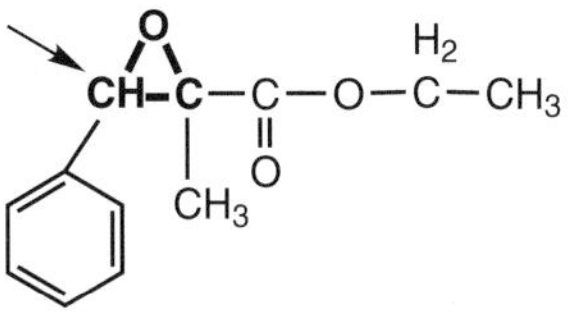

Ethyl methyl phenyl glycidate

$C_{12}H_{14}O_3$

FW = 206.24
logP = 1.97
MR = 55.39

Figure 5.11: Epoxy esters.

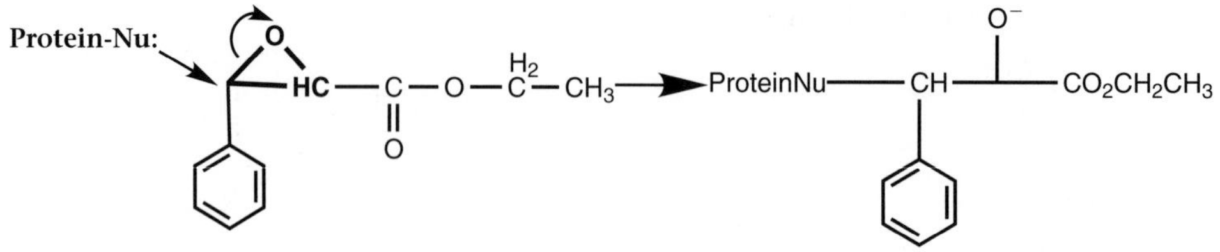

Scheme 5.16: Mechanism of protein nucleophilic addition to epoxides.

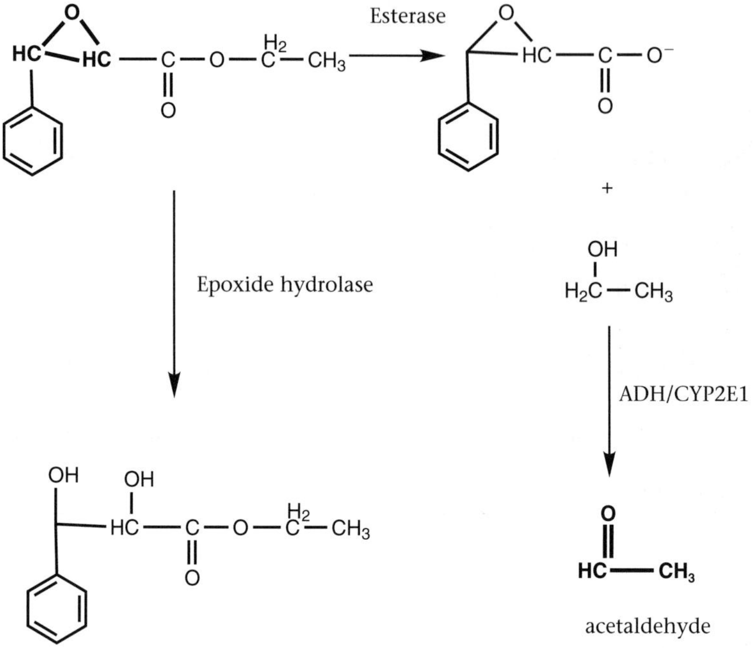

Scheme 5.17: Potential metabolism of epoxy esters.

5.3.6 Peroxides

5.3.6.1 Hydroperoxides

Organic hydroperoxides are chemicals that possess an R—OOH structure and are often generated as a product of air oxidation. The —OOH group is not electrophilic and is not protein reactive. It is thought that peroxides undergo one electron reduction in the skin (possibly by CYP) to $RO^{\bullet}$ and OH^-. $RO^{\bullet}$ (or other $RO^{\bullet}$-derived radicals) can act as haptens. Radicals can add to a C=C double bond in a protein residue such as Tyr, Phe or Trp or abstract a hydrogen from a protonated Lys or His residue (see Scheme 5.8 and Figure 5.2). In the presence of Fe(II), $RO^{\bullet}$ may also rearrange to form epoxides (see sec-

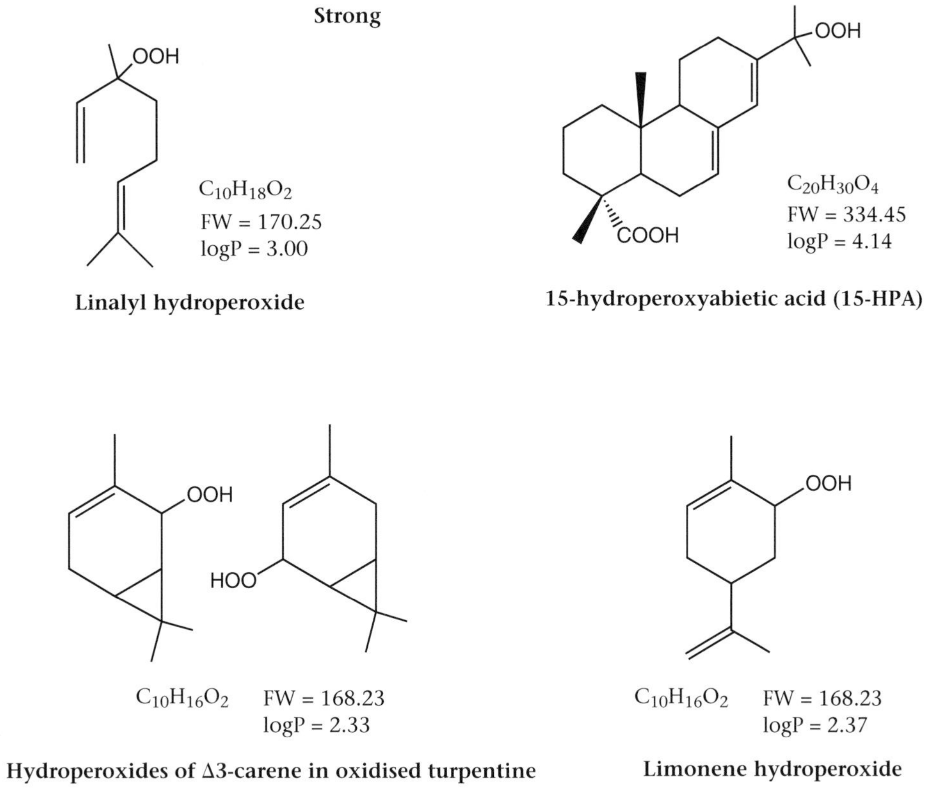

Figure 5.12a: Hydroperoxides.

tions 5.3.6.1 and 5.3.6.2 below). Figure 5.12a presents the chemical structures of some strong skin sensitising hydroperoxides.

Linalyl hydroperoxide is an allylic peroxide thought to be the sensitising agent in ylang ylang and lavender oils. Upon one electron reduction of linalyl hydroperoxide (Scheme 5.18), the resulting radical can bind to protein nucleophiles or can rearrange to a variety of epoxy products (as a result of the molecule containing two double bonds) (Scheme 5.18). In an attempt to distinguish whether a radical or an epoxide acts as the hapten in linalyl peroxide allergy, Bezard *et al.* (1997) synthesised the compounds shown in Scheme 5.18 and assessed their sensitisation potential and cross-reactivities using the murine LLNA and guinea pig Freund's complete adjuvant test.

Only the hydroperoxide and epoxylinalool were sensitisers and there was no cross reactivity between these compounds suggesting the formation of two different antigenic determinants by two sufficiently different hapten-protein binding mechanisms. Epoxylinalool (a) can bind to protein residues via an epoxy ring-opening mechanism (Scheme 5.16). The oxygen-centred radical intermediate of linalyl hydroperoxide could bind to protein residues as in Scheme 5.8. However, Bezard *et al.* (1997) could not detect any

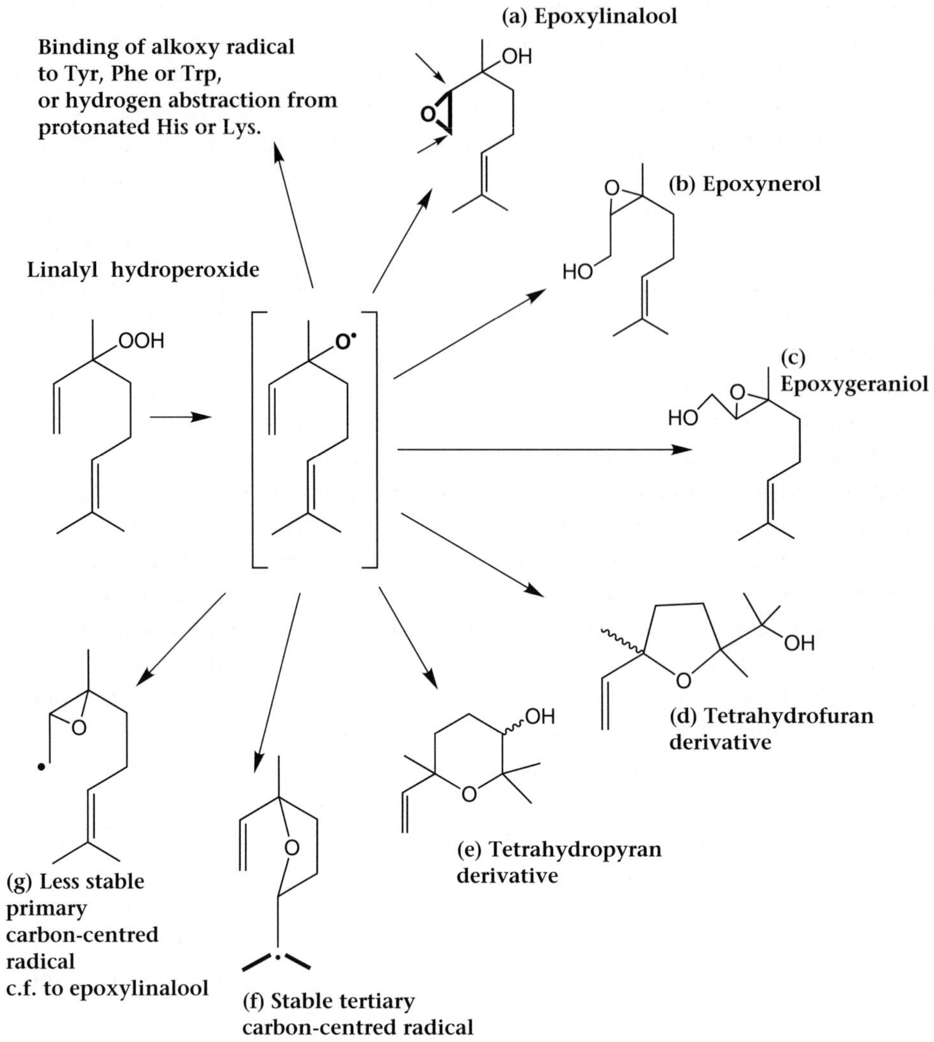

Scheme 5.18: Potential products of linalyl hydroperoxide rearrangement via an oxygen centred radical.

such radical adducts. They were able to detect, by electron paramagnetic resonance spectroscopy, a spin-trapped tertiary carbon-centred radical (formed by reaction of the oxygen-centred radical with the isoprenyl double bond (f)). Hence, Bezard *et al.* (1997) favour this carbon-centred radical as an intermediate in linalyl hydroperoxide sensitisation (Scheme 5.18).

Other examples of hydroperoxides acting as skin sensitising agents are 15-hydroperoxyabietic acid (15-HPA) in rosin (colophony) (Karlberg *et al.*, 1988; Karlberg, 1991;

Farm, 1998), terpene hydroperoxides in oxidised turpentine (fresh turpentine is not allergenic, hence air oxidation of hydrocarbons to hydroperoxides is important here) (Hellerstrom *et al.*, 1955), and similarly *d*-limonene hydroperoxide, the oxidised by-product of *d*-limonene (a non-allergenic monoterpene) from citrus juice/oils (Karlberg *et al.*, 1994; Nilsson *et al.*, 1996; Karlberg and Dooms-Goossens, 1997) (Figure 5.12a). As with linalyl hydroperoxide, it is unknown as to whether a radical or an epoxide or both act as haptens for these hydroperoxides but hypotheses have been offered (Gäfvert *et al.*, 1994; Lepoittevin and Karlberg, 1994). In the case of 15-HPA in colophony, it was suggested by Gäfvert *et al.* (1994) that both mechanisms of oxygen-centred radical and epoxide protein binding can occur (Scheme 5.19). Cross-reactivity studies showed that 15-HPA sensitised guinea-pigs did not cross-react with 15-hydroperoxydehydroabietate (15-HPDA) (Scheme 5.19) but did cross-react with α- or β-epoxyabietates (Scheme 5.19). This suggests that an epoxide is the favoured hapten for 15-HPA.[21] Conversely, 15-HPDA sensitised guinea-pigs cross reacted with 15-HPA but not with α- or β-epoxyabietates. 15-HPDA cannot react via an epoxide route (presumably due to the additional electronic stability of the ring system), hence it is not surprising that this molecule does not cross-react with the epoxides.

15-HPDA must share a common protein-hapten binding mechanism with 15-HPA however, in order that these two molecules may cross react. The authors suggest that protein-radical adducts could act as the cross-reactive antigens and the relative levels of these antigens and subsequent memory T-cell population produced during sensitisation, may explain why 15-HPDA sensitised guinea pigs cross-react with 15-HPA but the reverse is not true. During 15-HPA sensitisation, certain relative proportions of both protein-radical and protein-epoxide adducts will be formed, thus creating two different antigens. If the protein-epoxide conjugate is the major adduct, there may not be a sufficient population of protein-radical adduct specific memory T cells present to effect an allergic reaction on challenge with 15-HPDA. However, during 15-HPDA sensitisation the major adduct is the protein-radical adduct and a significant population of memory T cells for this adduct may be generated. Upon challenge with 15-HPA, the levels of both cross-reactive protein-radical antigen and antigen-specific memory T cells present are enough to trigger an allergic reaction.

5.3.6.2 Benzoyl peroxide and peroxy acids

The structures of benzoyl peroxide and some selected peroxy acids are shown in Figure 5.12b. Peroxy acids are chemicals that possess a -CO(OOH) group.

Benzoyl peroxide, a commonly used component in topical medicaments, has been shown to be a skin sensitiser by the murine LLNA (Kimber *et al.*, 1998b) and also in humans (Lindemayr and Drobil, 1981; Greiner *et al.*, 1999). Few studies have been performed to investigate the mechanism of benzoyl peroxide allergy. It is hypothesised here that the oxygen atom marked in Figure 5.12b is a potential reactive centre.

The peroxy acids are not electrophilic and are non-sensitising. The presence of a neighbouring carbonyl group causes radical formation at the peroxy group to become unfavourable and also there is no opportunity elsewhere in the molecule for epoxides to form.

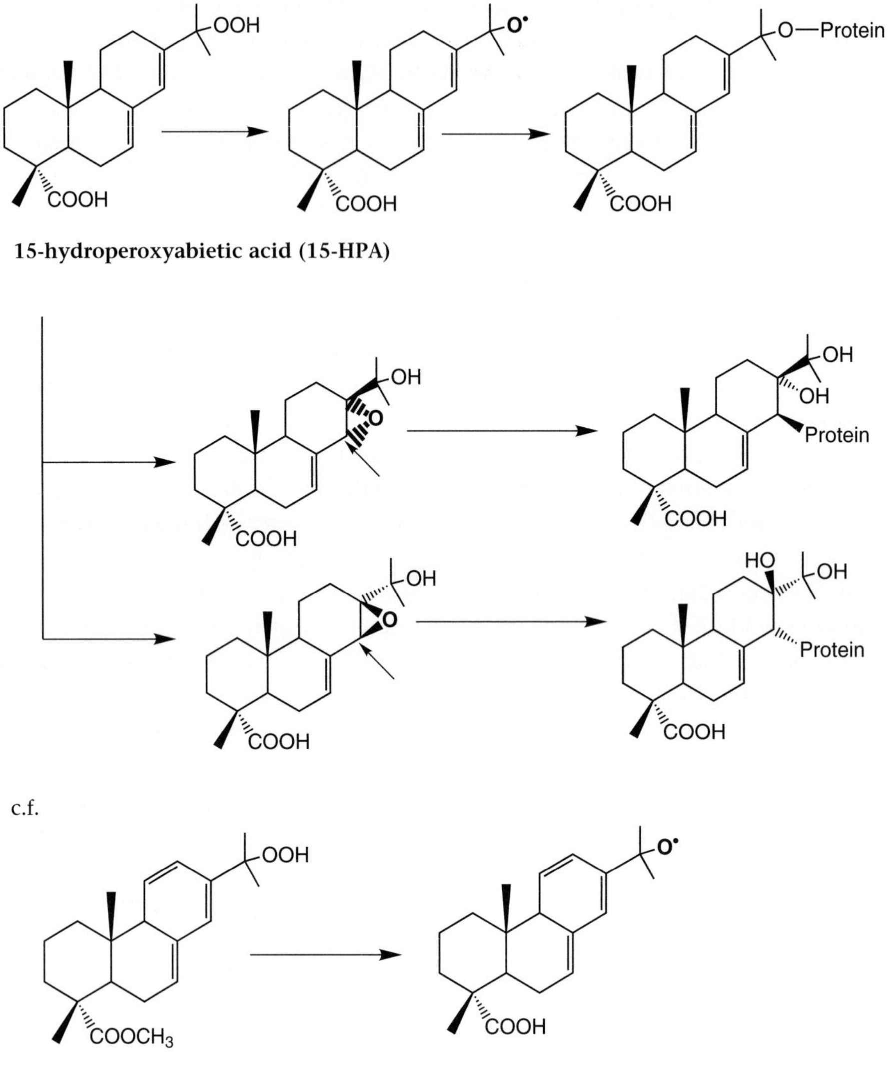

15-hydroperoxyabietic acid (15-HPA)

15-hydroperoxydehydroabietate (15-HPDA)

Scheme 5.19: Two possible mechanisms of protein-binding for 15-HPA.

5.3.7 Salicylates

The salicylate group itself, typified by salicylic acid (Figure 5.13b), is non-electrophilic. Those salicylates that are sensitisers, e.g. phenyl salicylate (moderate) (Figure 5.13a), possess other electrophilic functionalities.

Phenyl salicylate is in fact an activated ester similar to those shown in Figure 5.10a

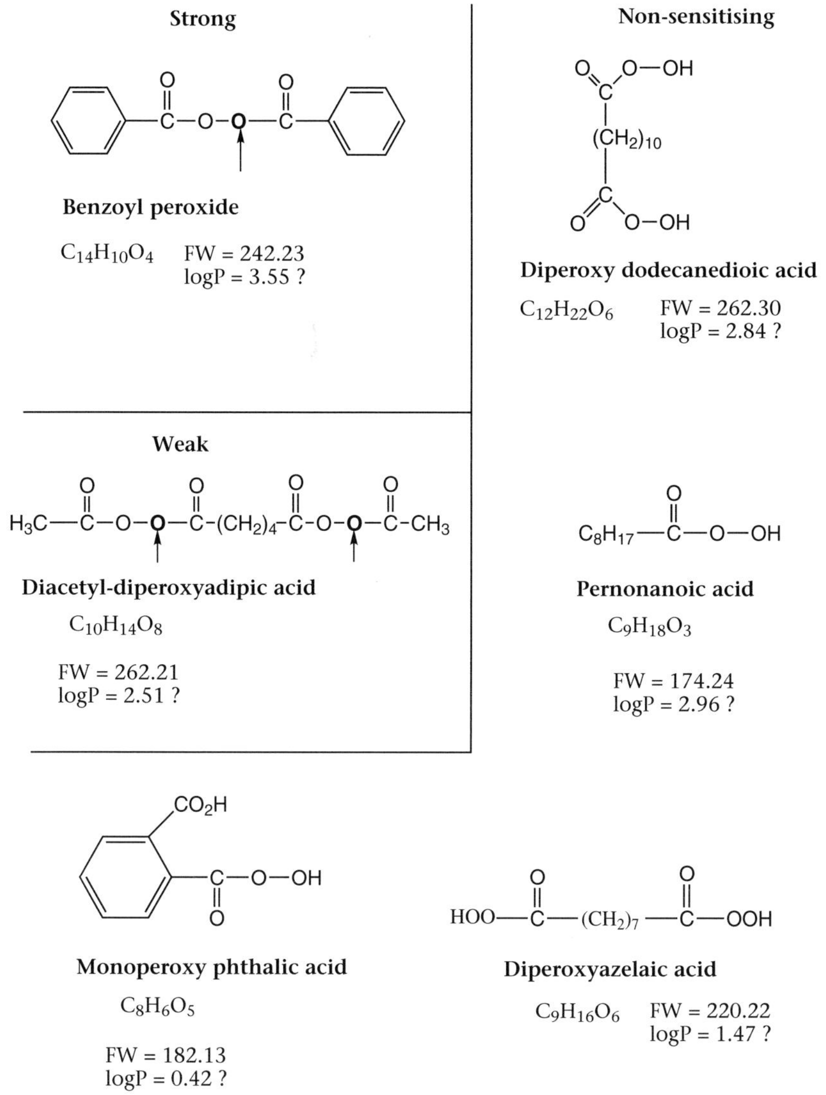

Figure 5.12b: Benzoyl peroxide and peroxy acids.

but in comparison to the latter, phenyl salicylate is only moderately sensitising. It is likely that intramolecular hydrogen bonding occurs between the phenolic hydrogen and the carbonyl oxygen, which would reduce the polarity of the carbonyl group and hence reduce the electrophilic character of the carbonyl carbon atom.

All of the salicylates in Figure 5.13b are non-sensitising, which is in agreement with the lack of electrophilic centres in these molecules and they are not likely to be actively metabolised. Methyl salicylate has been used in mechanistic studies on a number of

Moderate

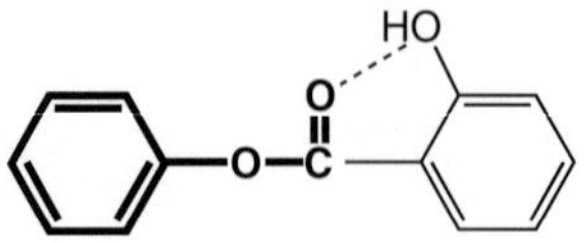

Phenyl salicylate

FW = 214.22
logP = 2.50
MR = 59.06

Weak

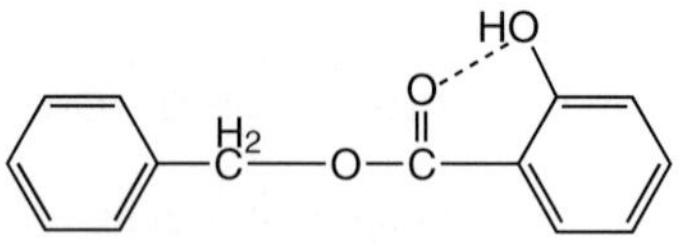

Benzyl salicylate

$C_{14}H_{12}O_3$ FW = 228.24
logP = 2.61
MR = 63.89

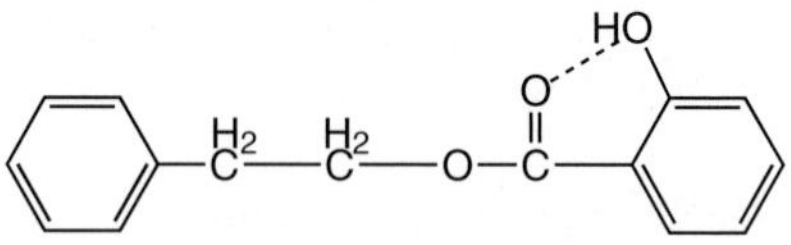

Phenyl ethyl salicylate

$C_{15}H_{14}O_3$ FW = 242.27
logP = 3.07
MR = 68.65

Figure 5.13a: Salicylates.

occasions as an example of a skin irritant without sensitising properties (Yokozeki *et al.*, 1995; Arts *et al.*, 1997).

5.3.8 Gallates

Propyl gallate is a strong sensitiser (but a potential prohapten) and could be oxidised enzymatically to an orthoquinone in a similar way to catechols (Scheme 5.10a). Thus quinone could then bind to protein nucleophiles by Michael addition. Alternatively, non-enzymatic keto-enol tautomerisation of propyl gallate (Scheme 5.20) could lead to the formation of an α,β-dicarbonyl hapten that could react with arginine residues in the manner depicted in Scheme 5.15.

5.3.9 Coumarins and anhydrides

Coumarin and anhydride derivatives can exhibit very different sensitisation potentials depending upon the properties and substituents of the ring systems (Hausen and Berger, 1989). For example, coumarin itself and 6-methyl coumarin (Me-coumarin) are non/weak sensitisers, yet dihydrocoumarin (DH-coumarin) is a strong sensitiser (Figure 5.14).

Non-sensitising

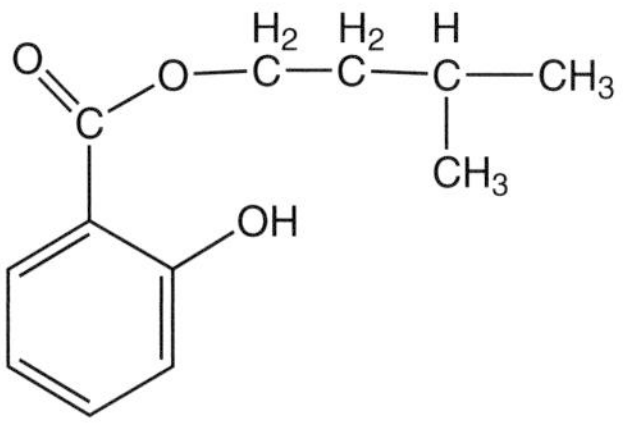

Amyl salicylate

$C_{12}H_{16}O_3$ FW = 208.25
logP = 2.71
MR = 57.70

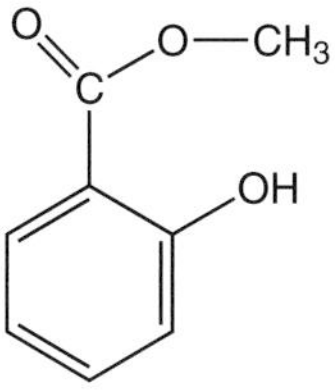

Methyl salicylate

$C_8H_8O_3$ FW = 152.15
logP = 1.30
MR = 39.28

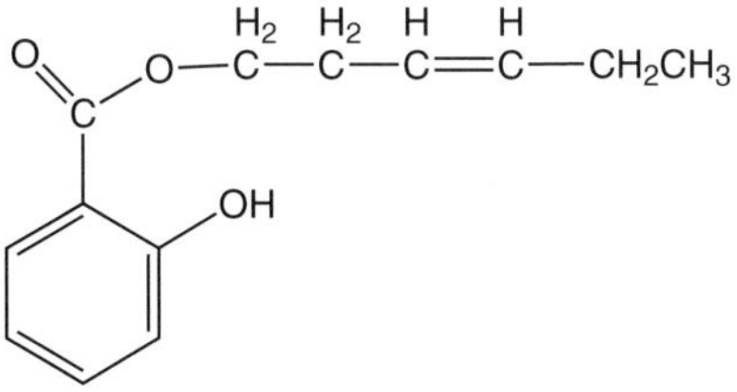

cis-3-hexenyl salicylate

$C_{13}H_{16}O_3$ FW = 220.26
logP = 2.70
MR = 63.47

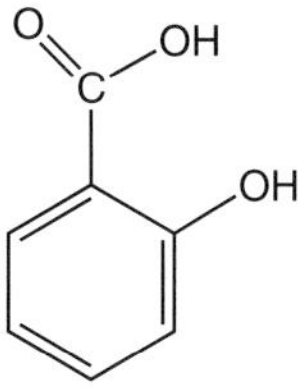

Salicylic acid

$C_7H_6O_3$ FW = 138.12
logP = 0.83
MR = 34.51

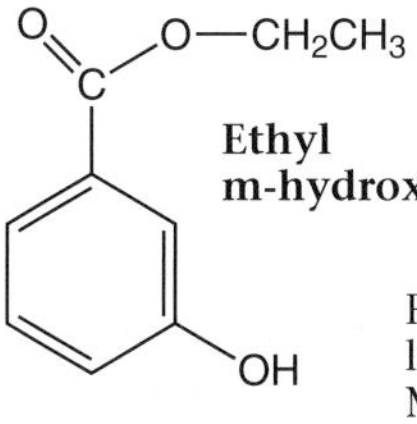

Ethyl m-hydroxybenzoate

FW = 166.17
logP = 1.59
MR = 44.03

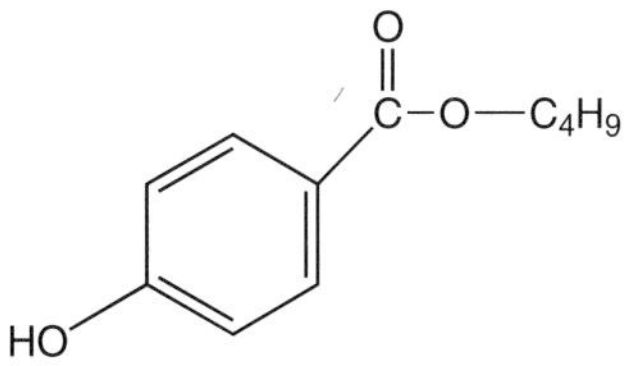

Nipabutyl/butylparaben FW = 194.23
$C_{11}H_{14}O_3$ logP = 2.50
MR = 53.15

and **Propylparaben** $C_{10}H_{12}O_3$

FW = 180.21
logP = 3.04
MR = 48.86

and methylparaben $C_8H_8O_3$

FW = 152
logP = 1.99
MR = 39.58

Figure 5.13b: Salicylates (cont.).

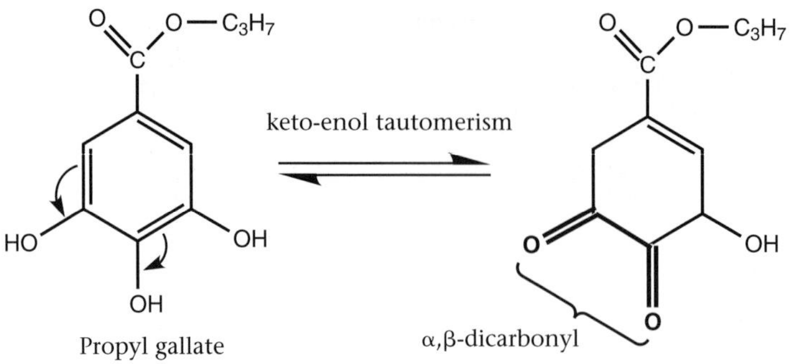

Scheme 5.20: Keto-enol tautomerism of propyl gallate.

DH-coumarin (Group I hapten) is an activated ester and the only point of nucleophilic attack in this molecule would be at the carbonyl carbon; nucleophilic attack would occur easily with the phenolic oxygen acting as a good leaving group (Figure 5.14). For Me-coumarin and coumarin, one possible theory as to why these potential haptens are non-sensitising could be that either Michael addition at the double bond adjacent to the carbonyl group or direct nucleophilic attack at the carbonyl carbon would disturb the partial aromaticity of the ring system, thereby increasing the activation energy. Also, a nucleophilic substitution reaction at the carbonyl carbon would be hindered by resistance to bond rotation in the ring system. Therefore in these molecules, reaction with protein nucleophiles is unlikely.

Octahydrocoumarin is likely to be non-sensitising for a different reason. This is not an activated ester or an aromatic molecule and the carbonyl group is neither sufficiently electrophilic nor provided with a good leaving group to react with protein, hence it is non-sensitising.

Phthalic anhydrides and acid anhydrides (e.g. trimellitic anhydride, TMA) (Grammer *et al.*, 1997; Kanerva *et al.*, 1997b) have been reported to cause immediate-type allergies that can result in asthma and contact urticaria, but are not typically associated with allergic contact dermatitis. In the local lymph node assay, phthalic anhydride is a strong sensitiser (see Appendix 1). It is a reactive acylating agent that possesses a good carboxyl leaving group and has the potential to react strongly with protein nucleophiles. A recent study has shown suspected simultaneous delayed and immediate allergenicity of methylhexahydrophthalic anhydride in an individual (Kanerva *et al.*, 1997b).

It is suspected that the lower logP, and hence reduced skin absorption, of the closely related compound, TMA (a respiratory sensitiser, and moderate contact allergen in the local lymph node assay) may contribute to the reduced level of sensitisation, in comparison to phthalic anhydride. It is conceivable that the presence of a carboxyl group on the aromatic ring may also affect/reduce the reactivity of the electrophilic centres, as the electrons in TMA are more delocalised than in phthalic anhydride. However, as anhydrides are unusual in that they can effect both immediate and delayed type allergy, it is likely that distinct mechanisms, at present unknown, lead to events that trigger the generation of either a Th2 cytokine profile observed in respiratory allergy or a Th1 cytokine profile observed in ACD.

Strong

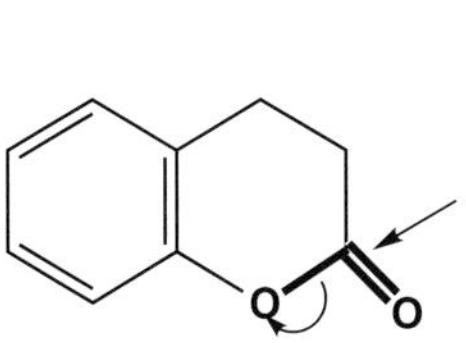

dihydrocoumarin

$C_9H_8O_2$

FW = 148.16
logP = 1.67
MR = 40.46

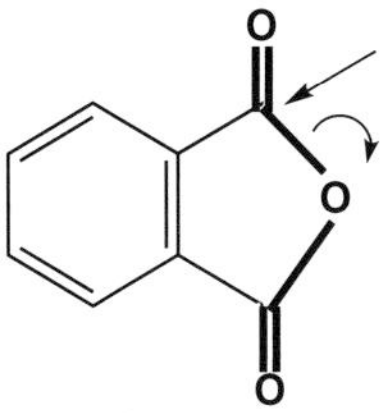

phthalic anhydride

$C_8H_4O_3$

FW = 148.12
logP = 1.43
MR = 36.37

Moderate

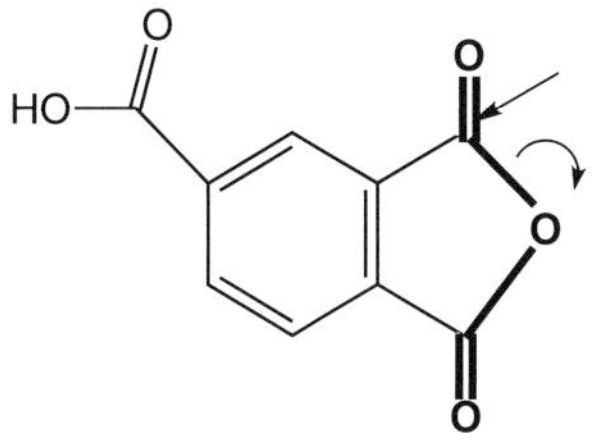

Trimellitic anhydride (TMA)
(1,2,4-benzenetricarboxylic anhydride)

$C_9H_4O_5$

FW = 192.13
logP = 0.99
MR = 43.13

Non-sensitising

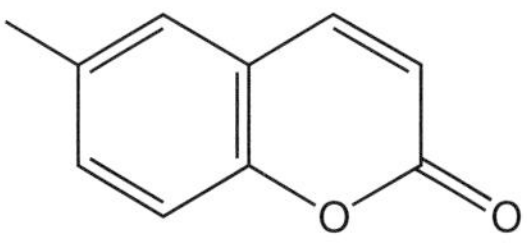

6-methylcoumarin

$C_{10}H_8O_2$

FW = 160.17
logP = 2.18
MR = 46.59

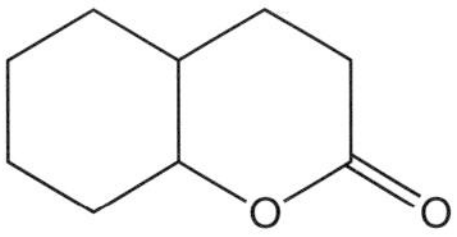

octahydrocoumarin

$C_9H_{14}O_2$

FW = 154.21
logP = 2.15
MR = 41.12

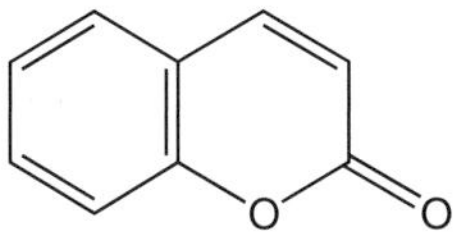

coumarin

$C_9H_6O_2$

FW = 146.14
logP = 1.76
MR = 41.55

Figure 5.14: Coumarins and anhydrides.

5.3.10 Amines and nitrobenzenes

5.3.10.1 Aliphatic amines

One observation, along with the early work on the catechol, urushiol (see section 5.3.1.2), which led to the original 'prohapten hypothesis' by Dupuis and Benezra (1982) was the fact that the aliphatic amine 1,2-diaminoethane (DAE, ethylenediamine) (Figure 5.15) is a sensitiser (Balato *et al.*, 1984; Babiuk *et al.*, 1987; English and Rycroft, 1989; Matthieu *et al.*, 1993; Corazza *et al.*, 1994), yet it is clearly not a protein-reactive compound. This went against all hypotheses that a small molecule had to be electrophilic and bind to protein nucleophilic residues to form a larger immunogenic complex in order for an allergic reaction to occur. Using their prohapten hypothesis (that non-electrophilic sensitisers, such as DAE, must be transformed within the skin into protein-reactive haptens) they proposed that DAE is oxidised/hydrolysed to the sensitising dialdehyde, glyoxal (Figure 5.7b) by the enzyme monoamine oxidase (see Figure 3.12). However, this theory remains to be proven.

5.3.10.2 Aromatic amines and nitrobenzenes

The aromatic amines in Figure 5.16a are also strong sensitisers but are prohaptens that require activation to haptens. It was originally suggested by Mayer (1954) and Dupuis and Benezra (1982) that 1,2- and 1,4-diamines are converted to ortho- and para-benzoquinones, respectively, via protonated intermediates (Scheme 5.21), and that this may account for the observed cross-reactivity between 1,2-diamines and 1,4-diamines. However, Basketter and Goodwin (1988) and later Lisi and Hansel (1998) suggest that benzoquinone (BQ) is neither the only, nor even the major, intermediate in cross-reactivity of *p*-amino groups and in fact a spectrum of antigenic determinants may result from a mixture of oxidation products. In two cross-reactivity human patch test studies with BQ and the commonly sensitising prohaptenic hair and skin dye component para-phenylene diamine (PPD; Conde *et al.*, 1995; Leino *et al.*, 1998; Wakelin *et al.*, 1998), only 3/10 (Basketter and Liden, 1992) and 4/22 (Lisi and Hansel, 1998) PPD-sensitised patients cross-reacted with BQ. None of the PPD-sensitised patients studied cross-reacted

Strong

1,2-diaminoethane

FW = 60.10
logP = −1.26
MR = 17.87

$C_2H_8N_2$

Figure 5.15: Aliphatic amines.

Strong

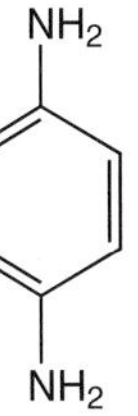

Paraphenylenediamine (PPD)

$C_6H_8N_2$ FW = 108.14
logP = 0.24
MR = 35.46

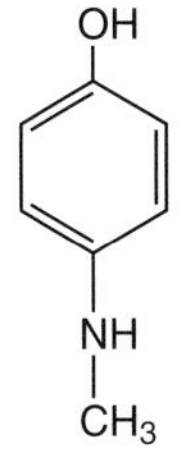

Metol
N-methyl-4-aminophenol

FW = 123.15 C_7H_9NO
logP = 1.40
MR = 37.95

cf. 4-methylaminophenol sulfate
p-aminophenol

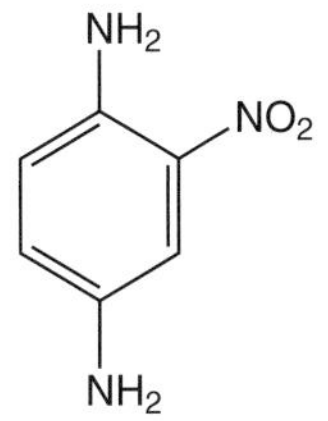

2-nitro-1,4-phenylenediamine

FW = 153.14 $C_6H_7N_3O_2$
logP = 0.20
MR = 36.74

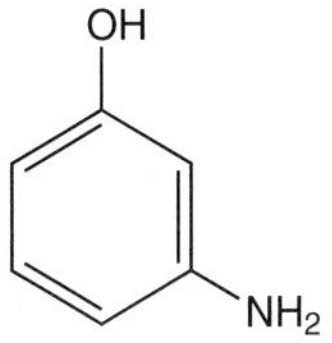

m-aminophenol

FW = 515.01 C_6H_7NO
logP = 0.66
MR = 32.45

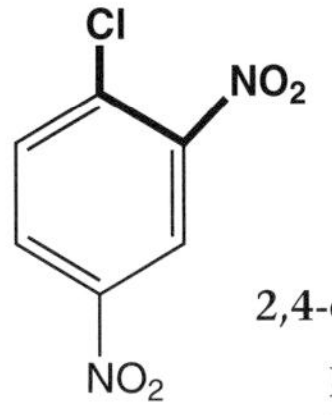

2,4-dinitrochlorobenzene (DNCB)

FW = 202.55 $C_6H_3ClN_2O_4$
logP = 2.40
MR = 46.31

Figure 5.16a: Aromatic amines and nitrobenzenes.

with hydroquinone (HQ) (which may be oxidised to BQ), in agreement with other studies on HQ (Picardo *et al.*, 1990). However, Picardo *et al.* (1990) suggested that the comparative rates of decomposition/oxidation to BQ of PPD (almost complete (pH 7.4) and 65% conversion (pH 5.5) at 24 h) and HQ (c.f. 35% (pH 7.4) and only 5% (pH 5.5) conversion at 24 h), may explain this observation. Given the acidity of the skin (pH 5.5), the low level of HQ conversion to BQ is not expected to be high *in vivo*.

It has also been postulated that PPD sensitisation could result from the formation of reactive semiquinone imine radicals (Scheme 5.21) and be influenced by oxidative stress mechanisms (Schmidt *et al.*, 1990; Picardo *et al.*, 1992; Picardo *et al.*, 1996). In the presence of 5–10 μg/ml PPD, keratinocyte proliferation in culture was seen to be enhanced (Picardo *et al.*, 1992). Above this level of PPD, cytotoxicity and lipid peroxidation damage were observed. The production of highly reactive superoxide, hydrogen peroxide and hydroxyl radicals in cell culture were also increased by PPD. In keratinocyte culture medium alone, however, PPD was seen to autoxidise, hence any oxidation seen in culture may not be representative of the situation *in vivo* where, in skin, reduction may be more favourable (Picardo *et al.*, 1992).

It has also been hypothesised that the substituent at the para position of an aromatic compound may influence chemical reactivity i.e. some substituents are activating (e.g. $-NH_2$, -OH and $-CH_3$) and some deactivating ($-NO_2$, SO_3 and -COOH) (Kleniewska and Maibach, 1980). To support this, Lisi and Hansel (1998) found that the incidence of sensitisation to compounds with a 2nd amine in the para position (e.g. PPD) was higher than that seen for compounds with an -OH (p-aminophenol), $-CH_3$ (p-toluenediamine) or -COOH (benzocaine and p-aminobenzoic acid) in the para position. However, they did not rule out the potential for differences in percutaneous penetration (logP) to affect allergic potential with these compounds.

A study has also been performed on whether there is a correlation between PPD sensitisation in humans and their ability to potentially detoxify PPD by acetylation performed by N-acetyltransferase (NAT) (Kawakubo *et al.*, 1997). These authors concluded that in PPD positive patients there were similar numbers of slow (5/9 patients) and rapid (4/9 patients) acetylator phenotypes, but non-PPD sensitive patients were predominantly rapid acetylators (63/76 patients). In comparison, a study by Schnuch *et al.* (1998b) also investigated this phenomenon with respect to individuals with ACD (resulting from a variety of chemicals) and also found a similar number of slow (25/52 patients) and rapid (27/52) acetylator phenotypes in these patients. Their control group, however, showed predominance (65/85 individuals) of slow acetylator phenotype in non-allergic individuals, which contrasts with the findings of Kawakubo *et al.* (1997) whose control group were mainly rapid acetylators. Perhaps it is a result of the small sample sizes analysed that these studies remain inconclusive as to whether there is a relationship between acetylator phenotype and susceptibility to ACD.

To corroborate their *in vivo* studies, Kawakubo *et al.* (1999) performed *in vitro* studies on PPD acetylation, in the presence of human skin cytosol and acetyl CoA, and detected monoacetyl-PPD and from this small amounts of diacetyl-PPD using HPLC methods. The K_m and V_{max} values for monoacetyl PPD formation were 1080 μM and 3.58 nmol/mg/min, respectively, and the corresponding values for diacetyl-PPD formation were 358 μM and 6.12 nmol/mg/min. Activities for PPD N-acetylation in seven humans ranged from 0.41–3.68 nmol/mg/min and correlated better with other known NAT1 substrate activities (e.g. 2-aminofluorene). NAT2-specific activities (e.g. sulphamethazine) could not be

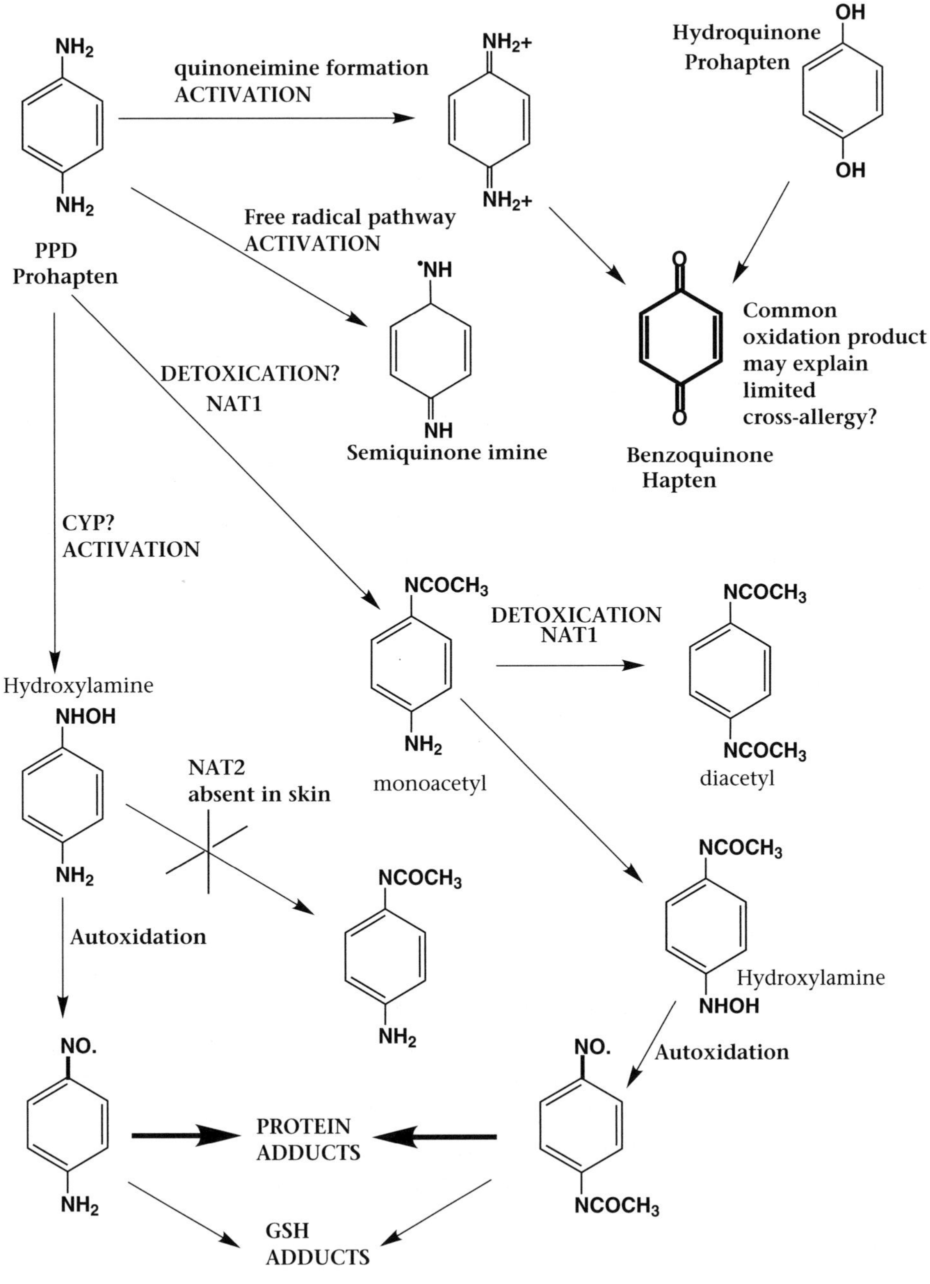

Scheme 5.21: Potential metabolism of para-phenylenediamine (PPD).

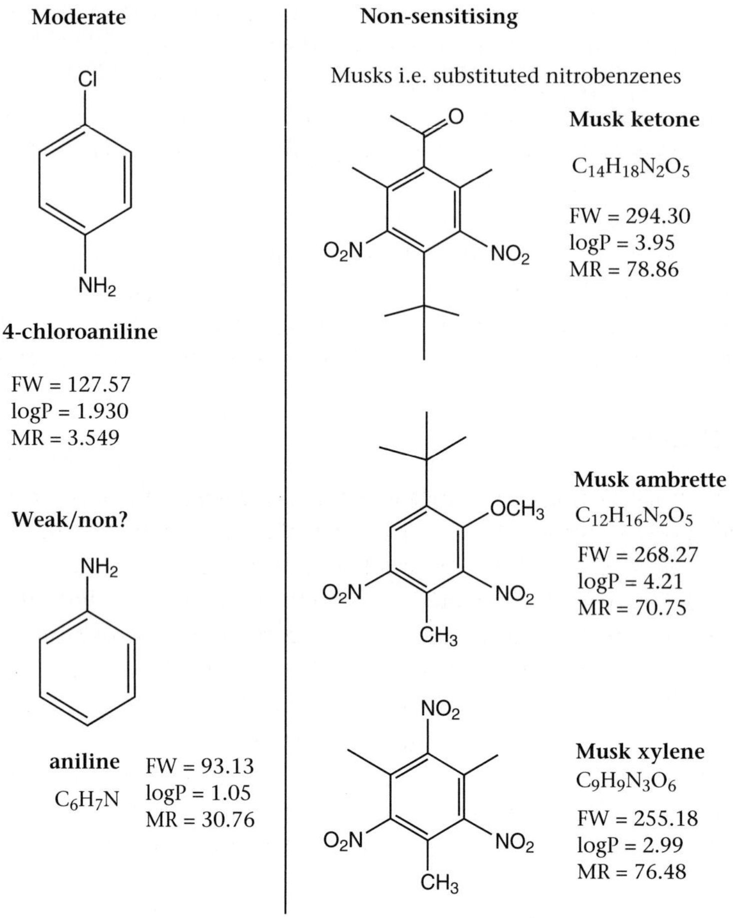

Figure 5.16b: Aromatic amines and nitrobenzenes (cont.).

detected in human skin cytosol. On using the NAT1 inhibitor, para-aminobenzoic acid, the degree of PPD N-acetylation could be inhibited by 74%. These findings have later been supported by the detection of mRNA for NAT1 but not NAT2 in human keratinocytes (Reilly *et al.*, 2000).[22] Therefore, these authors concluded that slow acetylating (hence poor detoxifying) capacity in some individuals may render them more susceptible to PPD sensitisation.

Possibly, a more likely alternative route of PPD activation would be enzymatic conversion to a hydroxylamine (Scheme 5.21), possibly via CYP N-oxidation (Scheme 3.6). Autoxidation of hydroxylamine would lead to a nitroso compound that is protein-reactive. Once a hydroxylamine was formed in the skin it is likely, in light of the aforementioned lack of NAT2 in the skin, that this could not be detoxified by the typical

NAT2 acetylation. The nitroso compound could also bind to GSH and be detoxified. The possibility of sulphation of PPD in skin has not yet been investigated.

Aniline (Figure 5.16b) is a non-sensitising aromatic amine that does not have the capacity to be converted to a quinone species, but can undergo acetylation. The nitrobenzene musks shown in Figure 5.16b are all non-sensitising.[23] None of these musks can be oxidised to ortho or para quinones and they are not electrophilic, hence they are non-sensitising.

2,4-Dinitrochlorobenzene (DNCB) (Group I hapten) is the classic strong skin sensitiser (Basketter *et al.*, 1996; Basketter *et al.*, 1997). This halogenated nitrobenzene can bind covalently to protein nucleophiles via an S_NAr mechanism, as shown in Scheme 5.1. DNCB is discussed in more detail in section 5.3.16 on halogenated compounds.

5.3.11 N-rings

All of the heterocyclic ring compounds in Figure 5.17a are strong sensitisers. Kathon CG and proxel possess isothiazolinone structures that are known to be sensitising in humans (Bjorkner *et al.*, 1986; de Groot and Weyland, 1988; Hasson *et al.*, 1990; Knudsen and Menné, 1990; Menné *et al.*, 1991; Toren *et al.*, 1997; Basketter *et al.*, 1999a) and they can undergo a variety of nucleophilic reactions (Group VI haptens) (Scheme 5.22). An S_NAr mechanism (Scheme 5.1) is possible for Kathon CG, with substitution of the chloride atom. Disulphide bond formation may be possible with reaction between the S atom of the ring and cysteine thiol groups.

Preventol a3 and glydant have electrophilic carbonyl groups neighbouring good nitrogen-containing leaving groups, and hence are susceptible to acyl transfer reactions. Dowicil breaks down to formaldehyde, which would act as the sensitising Group II hapten.

It is possible that tautomerisation can explain the sensitising properties of 2-mercaptobenzothiazole (MBT). As it is drawn in Figure 5.17a, MBT is not apparently electrophilic. However, it may equilibrate with an electrophilic tautomer (Scheme 5.23).

Isothiazolinone (Figure 5.17b) is only a weak sensitiser. It has the capacity to undergo all of the reactions in Scheme 5.22 but perhaps its low logP value hinders skin penetration.

All of the compounds in Figure 5.17c are unlikely to be able to penetrate the skin easily due to their low hydrophobicity. This is perhaps a reason for them being non-sensitisers as even though Intace B350 and valerolactam are non-electrophilic, the others (benzoylpyrrolidone, allantoin and acetyl caprolactam) are electrophilic. However, it may be that these chemicals are detoxified by metabolism into non-electrophilic species.

5.3.12 Dyes

The molecules in Figures 5.18a and b are all dyes, commonly used in the textile industry, but they have different functionalities that account for their sensitisation. Yellow 5HC and HC Red3 (Figure 5.18a) are both aromatic amine/nitro-containing compounds.

Strong

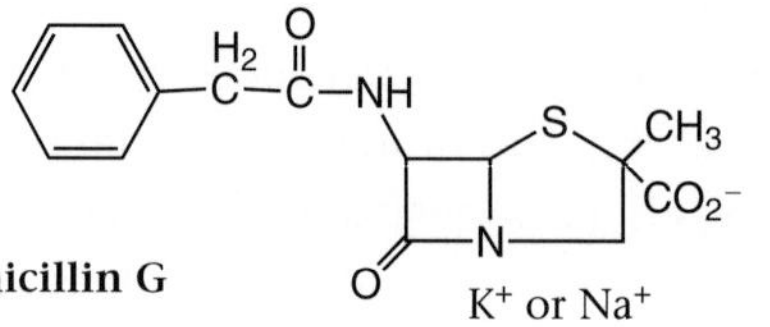

K+ or Na+

Penicillin G

$C_{15}H_{15}N_2O_4S^-$ FW = 319.36
logP = 0.552
MR = 83.56

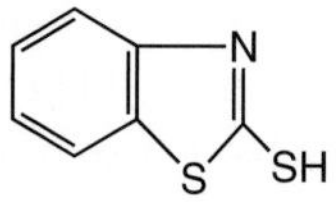

2-mercaptobenzothiazole

$C_7H_5NS_2$ FW = 167.25
logP = 3.42
MR = 46.75

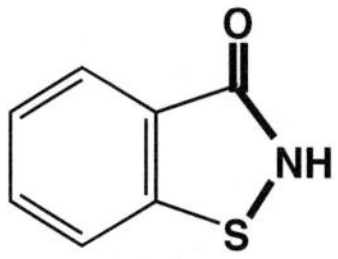

Proxel C_7H_5NSO
1,2 benzisothiazolin-3-one

FW = 151.19
logP = 1.57
MR = 41.05

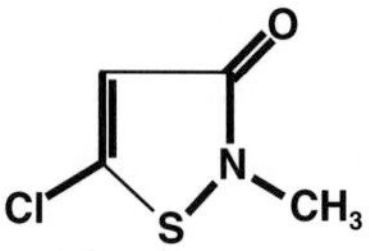

C_4H_4ClNSO
FW = 149.60
logP = NC
MR = 34.55

Kathon CG V. strong!
5-chloro-2-methyl-4-isothiazolin-3-one
NB. A mixture containing 20% non-chlorinated form. The chlorinated form is likely to be the potent sensitiser.

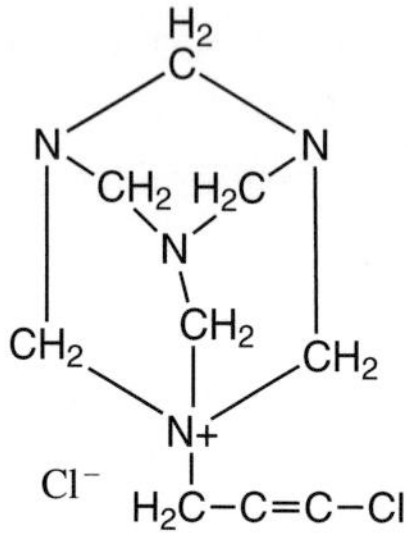

Dowicil

$C_9H_{16}N_4Cl_2$ FW = 251

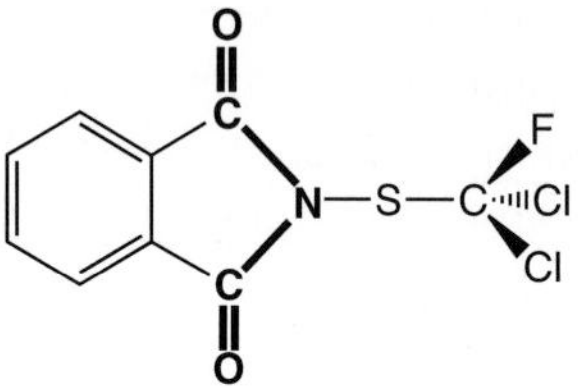

V. strong!

Preventol a3
N(Fluorodichloromethylthio)phthalimide

$C_9H_{16}N_4Cl_2$ FW = 280.10
logP = 3.90
MR = 60.76

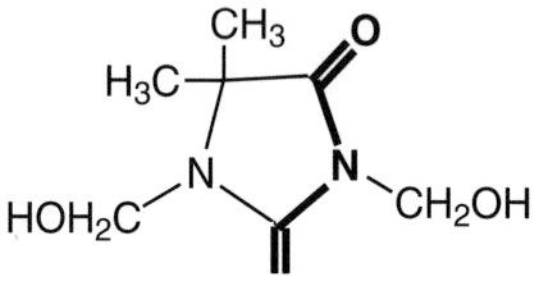

Glydant
Dimethylol 5,5 dimethyl hydantoin

$C_7H_{12}O_4N_2$ FW = 188.18
logP = −0.65
MR = 42.20

Figure 5.17a: N-rings.

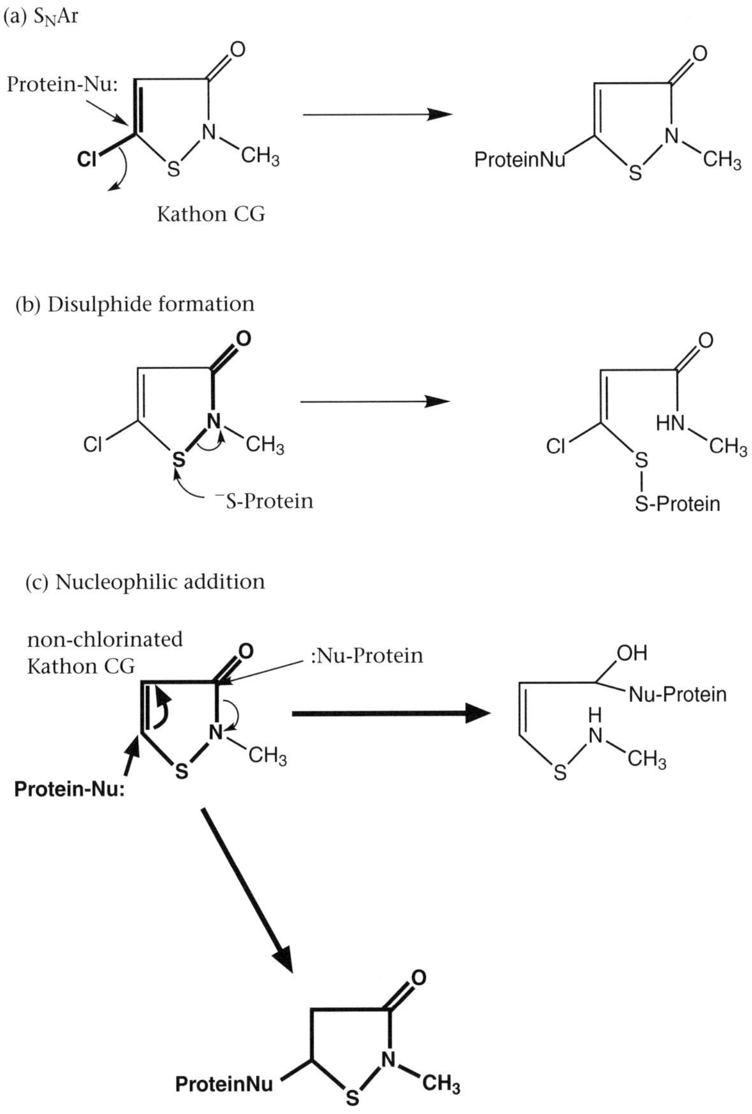

Scheme 5.22: Isothiazolinone reactivities.

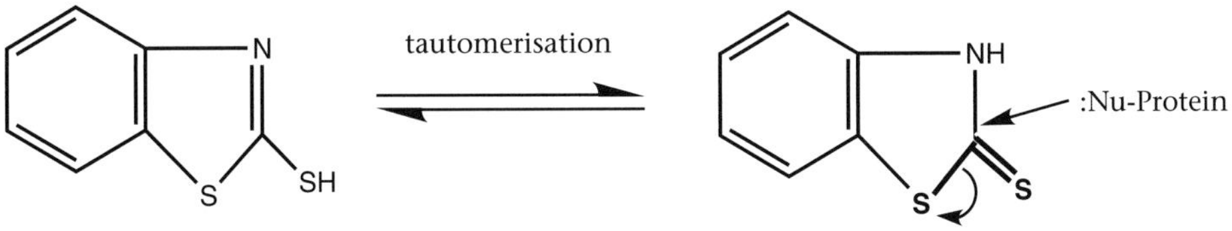

Scheme 5.23: Tautomerisation of 2-mercaptobenzothiazole.

Moderate

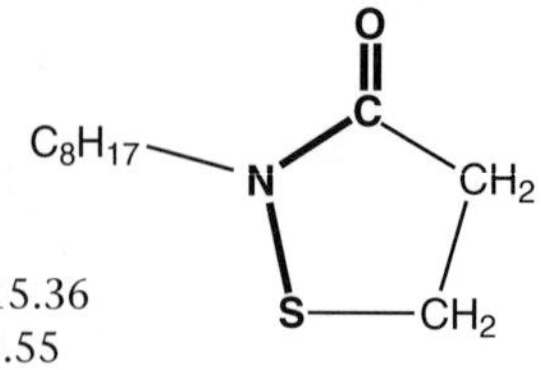

Kathon 893

$C_{11}H_{21}NOS$ FW = 215.36
logP = 3.55
MR = 62.10

Weak

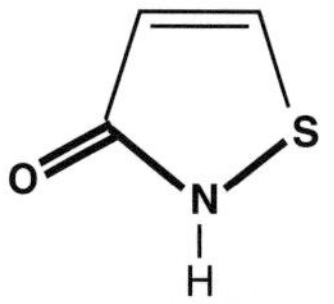

iso-thiazolone

C_3H_3NOS FW = 101.13
logP = 0.19
MR = 25.52

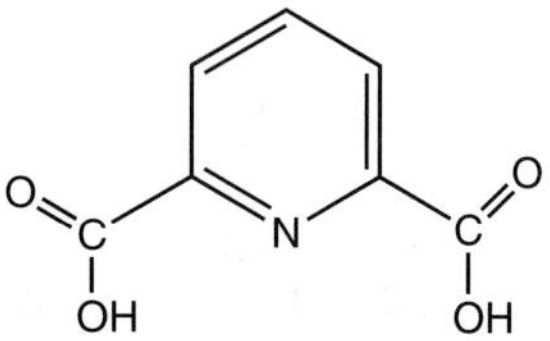

Pyridine 2,6-dicarboxylic acid

$C_7H_5NO_4$ FW = 167.17
logP = 0.66
MR = 36.67

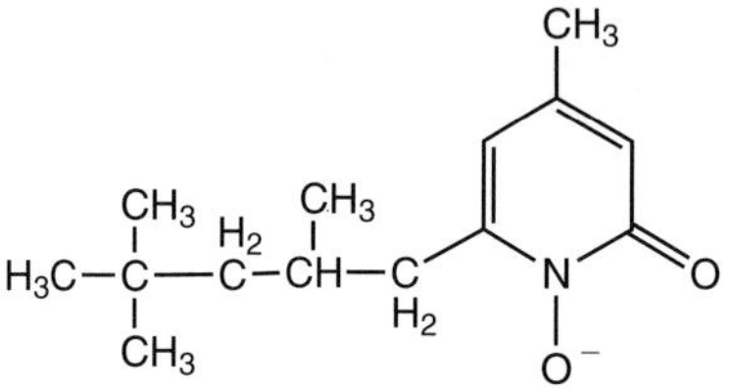

Octopirox

$C_{14}H_{22}NO_2^-$ FW = 236.33
logP = NC
MR = 84.67

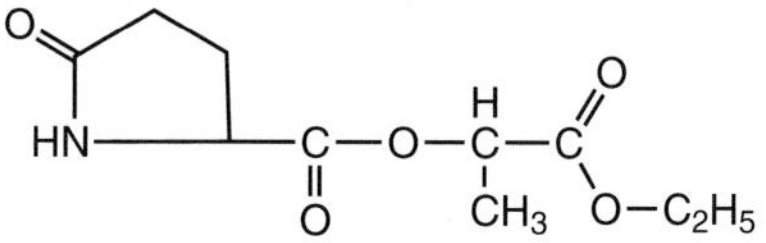

Ethyl lactyl PCA

$C_{10}H_{15}NO_5$ FW = 229.23
logP = −0.25
MR = 54.20

Figure 5.17b: N-rings (cont.).

One hypothesis that could account for the strong sensitisation of these compounds is illustrated in Scheme 5.24. Tautomerisation could lead to ethylene oxide release. The resulting amine groups could be converted to nitro groups via oxidative metabolism, which may ultimately lead to the generation of a reactive quinone species as shown.

Brilliant blue and Violet 2r cibacet are Group IV haptenic paraquinones. Disperse black is an azo dye that could be reduced by the MFO system or azo reductase (see Figure 3.17) to two amines, one of which is *p*-phenylene diamine (PPD) that could also be reduced to a quinone (Scheme 5.21). Cross-reactivity in dye-sensitised individuals with paraphenylene diamine has been reported (Nakagawa *et al.*, 1996; Seidenari *et al.*, 1997). Tautomerisation could also lead to a molecule that is also hydrolysable to a

Non-sensitising

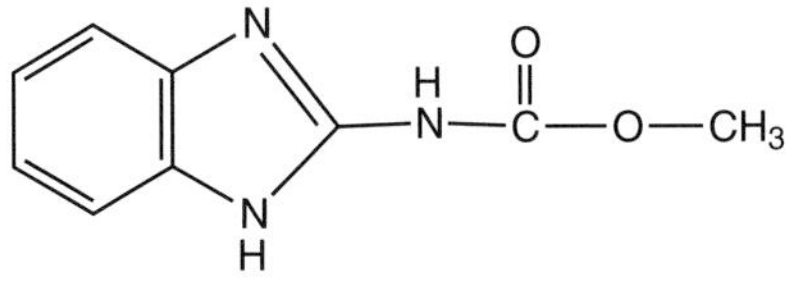

Intace B350 $C_9H_9N_3O_2$ FW = 191.19 logP = 1.29 MR = 49.10

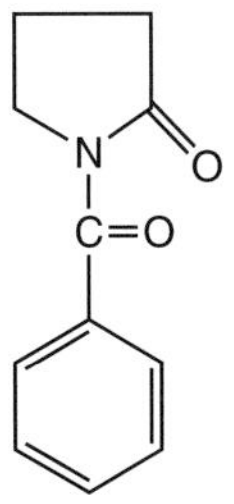

n-benzoylpyrrolidone $C_{11}H_{11}NO_2$ FW = 189.08 logP = 1.43 MR = 52.00

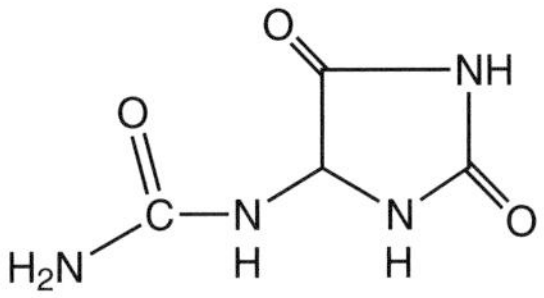

Allantoin $C_4H_6N_4O_3$ FW = 158.12 logP = −1.96 MR = 31.92

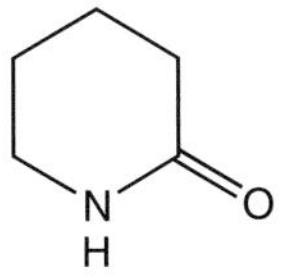

Valerolactam C_5H_9NO FW = 99.13 logP = 0.04 MR = 26.86

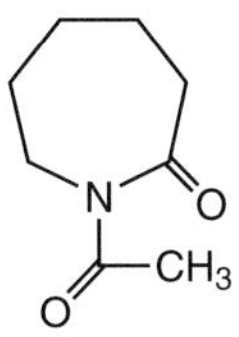

Acetyl caprolactam $C_8H_{13}NO_2$ FW = 155.19 logP = 1.05 MR = 41.03

Figure 5.17c: N-rings (cont.).

quinone species (Scheme 5.25). (Red oil (Figure 5.18b) can also be reduced to PPD in a similar fashion but it may only be moderately sensitising due to its higher level of hydrophobicity and hence reduced absorption.)

In fact, all of the above mechanisms suggest that a reactive quinone may be a common hapten for all of the strongly sensitising dyes in Figure 5.18a. Quinones are notorious for forming stable, long-lived radicals that will bind covalently to biological macromolecules and hence radical mechanisms may also play a role in the toxicity of these compounds.

It may be the case that the variability in reactivity of the amine products of azo reduction for the compounds shown in Figure 5.18b, accounts for the differences in

Strong

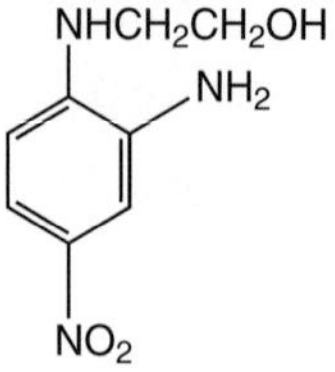

Yellow 5HC
N-2-hydroxyethyl-4-nitro-o-phenylenediamine

$C_8H_{11}N_3O_3$ FW = 197.19
logP = 0.37
MR = 52.32

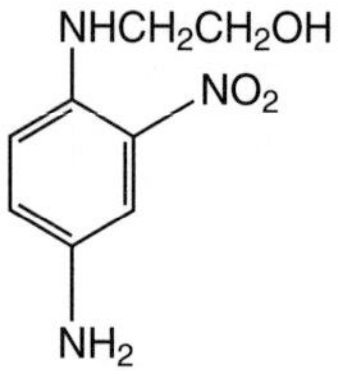

HC Red 3
N-2-hydroxyethyl-2-nitro-p-phenylenediamine

$C_8H_{11}N_3O_3$ FW = 197.19
logP = 0.84
MR = 52.32

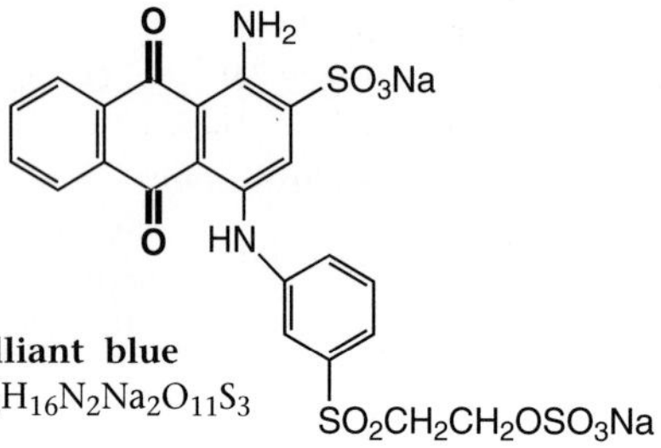

Brilliant blue
$C_{22}H_{16}N_2Na_2O_{11}S_3$

FW = 626.55

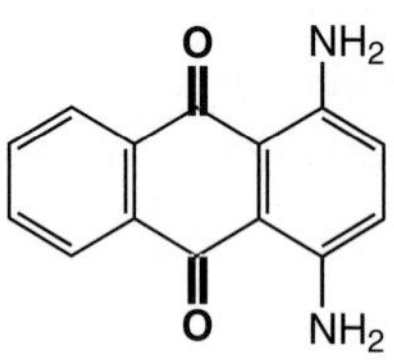

Violet 2r Cibacet

$C_{14}H_{10}N_2O_2$ FW = 238.24
logP = 0.81
MR = 70.55

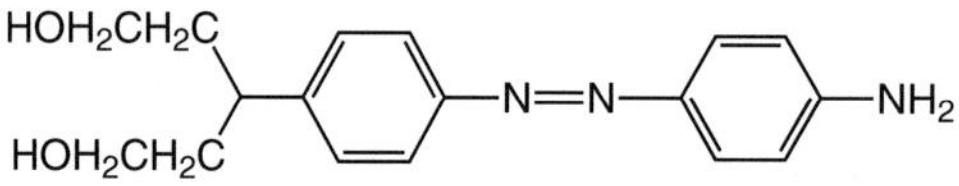

Disperse black

$C_{17}H_{21}N_3O_2$ FW = 299.37
logP = 3.34
MR = 92.33

Figure 5.18a: Dyes.

observed sensitisation. The weak or non-sensitising compounds in Figure 5.18b are neither electrophilic nor are they able to be metabolised to quinones.

5.3.13 Substituted 5 atom rings

2-Pentylcyclopenta-1,3-dione (Figure 5.19) is a strong sensitiser. It is electrophilic (Group II hapten) and can bind to protein nucleophiles via a Schiff base mechanism at

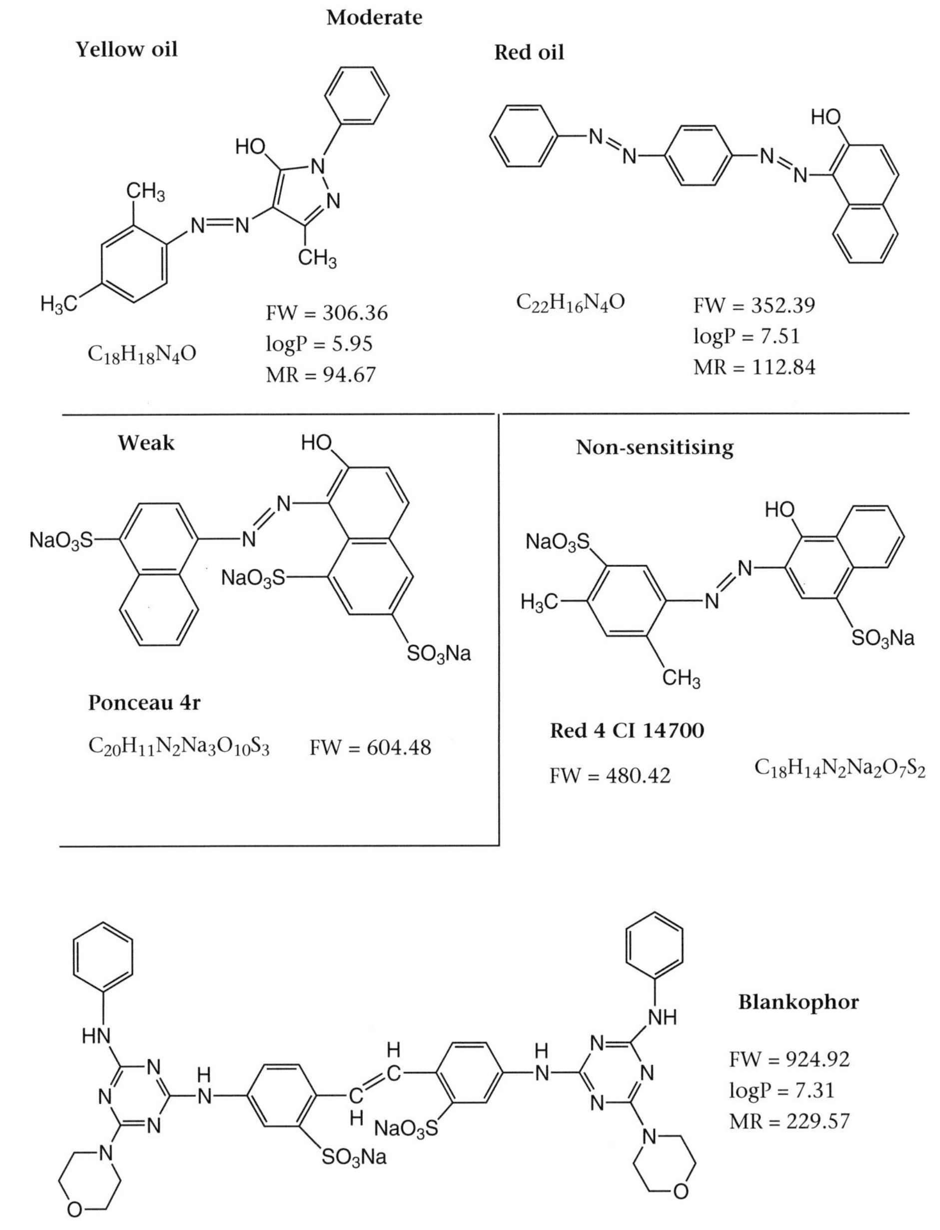

Figure 5.18b: Dyes (cont.).

either carbonyl carbon atom (Scheme 5.2). 2-Pentylcyclopent-2-enone and 2-pentylidene cyclopentanone (Figure 5.19) are both weak sensitisers that can act as Michael acceptors at the β-carbon atom. The presence of an electron-donating alkyl chain on the unsaturated double bond in both of these molecules lessens the reactivity of the Michael

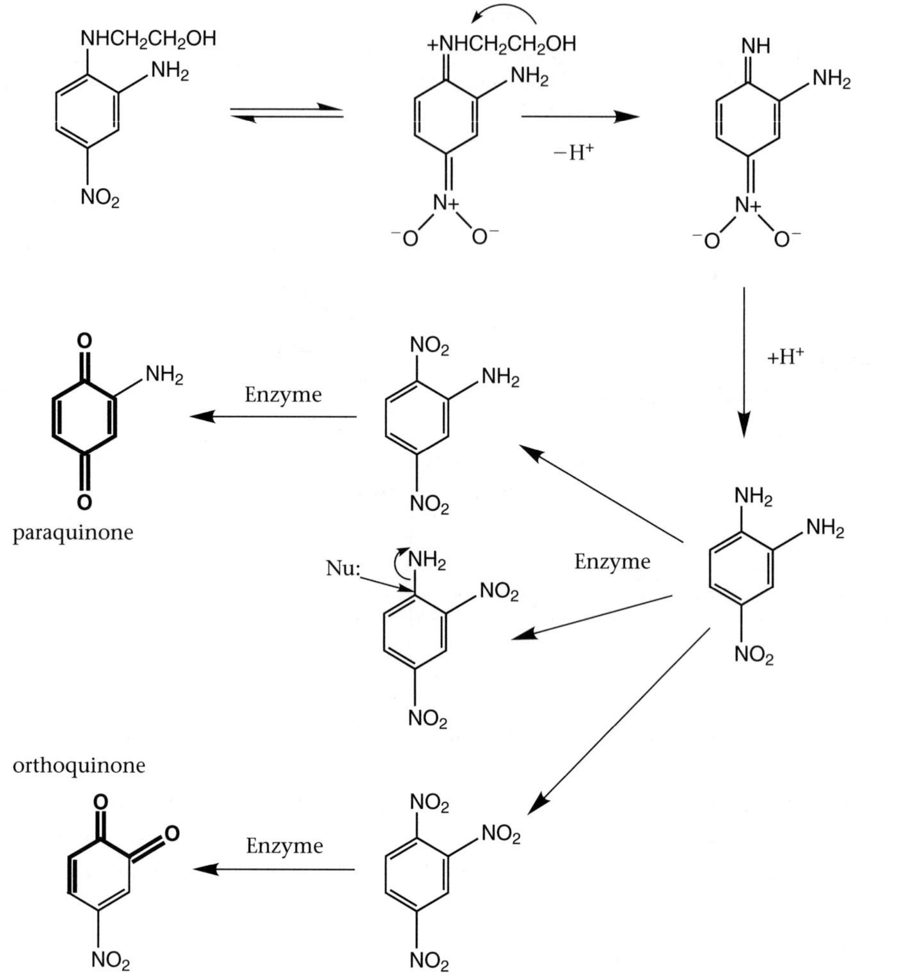

Scheme 5.24: Potential conversion of Yellow 5HC to ortho and/or para quinones.

acceptor in a similar fashion to that described for the α-substituted derivatives of cinnamaldehyde (see section 5.3.2.2.3).

There are no apparent reasons as to why 2-n-hexylcyclopentanone should be a weak sensitiser as it is non-electrophilic. It may be the case that an impurity derived from its synthesis is responsible for the observed sensitisation in the LLNA. Octalactone is not electrophilic and hence is non-sensitising.

5.3.14 Saturated 6 atom rings

2,4-Dimethylcyclohexene-3-carbaldehyde and cyclal C are both reactive aldehydes

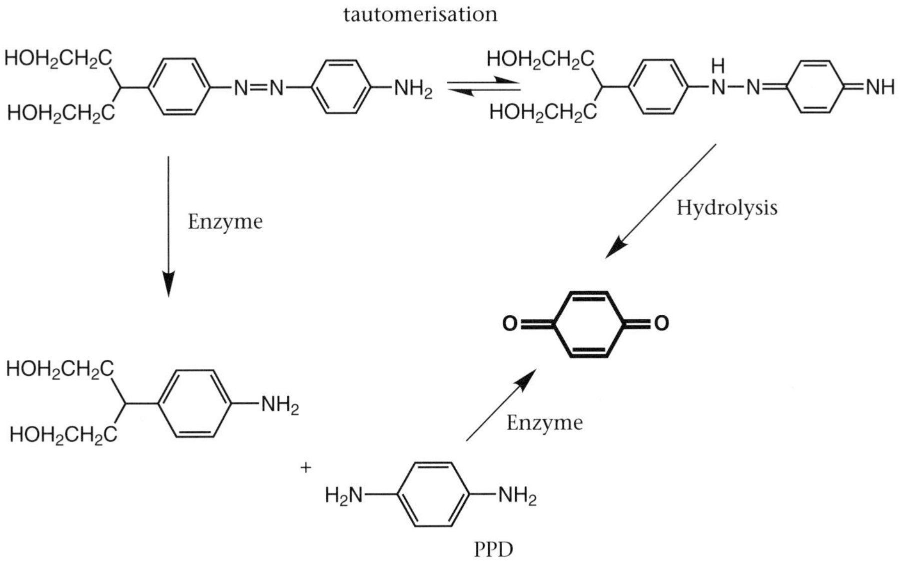

Scheme 5.25: An example of azo dye metabolism.

(Group II haptens) and can react with protein nucleophiles via a Schiff base mechanism (Scheme 5.2).

Dihydrofluorifone is an α,β-unsaturated compound (Group IV hapten) that can react by Michael addition at the position shown. Limonene extra is non-sensitising as it is not electrophilic (however, its peroxides are sensitising — see section 5.3.6 above).

5.3.15 Sulphonates and sulphanilic acids

The sulphonated compounds in Figure 5.21a are all sensitisers. It has been hypothesised (personal communication with David W. Roberts) that, via sulphoconjugation, SO_3^- substituents can be as activating as NO_2 or CN groups. For example, phenyl benzoate (PB) (c.f. benzyl benzoate Figure 5.10b) and 4-sulphophenyl benzoate (SPB) (Scheme 5.26) are cross-reacting sensitisers. From their logP values and poor SO_3Na reactivity it would be predicted that PB is a stronger sensitiser than SPB. However, this is not the case and SPB is stronger than PB. *In vivo,* when ATP reacts with sulphate anions (SO_4^{2-}) a sulphoconjugate (3′-phosphoadenosine-5′-phosphosulphate, PAPS) is produced. It is proposed that Ar-SO_3^- can mimic a sulphate group and a PAPS-like conjugate to ATP can be formed. This sulphoconjugate substituent can then be electron-withdrawing and activate other substituents on the aromatic ring, in a similar manner to the activation by nitro substituents in DNCB (Figure 5.16a). Hence, norbornanacetyloxy-4-benzene sulphonate and benzyl phenol-2,4-disulphonic acid (Figure 5.21a) would both become activated esters and an S_N2 reaction would then be possible at the ester carbonyl.

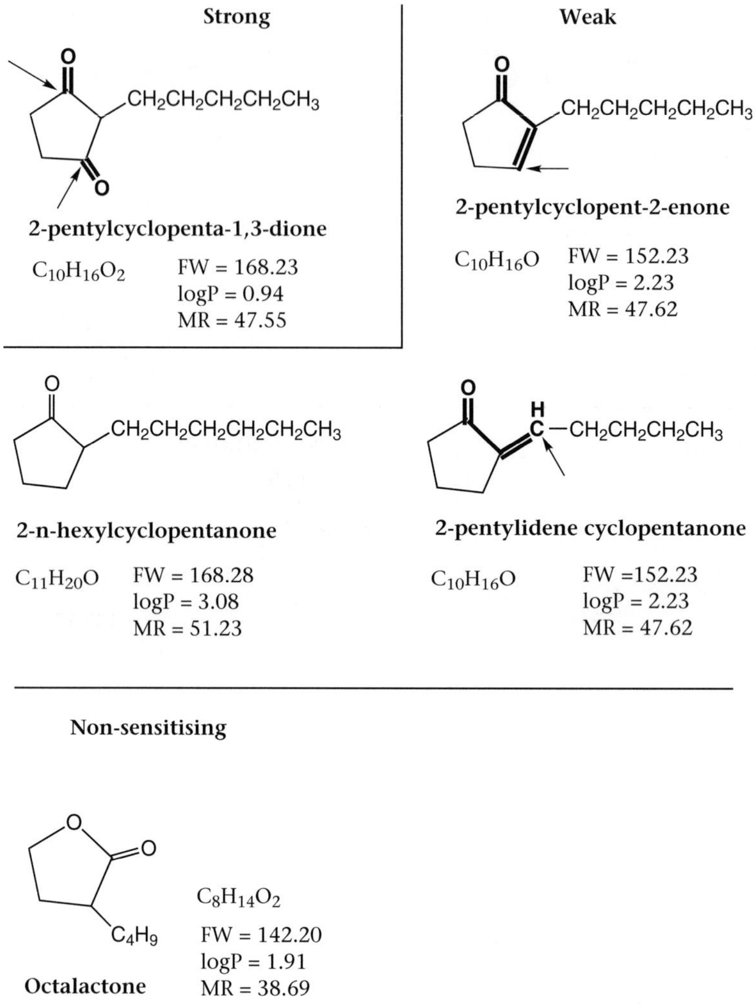

Figure 5.19: Substituted 5-atom rings.

It is expected that 1,2-dihydroxy-3,5-benzene disulphonate would undergo classical oxidation to an orthoquinone, similar to eugenol, isoeugenol and other catechols.

Sodium lauryl sulphate (SLS) and sodium p-phenolsulphonate do not possess any electrophilic centres that could be activated by sulphoconjugation. These compounds are non-sensitising, however, SLS is a known irritant and is typically used in experiments designed to investigate the mechanisms of skin irritation.

Strong

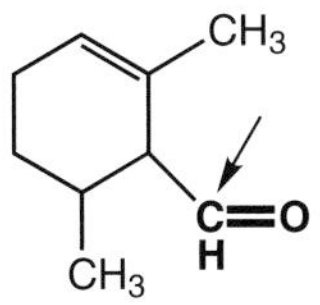

2,4-dimethylcyclohexene-3-carbaldehyde

$C_9H_{14}O$

FW = 138.21
logP = 1.21
MR = 42.87

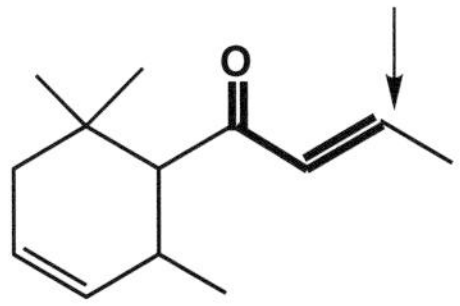

Dihydrofloriflone $C_{13}H_{20}O$

1-(2,6,6-trimethyl-3-cyclohexene-1-yl)-2-buten-1-one

FW = 192.30
logP = 3.38
MR = 62.52

Moderate

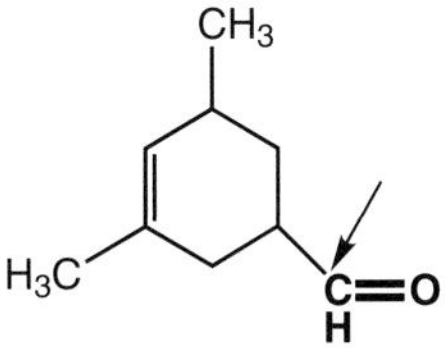

Cyclal C

$C_9H_{14}O$

FW = 138.21
logP = 1.21
MR = 42.87

Non-sensitising

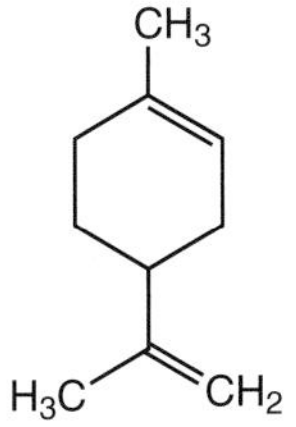

N.B. Racemic

Limonene extra

$C_{10}H_{16}$

FW = 136.23
logP = 2.41
MR = 46.48

Figure 5.20: Saturated 6-atom rings.

5.3.16 Halogenated compounds

A selection of strongly sensitising halogenated compounds are shown in Figure 5.22. The classical strong sensitisers used in many seminal studies related to ACD have been the 2,4-dinitrohalobenzenes (Nishioka *et al.*, 1971; Nakagawa and Tanioku, 1972; Polak and Macher, 1974; Dupuis and Benezra, 1982; Carr *et al.*, 1984; Basketter *et al.*, 1996; Basketter *et al.*, 1997). LLNA results for 2,4-dinitroiodobenzene (DNIB), 2,4-dinitrobromobenzene (DNBB), 2,4-dinitrochlorobenzene (DNCB) and 2,4-dinitrofluorobenzene (DNFB) suggest, theoretically, that electrophilicity/protein reactivity correlates with sensitisation potential (Basketter *et al.*, 1997). Hence, this data supports that dinitrohalobenzenes are direct acting haptens.

Halogens act as a good leaving group when bonded to a sufficiently electrophilic centre. This is the case for the strong sensitisers picryl chloride and 2,4-dinitrochlorobenzene (DNCB), where the C—Cl bond is activated by the electron-withdrawing

Strong

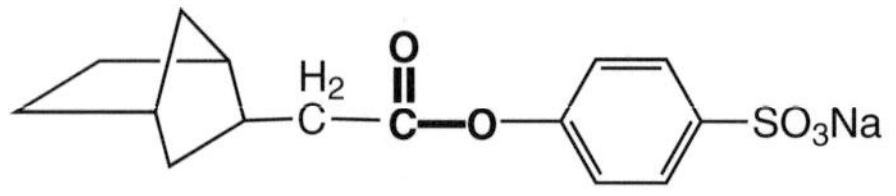

Norbornanacetyloxy-4-benzene sulphonate

$C_{15}H_{18}O_5S$ FW = 310.37

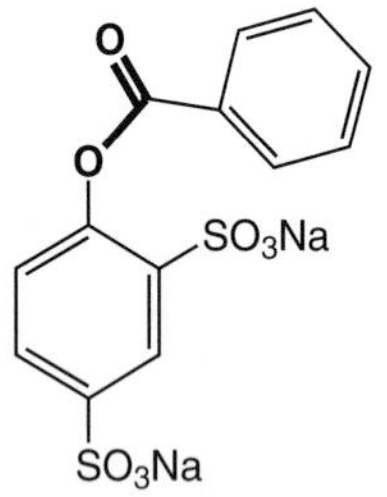

Benzyl phenol 2,4-disulphonic acid

$C_{13}H_{10}O_8S_2$ FW = 402.31

Moderate

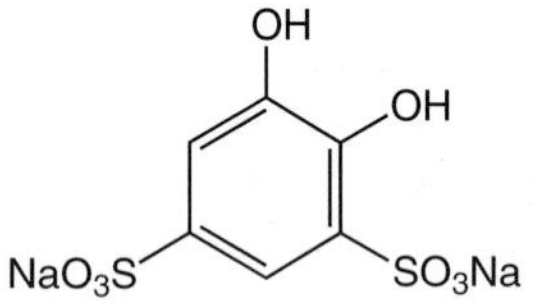

1,2-dihydroxy-3,5-benzene disulphonate

$C_6H_6O_8S_2$ FW = 270.24

Figure 5.21a: Sulphonates and sulphanilic acids.

nitro substituents (Figure 5.22) and an S_N2 reaction is possible. The same situation also occurs in dansyl chloride (Figure 5.22), where nucleophilic attack occurs at the S atom.

DNCB is also known to deplete glutathione (presumably by Phase II conjugation) in rat skin (Summer and Goggelmann, 1980) (at a rate of 34.7 nmol/min/mg protein) and following epicutaneous application in mouse skin (Schmidt and Chung, 1992); the dose and GSH availability affected the level of metabolism (Jewell *et al.*, 1996; Agarwal *et al.*, 1992; Hotchkiss, 1998). Hence, GSH conjugation may aid in the detoxication of DNCB in skin.

As well as investigating the role of GSH in dinitrohalobenzene sensitisation, Schmidt and Chung (1992) have also proposed, controversially, that a cutaneous NADPH-dependent reductase may be able to metabolise DNCB, DNBB and DNIB (and at the same time generate superoxide and hydrogen peroxide). A yellowing of the tissue following epicutaneous application to mouse skin (indicative of haptenation by

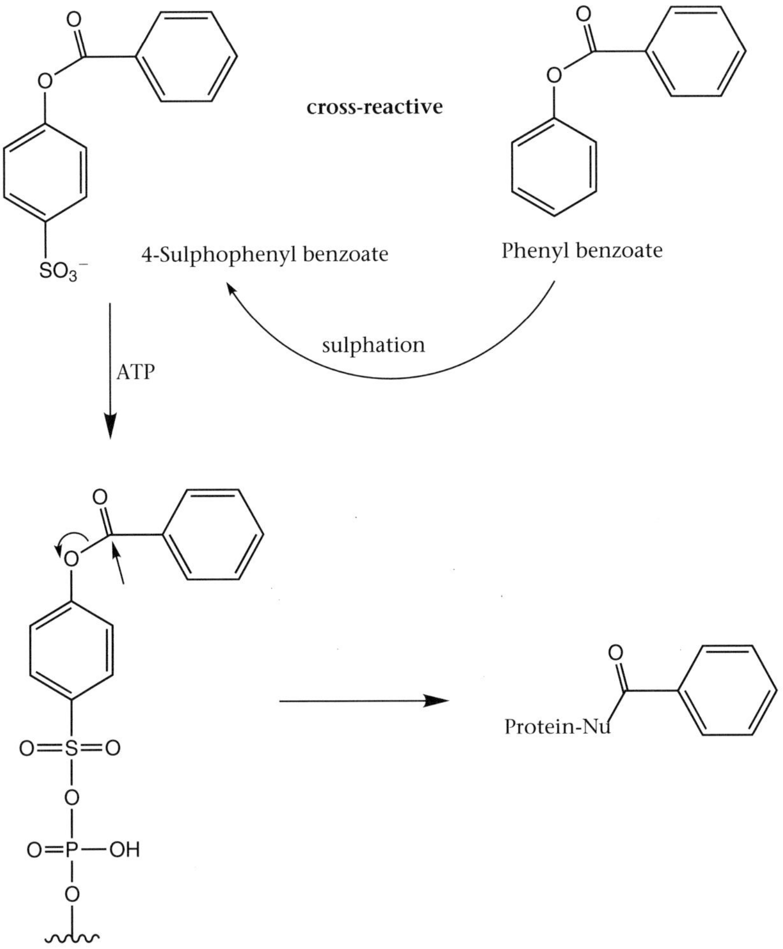

Scheme 5.26: Potential activation of aromatic xenobiotics via sulphoconjugation.

dinitrophenyl adduct formation to proteins, via an S_N2 reaction displacing the Cl group) was not observed with these three compounds, although it was observed for DNFB. Hence, they propose that DNCB, DNBB and DNIB could be prohaptens and sensitisation arises as a result of radical formation via metabolic activity. NADPH dependent oxygen usage in mouse and rat liver was measured for all the dinitrohalobenzenes, and was seen to decrease in the order DNIB > DNBB > DNCB > DNFB.

5.3.17 Corticosteroids

Skin sensitisation to corticosteroids may be a problem when they are administered topically as drugs (Lauerma *et al.*, 1993; Dooms-Goossens *et al.*, 1994; Freeman, 1995;

Non-sensitising

$H_3C(H_2C)_{11}$—O—SO_3Na

sodium lauryl sulphate

$C_{12}H_{25}NaO_4S$
FW = 288.38

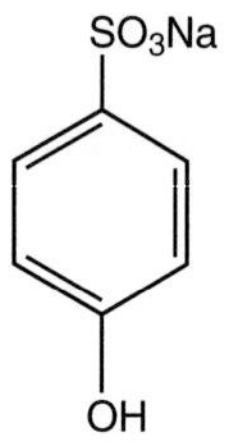

sodium p-phenolsulphonate

$C_6H_5NaO_4S$ FW = 196.16

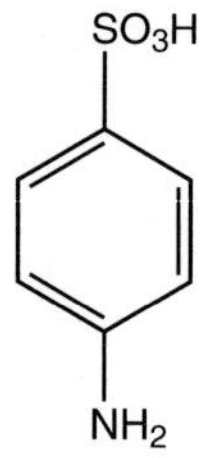

Sulphanilic acid

$C_6H_7NO_3S$

FW = 173.19
logP = 0.39
MR = 41.09

Figure 5.21b: Sulphonates and sulphanilic acids (cont.).

Strong

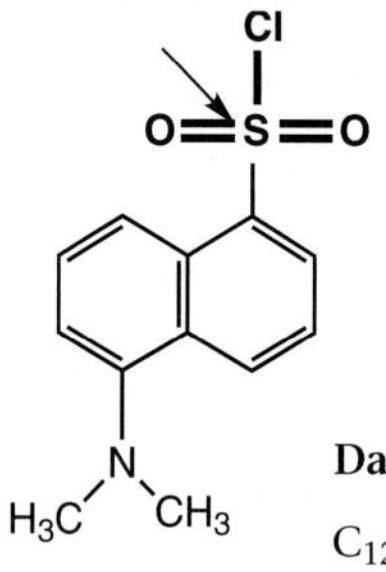

Dansyl chloride

$C_{12}H_{12}ClNO_2S$

FW = 269.75
logP = 3.05
MR = 71.13

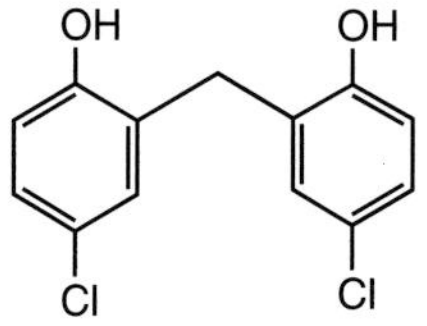

Dichlorophen

FW = 269.13
logP = 5.045
MR = 69.53

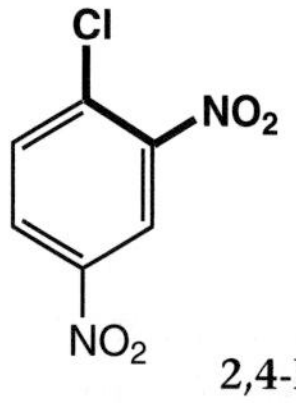

2,4-Dinitrochlorobenzene (DNCB)

FW = 202.55 $C_6H_3ClN_2O_4$
logP = 2.40
MR = 46.31

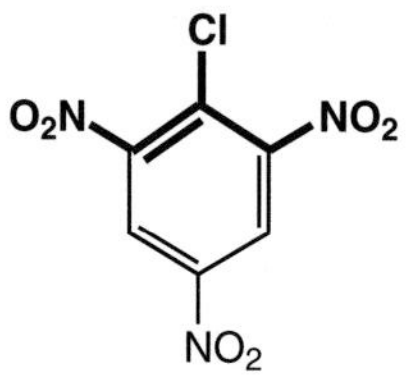

Picryl chloride

FW = 247.55 $C_6H_2ClN_3O_6$
logP = 2.37
MR = 46.31

Figure 5.22: Halogenated compounds.

CLASS A — no substitution on the D ring or C20/C21 side chains

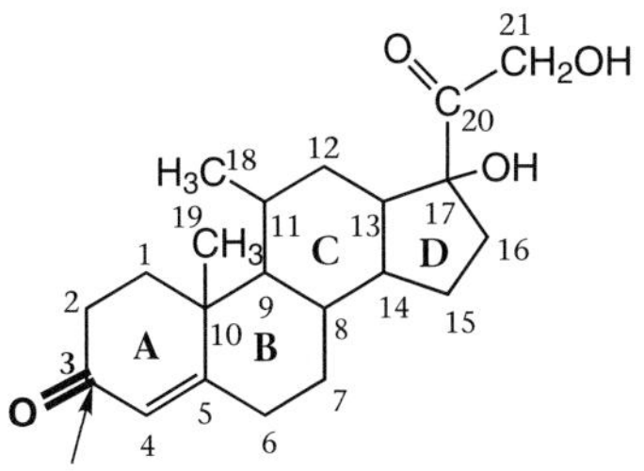

Hydrocortisone

$C_{21}H_{30}O_5$ FW = 362.46
logP = 0.50

(others include prednisolone, prednisone and tixocortol)

CLASS B — C16/C17 cis-ketal or diol

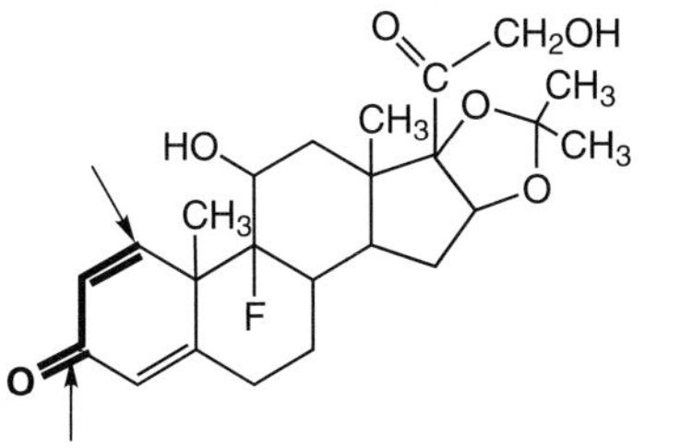

Triamcinolone acetonide

$C_{24}H_{33}FO_6$ FW = 450.54
logP = 0.71

(others include budesonide, amcinonide and halcinonide)

CLASS C — C16 methyl substitution

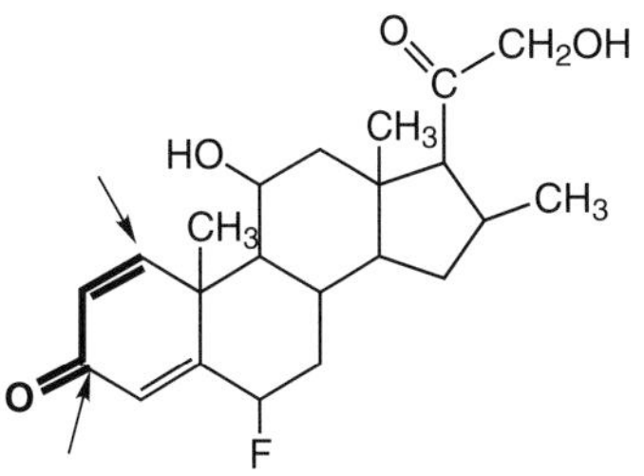

Fluocortilone

$C_{22}H_{29}FO_4$ FW = 376.46
logP = 1.18

(others include betamethasone and dexamethasone)

CLASS D — C17 and/or C21 long-chain esterification, with or without C16 methyl

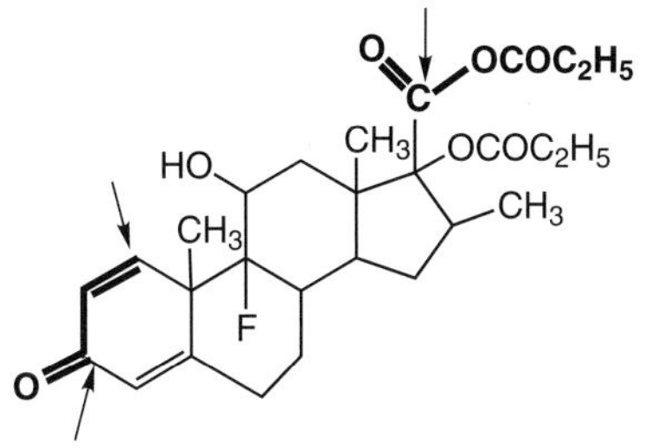

Betamethasone dipropionate

$C_{26}H_{33}FO_7$ FW = 490.56
logP = 3.09

(others include hydrocortisone-17-butyrate and hydrocortisone-17-valerate)

Figure 5.23: Corticosteroids.

Amkraut *et al.*, 1996; Lutz and El-Azhary, 1997). There are four classes of corticosteroids (A–D), all of which can react with hard protein nucleophiles via a Schiff base mechanism at the C3 atom. Classes B, C and D can react with soft nucleophiles by Michael addition across the C1–C2 double bond.

The identical C20 side chains of hydrocortisone (the prototypical class A corticosteroid), triamcinolone acetonide (an example of a class B steroid) and fluocortilone

■ CHAPTER 5 ■

(a class C steroid) can also be metabolised by dehydration to 21-dehydro-17-deoxy-hydrocortisone or by oxidation to 21-dehydro-hydrocortisone (Figure 5.7b), both of which are α,β-diketones that can react with arginine residues (Scheme 5.15) (Roberts *et al.*, 1999). It is anticipated that this conversion of prohapten alcohol to haptenic diketone could be performed by a CYP enzyme. The class D corticosteroid, betamethasone dipropionate, possesses a strongly electrophilic anhydride side chain, which also provides this molecule with a third opportunity to act as a hapten.

5.3.18 Quaternary ammonium salts

Of the quaternary ammonium salts shown in Figure 5.24, the haptenic part of the molecule is likely to be the non-charged, electrophilic region of the molecule. TMATCC and TMATMMSC (Figure 5.24) possess reactive amides that are activated by a carbonyl group or by SO_2Me, respectively. However, in their charged state it is unlikely that TMATCC and TMATMMSC can penetrate the skin. Possibly, the $+NME_3$ group is lost on the surface of the skin?

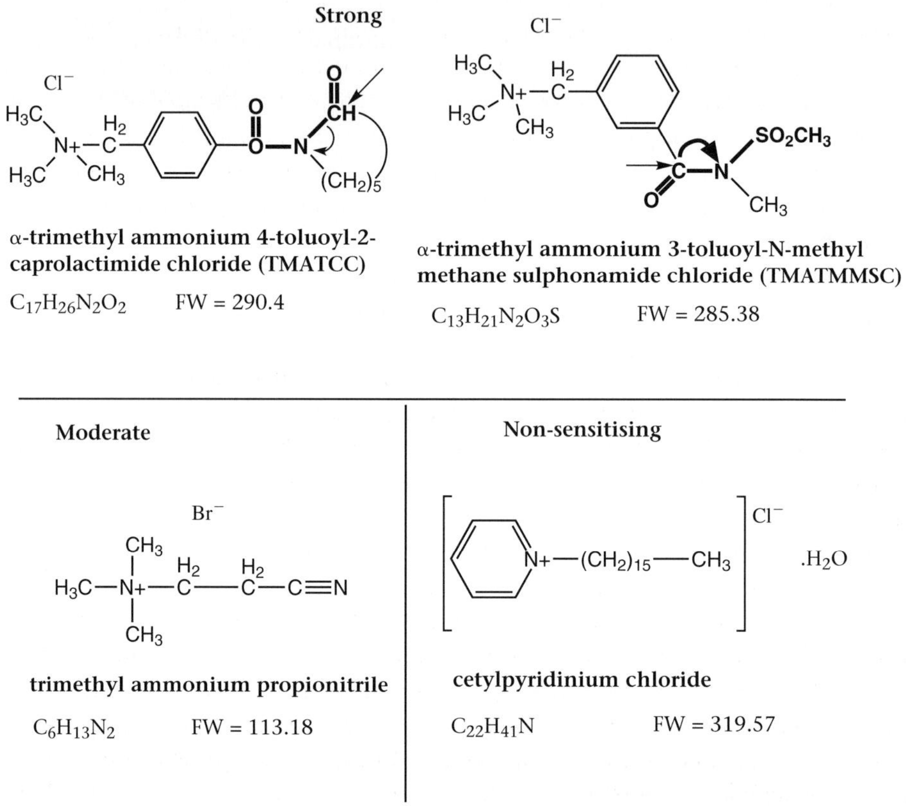

Figure 5.24: Quaternary ammonium salts.

It is anticipated that trimethylammonium propionitrile (Figure 5.24) can easily break down by loss of $+NMe_3$ to acetonitrile, which is a good Michael acceptor.

Cetylpyridinium chloride (Figure 5.24) is an example of a quaternary ammonium salt that contains no electrophilic centres and this is a non-sensitiser. It can only bind to charged protein residues via electrostatic interactions. Therefore, it appears that ionic bonding is not a mechanism via which sensitisation can occur.

5.4 PREDICTING HAPTEN FORMATION IN SKIN AND EVALUATING SENSITISATION POTENCY *DE NOVO*

The above section (5.3) contains mechanistic hypotheses, which are based upon current knowledge of chemistry and metabolism, as to why some molecules are sensitising and others are not. The focus has been on hazard identification i.e. evaluating the protein-binding reactivity of chemicals and their potential metabolites. However, all of these hypotheses are retrospective i.e. we know already from *in vivo* studies whether these molecules are non-sensitising or sensitising and we are attempting to explain the observations mechanistically for each compound. We even have reasonable estimates of potency for some of these chemicals from *in vivo* data (see Appendix 1). The situation becomes much more difficult when attempting to predict the sensitisation potential of an unknown entity. With the inevitable future eradication/reduction of skin sensitisation testing in animals, predicting toxicity from *in vitro* data will become increasingly more of an issue, especially for industry. At present, the prediction of whether or not a low molecular weight compound will act as a skin sensitiser is hampered by the inability to entirely predict its fate within the skin.

5.4.1 Predicting and evaluating chemical properties

Many factors pertaining to the chemical (including molecular volume, logP, pKa chemical reactivity, solubility (molar refractivity, MR), volatility, levels of exposure etc.) can be analysed and relatively easily incorporated into rule-based expert systems such as DEREK (Deductive Estimation of Risk from Existing Knowledge) to relate families of compounds (Barratt *et al.*, 1994; Barratt and Langowski, 1999). Such expert systems can be used for potential hazard identification by detecting the presence of a 'structural alert' in a compound i.e. a chemical group that is electrophilic and has the capacity to react with protein. However, an assessment of chemical reactivity (electrophilicity) alone (although causative in the formation of a macromolecular immunogen/antigen), is not a good predictor of sensitisation potency or threshold levels within the skin.

The applied dose of a compound and the absorption/partitioning properties of a chemical can contribute towards its availability to bind to skin protein and act as a sensitiser (Bronaugh *et al.*, 1994b). In attempting to correlate the electrophilicity, dose and absorption properties of a molecule with its observed sensitisation properties (e.g. from LLNA results) by a QSAR/dose response model, all of these properties can be taken into account using the relative alkylation index (RAI) (Roberts and Williams, 1982; Roberts and Basketter, 1990; Roberts *et al.*, 1991). The general formula is as follows:

$$\mathrm{RAI} = \log D + a \log k_{rel} + b \log P_{ow}$$

where D is the % concentration applied divided by molecular weight, k is the measured rate constant for a particular reaction and P_{ow} is the n-octanol/water partition coefficient. High correlations have been observed between the RAI of a molecule and measures of sensitisation or elicitation potential (Franot *et al.*, 1994; Roberts *et al.*, 1999) suggesting that in the future such models may contribute in predicting the sensitisation properties of unknown chemicals.

5.4.2 Predicting metabolism

One of the most difficult factors to determine is whether cutaneous metabolism of a xenobiotic contributes to the level of observed sensitisation. Metabolising enzymes are present in the skin (see Chapter 4) but there are only a few studies that have determined the activity of these enzymes with respect to a range of sensitising xenobiotic substrates. In addition to enzyme-substrate variability, xenobiotic metabolism (and absorption) could be affected by inherent and acquired factors relating to the individual (for example, inter-individual variability in enzyme expression, age, race, sex, anatomical site of exposure etc.) (Robinson, 1999). These individualistic factors are more difficult to incorporate into expert systems, but may be equally as important in determining the occurrence and severity of ACD in an individual.

Care should always be taken when directly extrapolating data from animal models to humans. Although animal models, such as the LLNA and GPMT etc., have proved to be useful tools in estimating the relative potencies of different sensitising chemicals, these models can also lead to the generation of false positive and false negative results in relation to human data. For example, geraniol and benzyl alcohol (section 5.3.1) are both sensitisers in humans but are non-sensitising in animal models (Cardullo *et al.*, 1989; Catanzaro and Smith, 1991; Corazza *et al.*, 1996; Verecken *et al.*, 1998; Podda *et al.*, 1999). It may be that in humans but not in rodents, geraniol is metabolically activated to geranial and that 1,2-propanediol is metabolised to 1,2-propanedione and these are the sensitising haptens. A recent study has indicated that the class 2 form of alcohol dehydrogenase (ADH 2) is present in human skin but not rodent skin (Cheung *et al.*, 2000b) and that aldehyde dehydrogenase 3 (ALDH3) is present in human, mouse and rat skin but is not in guinea-pig skin. Such absences of expression (or variations in enzyme activity) in rodents may underpin differences in observed sensitisation for some compounds between species.

The field of skin metabolism in relation to ACD is in its infancy and more investigations on the inter-individual and interspecies variability in expression, induction and activity of cutaneous enzymes are required for a diverse range of sensitising and non-sensitising compounds. In particular, it is important to understand potentially activating cutaneous metabolism for those compounds that are considered to be prohaptens and might otherwise be predicted as non-sensitising by expert rule-based systems. The prediction of false positives often invokes the 'Precautionary Principle' and leads to the recommendation that 'this compound may be sensitiser'. However, predicting false negatives from both animal and theoretical models could lead us into a false sense of security with some chemicals. When sufficient human cutaneous metabolism data are available, then perhaps, such data can be incorporated into expert systems to aid in more effective predictions of sensitisation, especially for prohaptens, and go towards eliminating false negatives.

5.4.3 Evaluating sensitisation potency

As eluded to in the previous section, the murine local lymph node assay (Kimber *et al.*, 1986) has been extensively validated during the past 15 years as a robust and reproducible animal model for use in assessing the relative potency of sensitising compounds. In brief, this assay exploits the end point of T-cell proliferation in the auricular lymph nodes as a measure of sensitisation potential. A stimulation index for each compound tested is calculated by measuring T-cell count from treated mice divided by T-cell count from non-treated control mice. The dose that yields a stimulation index of 3 is termed the EC3 value. Above a stimulation index of 3, a xenobiotic is regarded as a sensitiser (Basketter *et al.*, 1999b).

Traditionally, test concentrations and hence EC3 values are calculated as % w/v and for compounds that are of similar molecular mass, these values provide reliable estimations of relative potency. However, sensitisation is a process that is likely to require that a certain number of molecules or antigens be recognised by a certain number of molecules on the surface of Langerhans' cells (and threshold concentrations are known to exist whereby below a certain low dose/cm^2 a compound may be non-sensitising and above a high dose it may act as an irritant). Hence, when relating data for compounds of significantly different molecular mass, it may be more accurate to calculate the dose in moles/cm^2 skin. This point is illustrated in Figure 5.25, using known EC3 data for a selection of compounds ranging in molecular mass from 83–318 g/mol. Rank order of relative potency is changed when the EC3 is considered in moles rather than %.

5.5 SUMMARY

In agreement with Roberts and Lepoittevin (1998) a good indicator of whether a molecule has the capacity to act as a sensitiser can be the presence of electrophilic characteristics in its structure. The problem, however, comes with false negatives, when a molecule appears not to have any electrophilic potential and yet is a sensitiser. Then an investigation of potential activating metabolism for these chemicals should be performed.

This chapter has related observed levels of sensitisation (generically classified as non, weak, moderate or strong from the available *in vivo* data) purely to the chemical reactivity

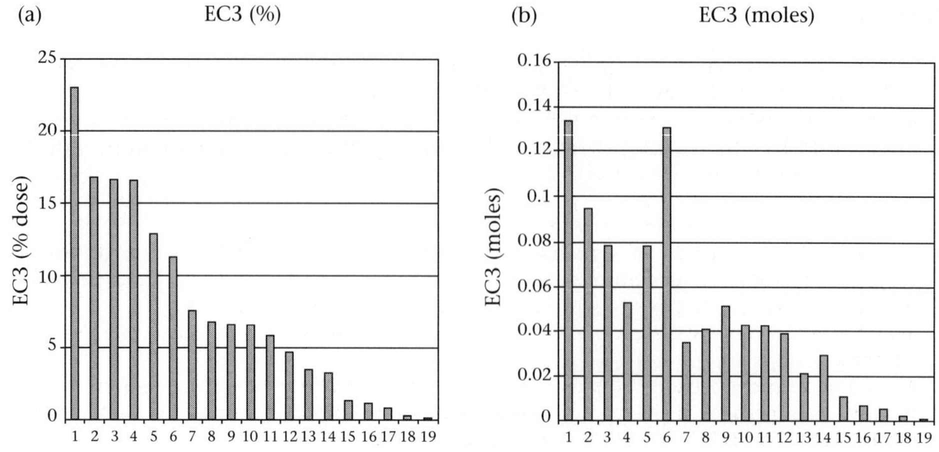

1 Hydroxycitronellal
2 Methyleugenol
3 Benzylbenzoate
4 Penicillin G
5 Eugenol
6 Butane-2,3-dione
7 Hexylcinnamaldehyde
8 Dihydroeugenol
9 4-Chloroaniline
10 Citral
11 2-Methoxy-4-methylphenol
12 Phenylacetic aldehyde
13 Isoeugenol
14 m-Amino phenol
15 Cinnamaldehyde
16 Linalyl hydroperoxide
17 Kathon CG
18 *p*-Phenylene diamine
19 2,4-Dinitrochlorobenzene

Figure 5.25: Evaluating rank order sensitisation potency using local lymph node assay EC3 values. EC3 is the effective concentration of dosing solution that yields a three-fold stimulation of T-cell proliferativity in the auricular lymph nodes of mice (when compared to control animals) following challenge with a skin sensitiser (Kimber *et al.*, 1986). Graph (a) shows the rank order of potency for 19 chemicals by plotting their EC3 values as % w/v. Graph (b) illustrates the same data when the EC3 values are calculated in moles. This takes into account the molecular weights of the compounds. The chemicals are listed in the same order as in graph (a) but the rank order of potency has changed.

and hypothetical metabolism of small molecules. However, the immune recognition mechanisms of skin sensitisation are expected to be highly specific for each allergenic compound. Protein-binding capacity appears to be a requirement for sensitisation but general protein-xenobiotic binding cannot define why a compound is allergenic in certain individuals and not others. It is expected that immunocompetency in an individual will be a contributing factor. A discussion of some of the more specific molecular recognition aspects that may be involved in specific DTH immune responses to low molecular weight compounds will be discussed in Chapter 6.

NOTES

1 The levels of sensitisation for selected compounds have previously been determined and classified (as published in Cronin and Basketter (1994) and also personal communication with D. Basketter, SEAC Toxicology, Unilever, Colworth House, Bedford) using *in vivo* methods such as the murine local lymph node assay (Kimber *et al.*, 1986) and guinea pig maximisation test (Magnusson and Kligman, 1969; Sato, 1985).
2 This may have relevance to the proposed reaction of α,β-dicarbonyl compounds with the guanidino group of arginine in proteins (Scheme 5.15).
3 It should therefore be noted that soft xenobiotic electrophiles can be toxic by binding to protein-Cys residues or detoxified, perhaps, by binding to glutathione (GSH), although binding to GSH has also been implicated with toxic mechanisms (see section 3.3.2.5).
4 3D small molecule crystal structures of xenobiotics are available from the Cambridge Structural Database.
5 As well as such endogenous radicals interacting with protein residues, these radicals may also modify, and perhaps activate, xenobiotics either by enzyme-mediated or non-enzymatic mechanisms. This is briefly discussed in section 5.4.
6 The infrequent occurrence of cross-reactivity between parent molecules that appear chemically unrelated may then be rationalised on the basis that a common metabolite acts as the sensitising hapten.
7 Some studies have shown that compounds in mixtures can have synergistic effects on elicitation responses (Johansen *et al.*, 1998).
8 It has been shown by site directed mutagenesis of the recombinant human class 3 ADH that a Thr48Ala exchange leads to an almost complete loss of alcohol dehydrogenase activity (Estonius *et al.*, 1994), suggesting that threonine is the active site nucleophile responsible for the alcohol to aldehyde conversion.
9 It should be remembered that the diagrammatic notation used in the figures of this chapter is not truly representative of the real 3D structure of a xenobiotic, which will contribute to its reactivity and suitability for enzyme active-site binding.
10 This hypothesis may also be relevant for aromatic alcohols such as cinnamic alcohol (see section 5.3.1.2.4).
11 Benzyl alcohol has also been reported to be a sensitiser in humans (see section 5.3.1.2).
12 It is also conceivable that skin surface bacteria may contain such an enzyme that could convert catechols to aldehydes on the skin surface.
13 Given that methylation at different positions would selectively alter the reactivities of eugenol and isoeugenol and alter the stability of any intermediates formed.
14 Given that the ε-amino group of Lys is expected to be protonated at physiological pH, the N-terminal amine may be a major nucleophile *in vivo*.
15 Studies relating to the reactivity of cinnamaldehyde are discussed in section 5.3.2.2.3 and it is expected that the considerations relating to the α,β-unsaturated carbonyl in cinnamaldehyde may also apply to citral.
16 Rabbit serum albumin.
17 α-substituents on cinnamaldehyde may sterically hinder the molecules from being suitable substrates for these enzymes.
18 Hexylcinnamaldehyde has been recommended as a weak positive test reagent in the European Standard Patch Test series of chemicals and has recently been used in validating the LLNA for weak allergens (Loveless *et al.*, 1996; Dearman *et al.*, 1998).
19 At physiological pH, arginine residues may be essentially all protonated.
20 Cinnamaldehyde is a stronger sensitiser and the α-alkyl substituted cinnamaldehyde derivatives.
21 It is not known as to whether cytochrome P450 in skin can oxidise 15-HPA in colophony to epoxides. However, abietic acid gives no significant level of sensitisation in animals (Karlberg *et al.*, 1985) and hence it is thought that levels of *in vivo* cutaneous epoxidation alone is not sufficient to induce sensitisation.
22 Reilly *et al.* (2000) investigated the acetylation (detoxification) of sulfamethoxazole, a cause of the severe cutaneous reactions that occur in Stevens-Johnson Syndrome.
23 Although musks are non-sensitising in standard allergen tests, they can be photosensitisers.

CHAPTER

6

Protein-hapten Binding and Immunorecognition Events During the Sensitisation and Elicitation Stages of ACD

Contents

Since the 1930s (Landsteiner and Jacobs, 1936) it has been widely accepted that small chemical allergens cannot stimulate a DTH response until they modify self-proteins/peptides (thus acting as a hapten) to form a macromolecular immunogen. However, the precise molecular mechanisms of hapten-protein modification and the identities of the immunologically relevant self-proteins/peptides that are modified and lead to the generation of antigenic epitopes remain largely speculative almost seventy years on. The nature of antigen formation is believed to be highly specific for each chemical family of allergenic electrophilic xenobiotics (e.g. aldehydes, aromatic esters, halogenated compounds etc.) (Lepoittevin and Leblond, 1997; Lepoittevin and Goosens, 1998) and protein modification is expected to be confined to certain crucially placed nucleophilic amino acid residues necessary for optimal recognition by T cells (Cavani *et al.*, 1995).

During sensitisation (see Chapter 1) naïve $CD4^+$ T cells recognise specific antigens in complex with class II major histocompatibility complexes (MHC). Hence, it is postulated in this chapter, that an individual's susceptibility to suffering from ACD to a particular chemical is largely governed by their immunocompetency and in particular, their ability to form covalently-modified specific MHC-restricted antigens that are recognised as modified-self molecules by their T-cell repertoire. The physico-chemical properties of an absorbed xenobiotic (although causative of inducing ACD by defining whether a molecule is sufficiently protein-reactive) are universal and covalent binding to a diverse spectrum of either extracellular or intracellular skin proteins/peptides is expected to occur. Such diverse protein-xenobiotic binding alone cannot define allergenic specificities and susceptibilities that arise in the human population from exposure to xenobiotics that are present in both natural and synthetic substances. An individual's capacity to actively metabolise a 'prohapten' (i.e. a compound that is an allergen but not protein-reactive e.g. cinnamic alcohol (Weibel and Hansen, 1989b; Basketter, 1992; Smith *et al.*, 2000a) and paraphenylenediamine (Picardo *et al.*, 1992; Picardo *et al.*, 1996; Lisi and Hansel, 1998)) to a hapten within the skin or, conversely, to detoxify a hapten to an unreactive species, may also contribute to allergenic susceptibility (see Chapters 4 and 5). Nevertheless, the specificity underlying ACD can only be determined by the individual's unique T-cell and MHC allele repertoires and their ability to recognise specific haptenated MHC-binding peptides. In addition, not all MHC-binding peptides can act as carrier molecules for haptens and those that can, are expected to be different for different families of chemicals. Only those peptides that possess a centrally located nucleophilic residue flanked by MHC-binding motif residues will be able to act as a carrier peptide. Hence, ACD is a condition that is underpinned by both xenobiotic chemistry and immunorecognition.

This chapter focuses in more detail on potential pathways that could be involved in the formation of hapten-modified self-peptides and their recognition by molecules of the T-cell mediated immune system during both the sensitisation and elicitation stages of ACD (as described in Chapter 1).

6.1 PEPTIDE-HAPTEN ANTIGEN FORMATION AND IMMUNE RECOGNITION MECHANISMS

In order for a small molecule xenobiotic to cause the adverse clinical symptoms associated with allergic contact dermatitis (Chapter 1), xenobiotic-specific sensitisation of the individual must occur i.e. initial priming of the immune system by the xenobiotic for recognition upon subsequent encounter (see Figure 1.2). The body does this by generating a population of antigen-specific memory T cells during sensitisation that circulate in the blood and lymph and are ready to recognise newly formed xenobiotic-specific antigens upon subsequent challenge at any region of the body with the same xenobiotic.[1] The precise molecular mechanisms that occur between initial absorption of the xenobiotic into the skin and the generation and proliferation of this population of memory T cells are unknown. However, it is known that ACD is a disease that is T-cell mediated and not antibody-mediated. Hence, it is expected that sensitisation involves the formation of a peptide-hapten antigen that is recognised by MHCs.

6.1.1 Possible mechanisms of peptide-hapten antigen formation

As shown in Chapter 5, there are a variety of possible mechanisms by which a xenobiotic electrophile can bind to a protein nucleophile (Schemes 5.1–5.23). However, the existence of limited selectivity in the binding of a diverse range of xenobiotics to only a few types of nucleophilic amino acids (or possibly the N-terminal amine) will result in many similarities in the sites of protein-binding for different xenobiotics. It is likely that the same limited set of protein/peptide sequences can act as carrier peptides for a multitude of xenobiotics, ultimately leading to the generation of a diverse array of xenobiotic-specific antigenic peptides (Germain and Margulies, 1993). The binding of the hapten to either full length, folded self proteins (that are subsequently processed into peptides by proteases) or short self peptides (that have evaded proteolysis into their constituent amino acids) (Craiu *et al.*, 1997; Baumeister *et al.*, 1998; Rock and Goldberg, 1999) could occur either extracellularly or intracellularly. The exact sub-cellular locations of protein-hapten binding that contributes to ACD are unknown at present but the possibilities are illustrated in Figure 6.1 (see colour section).

6.1.1.1 Extracellular protein-hapten binding

A number of extracellular protein-hapten binding mechanisms could occur upon skin absorption of a xenobiotic (Figure 6.1a):

- i the hapten may bind to extracellular proteins and the complexes generated could be recognised by cell surface molecules on APCs and internalised;
- ii the hapten may bind to extracellular proteins and the complexes generated could be actively transported into APCs by membrane-bound transport proteins;
- iii the hapten could bind to membrane-bound proteins on the surface of APCs and the binding could signal the internalisation of the haptenated protein.

6.1.1.2 Intracellular protein-hapten binding

An alternative mechanism of protein-hapten binding is that the xenobiotic hapten gets inside the cell and binds to intracellular proteins (Figure 6.1b). The hapten could either undergo

i active transport; or
ii passive diffusion

from the extracellular space, through the cell membrane and into the cytosol of APCs, with subsequent binding of the hapten to intracellular skin protein (or peptide).

The protein (or peptide) is likely to be a 'self' molecule in both extracellular and intracellular scenarios. However, it is feasible that viral proteins or peptides, which could potentially invade the body and co-exist in a parasitic fashion without harmful effect to the individual, may be present to bind to hapten.

6.1.1.3 Effect of pH on protein-hapten binding

One factor that will be important in determining the location of protein-hapten binding in the skin (i.e. whether it occurs to extracellular or intracellular proteins/peptides) is the varying pH in different compartments of the skin. As a molecule travels through the skin (from first absorption through the stratum corneum into the epidermis, through the dermis and finally into the blood stream) it experiences a pH change from approximately pH 5.5 of the outer layers of the skin to physiological pH of the blood (pH 7.4) (Gawkrodger, 1997). The kinetics of some reactions of xenobiotics with amino acid nucleophiles may be more favourable at acidic pH. For example, this would be the case for both Schiff base formation and Michael addition reactions for aldehydes (see section 5.3.2). Hence, the local pH may be a dominant factor in determining the tissue location of protein/peptide modification by a sensitising xenobiotic.

6.1.1.4 Limitations of hapten modification of globular proteins

There are some limitations with respect to the covalent modification of full-length, folded proteins, irrespective of whether haptenation occurs in the extracellular or intracellular space. The three-dimensional structure of the protein will limit the extent of exposed molecular surface area and the types of residues that exist on the surface of the protein (Branden and Tooze, 1991). By nature of protein folding, the exterior residues of proteins existing in aqueous environments will be predominantly polar or charged and the interior residues hydrophobic. Membrane-bound proteins may have extracellular and intracellular polar regions of the molecule, but possess a predominantly hydrophobic membrane-buried core. In order for a xenobiotic to react with a protein, a suitable nucleophilic side chain must be facing the exterior of the molecule and the pH of the environment in which it resides must be favourable (Roberts and Lepoittevin, 1998). Therefore, analysing a protein sequence alone would tell little about the availability of xenobiotic-binding residues within that protein *in vivo*. Only structural analyses of proteins will reveal where xenobiotic binding can actually occur on a folded protein and, in fact, appropriate nucleophilic xenobiotic-binding residues may be relatively few in number in folded proteins. This is especially true for xenobiotics that show a preference for binding to cysteine residues, very few of which exist on the surface of proteins and are more likely to be involved in internal disulphide bridges, which provide stability for the molecular architecture (Branden and Tooze, 1991).

6.1.1.5 Intracellular processing of haptenated proteins

Processing of a haptenated globular protein into antigenic peptides (Germain and Margulies, 1993) would be required for a DTH response to be generated irrespective of whether the protein arrived inside the cell via an extracellular route (e.g. by endocytosis) or was a hapten-modified intracellular protein. However, the mechanisms of proteolysis may be different depending upon whether initial extracellular or intracellular protein-hapten binding occurs. Proteolytic processing can occur within acidic endosomal compartments within the APC (Girolomoni *et al.*, 1990), as may be the case for an extracellular protein that has been hapten-modified and subsequently internalised by endocytosis. This would lead to the generation of internalised haptenated peptides in vesicles formed within the cell and it is most likely that these peptides will be recognised and presented by MHC class II molecules (Germain and Margulies, 1993). However, release of these peptide-hapten complexes into the cytosol could be effected by vesicle disruption, and transport of antigenic peptides from the cytosol to the endoplasmic reticulum, where MHC class I molecules reside, could also occur.

Intracellular self-proteins are continually being degraded into peptides by the 20S/26S proteosome (Baumeister *et al.*, 1998; Fruh and Yang, 1999) and these peptides are rapidly broken down by peptidases to the constituent amino acids. Proteins are targeted for rapid proteosomal degradation upon binding a chain of ubiquitin (a polypeptide) molecules. Ubiquitination occurs via isopeptide bond formation to the ε-amino group of lysine residues within either the target protein or a previously bound ubiquitin molecule. In this manner the cell can selectively degrade specific proteins whilst sparing others (Ciechanover, 1994).

It is thought that the proteosome contributes to the generation of antigenic peptides as two of the β-type subunits of the proteosome, LMP2 and LMP7, are present within the MHC locus (Brown, Driscoll and Monaco, 1991; Glynne *et al.*, 1991; Martinez and Monaco, 1991). Both of these subunits are upregulated by interferon-γ (IFN-γ) (a cytokine that is released by T_H1 cells and effector $CD8^+$ T cells selectively during contact hypersensitivity (Dearman *et al.*, 1996; Xu *et al.*, 1997; Dearman and Kimber, 1999)). If intracellular proteins are haptenated, peptide-hapten complexes that result from proteosome degradation could be formed in the cytosol. These complexes may be produced in a form already able to bind to MHC molecules or they may require further processing into antigenic peptides of the required amino acid length (8–10 amino acids for MHC class I or 13–20 amino acids for MHC class II) (see section 3). It is known that distinct proteolytic pathways are involved in the generation of defined N- and C-termini of antigenic peptides (Craiu *et al.*, 1997). The N-terminal degradation of cytosolic peptides can be effected by aminopeptidases, such as the IFN-γ-induced leucine aminopeptidase (Beninga *et al.*, 1998). However, if the N-terminus is modified by acetylation (or perhaps by xenobiotic-binding), aminopeptidase degradation/peptide trimming could be blocked (Rock and Goldberg, 1999). Very little carboxypeptidase activity has been observed in studies of antigen formation; the C-terminus is thought to be defined largely by proteosomal action (Craiu *et al.*, 1997). One challenge of understanding peptide-hapten antigen formation is to elucidate how such antigens evade rapid degradation by cytosolic proteolysis, as is the fate of most peptides generated by the proteosome (Baumeister *et al.*, 1998; Rock and Goldberg, 1999). Antigenic peptides must be generated by highly specific proteolytic mechanisms at defined residues.

6.1.1.6 Extracellular processing of haptenated proteins

An alternative mechanism has been proposed for extracellular protein antigen processing in an acidic extracellular environment (such as that found within the outer layers of the skin) and in the presence of immature dendritic cells (such as Langerhan's cells in the skin) (Santambrogio *et al.*, 1999). Dendritic cells secrete proteases into the extracellular space, therefore if there are hapten-modified proteins formed extracellularly within the skin in the environment of a dendritic cell they are likely to be locally proteolysed in the extracellular space into peptide fragments. It is also possible that extracellular self proteins are proteolysed and then hapten binds to the generated self-peptide fragments directly.

6.1.1.7 Processing-independent binding of haptens to peptides

An alternative to the haptenation of folded proteins is that haptens could bind directly to short self-peptides (<20 amino acids in length) derived from processed self-proteins or those that exist as native short peptides. However, hapten binding to free peptides would have to be rapid in order that the peptide could evade proteolytic degradation (Baumeister *et al.*, 1998; Rock and Goldberg, 1999). Such peptides may be derived from both the intracellular or extracellular proteolysis (see sections 6.1.1.5 and 6.1.1.6 above) of non-haptenated self proteins. If this is the case, then the three-dimensional structure of the intact protein from which the peptides derive would bear little significance to the availability of possible xenobiotic-binding residues in these peptides. Those xenobiotics that preferentially bind to cysteine residues (which are normally buried within an intact protein) may have no trouble in doing so when the cysteine exists in a processed peptide.

6.1.1.8 Covalent and non-covalent association of xenobiotics with MHC bound peptides

Peptides could bind to the hapten initially and bind to an MHC molecule subsequently, as a peptide-hapten complex. Alternatively, as suggested by Pichler's group in Bern, Switzerland (Zanni *et al.*, 1998; von Greyerz *et al.*, 1998), the hapten could either covalently bind to or non-covalently associate itself with an already existing MHC-peptide complex on the cell surface. This latter mechanism of non-covalent association with an

MHC-bound peptide, thus forming a labile complex, has been postulated to occur for the non-protein-reactive sulfamethoxazole and lidocaine drugs, as they have been shown to be recognised by drug-specific αβ T cells and effect downregulation of TCR expression (Zanni *et al.*, 1998).

6.1.2 Major histocompatibility complexes

The principal functions of major histocompatibility complex (MHC) are the recognition of foreign peptide antigens, in particular distinguishing 'self molecules' from 'non-self molecules', and the regulation of T-cell immune responses. Endogenous self-peptides and exogenous peptides can bind to either MHC class I (in humans — human leukocyte antigen (HLA) classes A, B or C) or MHC class II (HLA class D) within or on the surface of an antigen-presenting cell (APC). The MHC-peptide binding characteristics depend upon the length and also the anchor motif residues of the peptide (Lechler, 1994; Jones, 1997; Buus, 1999). As knowledge on the native and viral peptide-binding properties of different MHC alleles is expanding at an enormous pace, an internet database (named the SYFPEITHI database) has been established recently for MHC ligands and peptide motifs (Rammensee *et al.*, 1999; http://www.uni-tuebingen.de/uni/kxi/). Humans possess 3–6 different MHC class I alleles (Abele and Tampe, 1999) and hundreds of MHC class II allelic variants (Zarutskie *et al.*, 1999).

Three-dimensional structures of human and mouse MHC-peptide complexes (both class I and class II) have been determined by X-ray crystallography (Fremont *et al.*, 1992; Brown *et al.*, 1993; Fremont *et al.*, 1995; Dessen *et al.*, 1997; Bouvier *et al.*, 1998; Scott *et al.*, 1998; Speir *et al.*, 1999). These structures reveal that MHC class I molecules bind to discrete 8–10mer peptides, with N-terminal and C-terminal residues being as important as centrally-located residues in recognition within the binding groove (Falk *et al.*, 1991; Hunt *et al.*, 1992a; Fremont *et al.*, 1995). There is a preference for the C-terminal residue to be basic and hydrophobic. Binding of peptides to MHC class I occurs predominantly in the endoplasmic reticulum (ER) of APCs (Rock and Goldberg, 1999). As such, MHC class I peptide ligands must be transported to the ER for recognition and this transport is effected by the transporter associated with antigen processing (TAP) protein (Abele and Tampe, 1999; Lankat-Buttgereit and Tampe, 1999).

In contrast, MHC class II molecules bind 13–20mer peptides (intracellularly or at the cell surface of an APC) in a more promiscuous fashion, with the central residues of the peptide being involved in MHC recognition (Hunt *et al.*, 1992b; Ghosh *et al.*, 1995; Murthy and Stern, 1997) (Figure 6.2, see colour section). Each of the hundreds of MHC class II alleles can bind a diverse spectrum of antigenic peptides with relatively high affinity ($K_d \sim 10^{-4}$–10^{-6} M) (Zarutskie *et al.*, 1999).

To date, no structural studies have been performed to analyse the interactions or conformational changes that occur within MHCs at the molecular level upon binding of peptide-hapten antigens. In general, recognition of peptide-hapten antigens by MHC and the surveillance of self-modification by xenobiotics in relation to allergy is little understood.

6.1.3 The roles of T-cell receptors

6.1.3.1 Recognition of MHC-peptide complexes by TCRs

T-cell recognition of the MHC-peptide complex, present on the surface of an APC, is performed principally by the T-cell receptor (TCR) in conjunction with a $CD4^+$ or $CD8^+$ molecule depending on the T-cell type involved. The crystal structures of MHC-peptide-TCR complexes have also been determined (Garboczi *et al.*, 1996; Garcia *et al.*, 1998; Hausmann *et al.*, 1999) (Figure 6.3, see colour section). However, no structural studies have been performed to date to investigate the precise contacts involved in TCR recognition of hapten-modified 'self' peptides at the molecular level. In contrast to MHCs, which can bind peptides promiscuously, TCRs on the surface of T cells are highly specific for the antigenic peptide presented by MHCs.

MHC molecules (in particular class II) are promiscuous, in that they can bind a wide variety of self and antigenic peptides. In the case of haptenated-peptides, it is postulated that more than one peptide-hapten antigen (containing different anchor residues for binding to different types of MHC alleles but also containing similar xenobiotic-binding sites) could be recognised by the same xenobiotic-specific T cells (Figure 6.4, see colour section). However, this would depend on the recognition elements between MHC-(peptide-hapten)-TCR complexes and would only be feasible if the xenobiotic entity alone, and no characteristics of the peptide, were recognised (as evinced by Martin and Weltzien, 1994).

Some studies on trinitrophenyl (TNP) modified peptides (formed by a similar mechanism to that depicted for dinitrophenyl adduction in Figure 5.1) have shown that the majority of TNP-specific $CD4^+$ T-cell clones selectively proliferated upon recognition of peptides with the hapten bound to a central lysine residue (Martin and Weltzien, 1994; Cavani *et al.*, 1995). In fact, it was shown that the sequence of the peptide was not the most important factor (Martin and Weltzien, 1994). As long as the peptide had a binding affinity for the MHC molecule and had a centrally located hapten-modified lysine residue, the affinity was modified but retained upon haptenation of the peptide and the peptide-hapten was able to stimulate $CD4^+$ T-cell proliferation. It is entirely feasible that the presence of the xenobiotic bound to a self-peptide can alter the molecular volume of the peptide significantly enough to be specifically recognised as foreign by the TCR. From the three-dimensional structures of MHC-peptide-TCR complexes it is clear that the interface between MHC and TCR is highly complementary (Garboczi *et al.*, 1996; Garcia *et al.*, 1998; Hausmann *et al.*, 1999; Reinherz *et al.*, 1999). The majority of the peptide antigen is buried deep within the MHC peptide-binding groove and only one or two key residues of the antigen extrude from the groove in order to interact with the TCR. The presence of the xenobiotic, altering what would normally be an unrecognised 'self' peptide, may cause a structural alteration in either or both the MHC and the T-cell receptor upon binding that leads to a cascade of events (i.e. such as tyrosine phosphorylation and release of cytokines, chemokines etc.).

6.1.3.2 MHC-peptide-TCR interaction affinity and memory T-cell selection in the thymus

Positive and negative selection of memory T cells in the thymus is known to be mediated by the avidity and affinity of the MHC-peptide-TCR interaction (Ashton-Rickardt *et al.*, 1994; Sebzda *et al.*, 1994; Hogquist *et al.*, 1995; Alam *et al.*, 1996; Hu *et al.*, 1997; Chiu *et al.*, 1999; Goldrath and Bevan, 1999). Strong MHC-peptide-TCR interactions lead to negative selection and weak MHC-peptide-TCR interactions lead to positive selection. As the MHC molecule is the same for both types of selection, but is promiscuous in the variety of peptides it can bind, it is thought that the precise recognition of antigenic peptides and their MHC-binding affinities play crucial roles in selecting for the proliferation of antigen-specific memory T cells. MHC-peptide binding interactions are predominantly defined by hydrogen-bonds and it has been demonstrated that the disruption of a single hydrogen bond can lead to 200-fold increases in MHC-peptide dissociation rates (McFarland *et al.*, 1999; Sant *et al.*, 1999). Cavani *et al.* (1995) showed that three MHC class II-binding peptides (DKGILQINSR (K53), DYGIKQINSR (K56) and DYGILQIKSR (K59)) exhibited differences from the native peptide MHC class II binding affinities when the lysine (K) residues in these sequences were modified by TNP hapten. TNP-modified peptides K53 and K59 showed reduced MHC-binding affinity and TNP-peptide K56 showed slightly increased affinity (with respect to the binding of the corresponding native peptides): TNP-peptide K56 was the only one of the three to significantly stimulate $CD4^+$ T-cell proliferation. It is highly likely therefore, that even small molecular changes by xenobiotic-modification of a self peptide can lead to significant changes in MHC-peptide-TCR interaction affinity, which could in principle generate overactive immune responses (e.g. hypersensitivities) via the inappropriate hyperproliferation of memory T cells.

6.1.3.3 Allergenic cross-reactivities

In the case of allergies to small molecules, a common problem associated with the inability to erradicate allergy completely in an individual by avoidance of the offending agent, is the existence of cross-reactivity with other structurally related molecules e.g. such is the case for the methylol phenols (Bruze and Zimerson, 1997).

TCR recognition of haptenated peptides appears not to be so finely tuned as to rule out potential cross-reactivity between structurally similar chemicals (providing that the same residue in the same position within the antigenic peptide is haptenated). Martin *et al.* (1992) have shown that, *in vitro*, TCRs can recognise TNP- and DNP-modified mouse K^b (MHC class I)-binding peptides (that have been modified at the same lysine position 4 in the peptide) with comparable efficiency. Yet, in mouse, there exists no cross-reactivity between trinitrobenzene sulphonic acid (TNBS) and dinitrobenzene sulphonic acid (DNBS) contact sensitisation. The authors propose that differing chemical properties/reactivities of TNBS and DNBS *in vivo* cause different lysine residues to be modified in the skin and hence different antigenic peptides to be generated.

If we accept that TCRs are capable of recognising the hapten alone on a carrier peptide, then cross-reactive small molecules must possess similar chemical functionalities (in order to be able to modify the same residue in similar carrier peptides) and similar molecular volumes (so that they can be recognised by the same T-cell clone). Nowhere has this been more exquisitely evinced than for the four different families (A–D shown in Figure 5.23) of cross-reactive corticosteroids (Coopman *et al.*, 1989; Lepoittevin *et al.*, 1995; Lepoittevin and Goosens, 1998). Epidemiological studies have shown that cross reactivities occur within each of these families but not between families. On analysing the three dimensional structures of the corticosteroids within each family, all cross-reactive members possess similar molecular shapes and volumes and all have similar propensities to be metabolised or bind to the same selective amino acid residues. These properties are different between families.

6.2 POTENTIAL DIFFERENTIAL IMMUNORECOGNITION MECHANISMS IN THE SENSITISATION AND ELICITATION STAGES OF ACD

ACD to xenobiotics is believed to involve recognition of peptides by MHCs and subsequent recognition of MHC-peptide complexes by TCRs on Thy 1^+ (T_H1) cells. Classically, MHC class II molecules are regarded as the immune system's mechanism of screening for invading exogenous agents. Conversely, MHC class I molecules survey the endogenous contents of the cell, for example, to check for the presence of viral proteins and malformed self-proteins within the cell. The modification of self-peptides by xenobiotics, which underpins ACD, is neither wholly exogenous nor wholly endogenous. It is known that the generation of ACD involves responses from two different types of T cells. MHC class II-restricted $CD4^+$ T cells are activated and proliferate during sensitisation (Dearman *et al.*, 1996; Fujisawa *et al.*, 1996; Gerberick, Cruse and Ryan, 1999) and may also regulate cytokine production during elicitation (Abe *et al.*, 1996). MHC class I-restricted $CD8^+$ cytotoxic T cells are thought to be predominantly involved during elicitation but may also be generated during sensitisation (Dearman *et al.*, 1996; Gerberick, Cruse and Ryan, 1999; Kalish and Askenase, 1999; Kehren *et al.*, 1999).[2] Consequently, ACD may involve both MHC class I and class II recognition mechanisms. Hence, the mechanisms of initial peptide-hapten antigen recognition by MHC would possibly involve two different sets of haptenated peptides (Figure 6.5).

6.2.1 Immune mechanisms of sensitisation

6.2.1.1 Studies on HLA-DR

The sensitisation stage of DTH is thought to depend upon the recognition of antigenic hapten-modified peptides by epidermal Langerhans' cells, which possess MHC class II, specifically human leukocyte antigen class DR (HLA-DR), on their surface and within the cell (Girolomoni *et al.*, 1990; Kleijmeer *et al.*, 1994; Verrier *et al.*, 1999). It is unknown as to whether these antigenic peptides, which must be 13–20 amino acids in

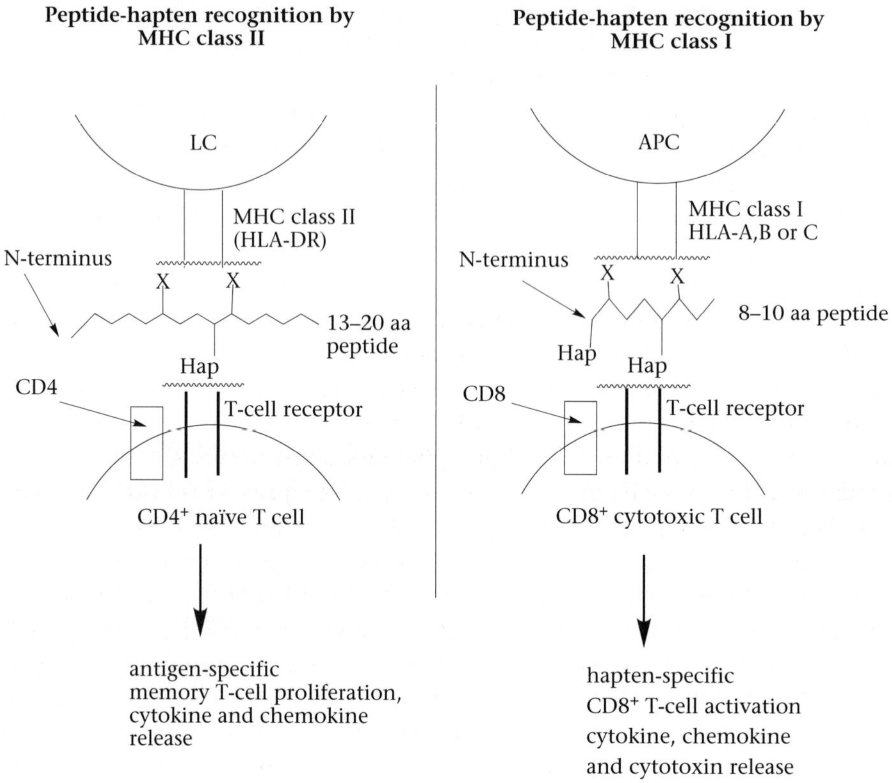

Figure 6.5: Schematic of the proposed hypothesis of differential peptide-hapten antigen recognition and presentation by MHC class II or MHC class I in the sensitisation and elicitation stages of DTH. It is expected that in the case of MHC class II-bound peptides, central haptenated residues (labelled Hap) may be the most important for recognition, and for MHC class I-bound peptides, both terminal and central residues are important. X represents anchor motif residues present in the MHC allele-specific self-peptide ligand.

length, are formed extracellularly or intracellularly. If peptide-hapten complexes are generated extracellularly, empty or peptide-receptive HLA-DR molecules could be loaded with antigenic peptide-hapten complexes directly on the LC surface (or by peptide exchange involving another class II MHC, HLA-DM, also on the surface of Langerhans' cells) without the haptenated complex ever entering the cell (Andersson *et al.*, 1998). Such extracellular generation of peptides and their binding to HLA-DR on the cell surface is intuitively the most rapid and efficient way that antigen recognition could occur during skin sensitisation but remains to be proven in the context of ACD. A recent study by Mommaas *et al.* (1999) has indicated that human epidermal Langerhans' cells have poor endocytotic and antigen processing capacities, which would support the notion of favourable extracellular binding of haptenated peptide to membrane-bound HLA-DR. Sherman *et al.* (1994) have demonstrated that peptide-binding to HLA-DR is influenced by the membrane environment and pH. They found that cell-surface binding of peptide to HLA-DR was optimal at low pH (~4) with virtually no binding at neutral pH. However, no pH effect on peptide binding to purified soluble HLA-DR was observed. Hence, from this study, it appears likely that the acidic pH of the skin may be favourable for membrane-bound MHC-peptide binding.

Although it is known that human MHC class II molecules (HLA class D) can bind peptides on the surface of an APC (Santambrogio *et al.*, 1999), it has also been shown that HLA-DR on the surface of freshly isolated Langerhans' cells can be internalised (Girolomoni *et al.*, 1990). Kleijmeer *et al.* (1994) performed a subcellular distribution study by probing intact normal human skin sections (that had been cryosectioned) and normal LC cultures with immunogold precipitation against the MHC class II α-chain. It was found that the LCs contained MHC class II-rich compartments (MIIC) (accounting for 44.2% of the immunogold staining), with significant levels of MHC class II in the endoplasmic reticulum (26.9%), vesicles (10.2%) and the plasma membrane (11.1%) and low levels in endosomes (3.5%), Golgi complex (3.0%) and Birkbeck granules (1.1%).

HLA-DR–peptide-hapten complexes, that are either formed intracellularly or have been internalised subsequent to extracellular peptide-binding, must ultimately be transported to the surface of the Langerhans' cell to be presented to MHC class II-restricted $CD4^+$ naïve T cells in the draining lymph nodes during sensitisation (Figure 1a). Two hypothetical scenarios are possible for signalling the trafficking of HLA-DR–peptide complexes within the cell. HLA-DR could 'blindly' bind a variety of peptides, both self and antigenic (that contain the required peptide binding motifs), and the act of peptide-binding signals the transport of the complex to the surface of the cell. Alternatively, HLA-DR–peptide complexes could only be transported to the surface of the cell if the peptide it carried was 'foreign', which would require an antigen-induced signalling event for trafficking. In the first scenario, if the HLA-DR binds to a self-peptide it may be trafficked to the surface but it should not stimulate immune mechanisms, i.e. the release of cytokines/chemokines, the migration of the Langerhans' cell to the draining lymph nodes and subsequent presentation to the T cell. However, if an antigenic peptide-hapten binds to HLA-DR and is trafficked to or is resident on the surface of the Langerhans' cell, then this binding will activate the Langerhans' cell and presentation to a $CD4^+$ T cell will result in an immune response. In the second scenario, the signal for trafficking to the surface of the Langerhans' cell may be a conformational change in the HLA-DR that only occurs upon antigenic peptide binding. Such conformational changes, from an open to a compact state upon peptide binding, have been observed in HLA-DR1 (Zarutskie *et al.*, 1999). The minimum length of peptide that could induce the compact conformation was as short as 2–4 amino acids (Sato *et al.*, 2000). However, it is unproven as to whether this peptide must be foreign or whether self-peptides can also effect this conformational change.

Some investigations into the nature of HLA-DR expression in the presence of sensitising chemicals have been performed. Upon 4 h treatment with sensitisers (isoeugenol, cinnamaldehyde, Bandrowksi base, 2,4,6-trinitrobenzene sulphonic acid and *p*-phenylenediamine), HLA-DR expression on the surface of a Langerhans' cell has seen to be decreased in a dose-dependent fashion, without a decrease in the number of HLA-DR positive cells, suggesting internalisation (Girolomoni *et al.*, 1990; Verrier *et al.*, 1999). However, a separate study by Manome *et al.* (1999) showed that HLA-DR expression in human monocyte-derived dendritic cells is augmented (along with expression of the cell surface receptor CD86). Stimulation of HLA-DR positive cells with sensitising chemicals (and not irritants) is known to induce tyrosine phosphorylation events, which may be a signal for Langerhans' cell activation (Kuhn *et al.*, 1998).

6.2.1.2 Translocation events associated with Langerhans' cells

If the antigen is bound to an HLA-DR molecule intracellularly, the complex must be translocated to the surface of the Langerhans' cell so that the peptide can be presented to the TCRs of $CD4^+$ naïve T cells. As well as this intracellular translocation of MHC-peptide complexes, the immature Langerhans' cell also matures to a dendritic cell as it is translocated from the epidermis to the dermis and eventually to the lymphatic system. It is here that it finally presents the MHC-peptide complex on its surface to the TCRs on $CD4^+$ naïve T cells. It is believed that when immunogenic peptides are recognised by the Langerhans' cell, the production of cytokines (such as interferon-γ (IFN-γ), interleukin-1β and TNF-α) and chemokines (such as IP-10, JE and KC), may promote the directional movement of Langerhans' cells from the skin to the draining lymph nodes (Enk and Katz, 1992; Flint *et al.*, 1998; Matsunaga *et al.*, 1998; Tang and Cyster, 1999; Wang *et al.*, 1999; Kimber *et al.*, 2000).

6.2.1.3 Attraction of T cells to LCs

It is anticipated that chemokines will play a major role in the attraction of T cells to Langerhans' cells once the latter have travelled to the lymph nodes and matured into dendritic cells. A recent study has identified the extraordinarily high expression of a CC chemokine (DC/B-CK) only expressed by mature murine Langerhans' cells and not by freshly isolated Langerhans' cells (Ross *et al.*, 1999). This chemokine is specific for attracting activated T cells and is believed to exert its effects on T cells over short distances, i.e. within the lymph nodes. Although many studies are currently being performed investigating the effects of cytokines and chemokines on sensitisation (too many to be discussed in this review) (Kondo and Sauder, 1995; Dearman and Kimber, 1999; Wang *et al.*, 1999; Kimber *et al.*, 2000), the exact mechanisms of the Langerhans' cell migration events remain unclear (Rambukkana *et al.*, 1995).

6.2.2 Immune mechanisms of elicitation

It is only in recent years that the modulatory role of $CD8^+$ T cells during elicitation has been observed (Hauser, 1990; Bour *et al.*, 1995; Abe *et al.*, 1996; Kehren *et al.*, 1999). In particular, a recent study by Kehren *et al.* (1999) has shown that hapten-specific cytotoxic activity, in DTH responses in mice to dinitrofluorobenzene, was exclusively mediated by MHC class I-restricted hapten-specific $CD8^+$ T cells. The activation of hapten-specific $CD8^+$ T cells stimulates the release of cytotoxins and cytokines (Kalish and Askenase, 1999). In particular, upregulation of the cytokine, interleukin 12 (IL-12), has been implicated in the elicitation of DTH in human skin (Yawalker *et al.*, 2000).

Although it is known that both $CD4^+$ and $CD8^+$ T-cell populations are increased in the epidermis and superficial dermis following elicitation (Garmann and Gollnick, 1995; Jorundsson *et al.*, 1999), it is unknown as to whether these cells are predominantly xenobiotic-specific or non-xenobiotic-specific. However, given the xenobiotic-specificity involved in the development of ACD following challenge with a xenobiotic, it is favoured that T-cell proliferation and/or recruitment will exhibit some degree of specificity. If xenobiotic-specific $CD8^+$ T cells are involved in elicitation, then the 8–10mer peptide-hapten complex that is presented by MHC class I, will be different (or may be a truncated version) from the 13–20mer peptide-hapten complex presented by MHC class II to $CD4^+$ T cells (Figure 6.5). In contrast to HLA-DR, MHC class I recognition of peptides also involves recognition of the N- and C-termini of the bound peptide (Falk *et al.*, 1991; Hunt *et al.*, 1992a; Fremont *et al.*, 1995). Therefore, covalent modification of a self-peptide N-terminus as well as modification of centrally-located residues by a xenobiotic could, hypothetically, be recognised as antigenic by an MHC class I molecule. The involvement of MHC class I molecules in ACD may necessitate the participation of the 20S/26S proteosome in antigen-generation and the transporter associated with antigen processing (TAP) protein, in the transport of peptide-hapten antigens from the cytosol to the endoplasmic reticulum (as mentioned in section 6.1.2).

6.3 SUMMARY

Two important differential mechanisms of self-peptide hapten-modification, involving the same hapten but different peptides, are hypothesised to play roles in the sensitisation and elicitation stages of delayed type IV T-cell-mediated immunity. However, the immunorecognition mechanisms underlying both of these stages remain unknown and many alternative mechanisms of peptide-hapten antigen formation are possible.

NOTES

1 In the case of cross-reactivity between molecules, elicitation may occur following challenge with close structural relatives of the sensitising xenobiotic.

2 $CD8^+$ T cells (following coupling of a xenobiotic to self) have also been implicated in the mediation of contact tolerance, which can occur upon exposure to doses too low to sensitise (Chase, 1982; Steinbrink *et al.*, 1999).

CHAPTER

7

Conclusion: The Future of In Vitro *Models and* De Novo *Prediction of Xenobiotic Skin Sensitisation, and an MHC-Peptide-Hapten Hypothesis*

Contents

It is anticipated that the study of the cellular and molecular mechanisms underlying ACD, together with the investigation of chemical properties of low molecular weight sensitisers, will be pivotal to the future understanding, prevention and management of contact allergic reactions to xenobiotics. From the information contained in Chapter 2 on percutaneous absorption of chemicals, Chapters 3 and 4 on activating and detoxifying metabolism, Chapter 5 on protein-binding capacity and propensity of chemicals to be metabolised by cutaneous metabolism, and Chapter 6 on the potential role of haptenated self-peptides in the T-cell-mediated immune system, it is apparent that there are many mechanisms that contribute to the condition, on which to focus future investigations.

7.1 ABSORPTION, CHEMICAL REACTIVITY, METABOLISM AND IMMUNOCOMPETENCY ALL CONTRIBUTE TO ACD

From our current state of knowledge in the field of ACD, we postulate that in order for a xenobiotic to act as a skin sensitiser in humans, it must:

i be readily absorbed into the skin following exposure to a sufficient but non-irritant dose (threshold doses will be compound specific due to differences in skin penetration, chemical reactivity etc.);
ii be sufficiently protein-reactive (i.e. an electrophilic hapten) or be activated by cutaneous metabolism from prohapten into a protein-reactive species;
iii not be entirely detoxified by cutaneous metabolism to an unreactive species;
iv bind to protein residues that are immunologically significant and hence form antigenic peptides that can be recognised by the MHCs and TCRs of the immune system.

For many known chemical sensitisers, it is possible to develop theoretical models based on the first two of the above criteria (using chemical and mathematical properties) that generate in-retrospect 'predictive' data that correlate well with observed *in vivo* levels of sensitisation. However, these models often reveal some chemicals that are anomalies and hence, these physicochemical models alone may be of little use in the *de novo* prediction of skin sensitisation for an unknown entity. It is expected that other metabolic and immunological factors, which may depend largely on the individual, must also be incorporated into future predictive sensitisation models to avoid the prediction of false positives and false negatives.

Xenobiotic metabolism in relation to ACD is an area that is little understood. As well as the lack of knowledge relating to the basic activation and detoxication mechanisms for skin sensitising chemicals, there is also very little known about the induction and down-regulation of cutaneous xenobiotic-metabolising enzyme expression. Inter-individual differences in enzyme expression, induction and activity for certain enzyme substrates may also contribute to a person's ability to generate/detoxify haptens and hence contribute to their susceptibility to a particular xenobiotic allergy.

Immunological mechanisms may also depend largely on the individual, i.e. the expression of various MHC alleles and the individual's T-cell repertoire. In addition to this, the subtle mechanisms involving the many different types of cytokines, chemokines and cytotoxins will also contribute to the observed level of sensitisation.

7.2 INCORPORATION OF IMMUNORECOGNITION MECHANISMS INTO AN MHC-PEPTIDE-HAPTEN HYPOTHESIS

Skin sensitisation is a complex phenomenon. However, we can form some fundamental hypotheses from which to focus on investigating the early molecular mechanisms underlying the condition of ACD. In the review by Dupuis and Benezra (1982), on hypothetical mechanisms relating to ACD to small chemicals, these authors highlighted that in order for a xenobiotic to act as a sensitiser, it must have the capacity to covalently modify proteins. For a range of known sensitisers and non-sensitisers (as detailed in Chapter 5), all previous *in vivo* sensitisation data support the hypothesis that protein-binding capacity is a requirement i.e. that the sensitising hapten is an electrophile that can bind to a protein nucleophile. Even for those molecules that are prohaptens, there is good evidence to support the postulate that activating metabolism converts them into protein-reactive haptens. Here, we take this fundamental hypothesis further (Figure 7.1) and incorporate that, in order for a xenobiotic to act as a sensitiser it must covalently modify a specific amino acid that is crucially placed within an MHC-binding peptide motif sequence, thus forming an MHC-restricted peptide-hapten antigen. This peptide-hapten could be formed in a number of ways as outlined in Chapter 6.

7.3 DEVELOPING *IN VITRO* ALTERNATIVES FOR THE HAZARD IDENTIFICATION OF SKIN SENSITISERS

In light of impending European Union requirements for *in vitro* alternative methods to be developed (for the hazard identification of skin sensitisers in the cosmetics and toiletries industries), we consider it vital that chemical reactivity, metabolism and immunorecognition specificity should be embodied into, at present, undeveloped *in vitro* assays. Protein/peptide-binding assays, together with studies on activating and detoxifying metabolism of sensitising chemicals within the skin, may be a basis from which to further the development of true *in vitro* assays for the future. Also, methods that embody the immunorecognition mechanisms outlined in Chapter 6 should also be developed. These biochemical and metabolic assays would complement methods of measuring immunological endpoints, such as T-cell proliferativity, and contribute to creating a battery of *in vitro* tests for skin sensitisation hazard identification. A long-term futuristic perspective would be that the data from these assays could be used by the clinician in conjunction with the genetic profile of an individual. The biochemical assays would show whether a xenobiotic could bind to particular protein residues in MHC-binding peptides. The metabolic assays would show whether a xenobiotic could be activated to a protein-reactive species or detoxified. The genetic profile could reveal whether

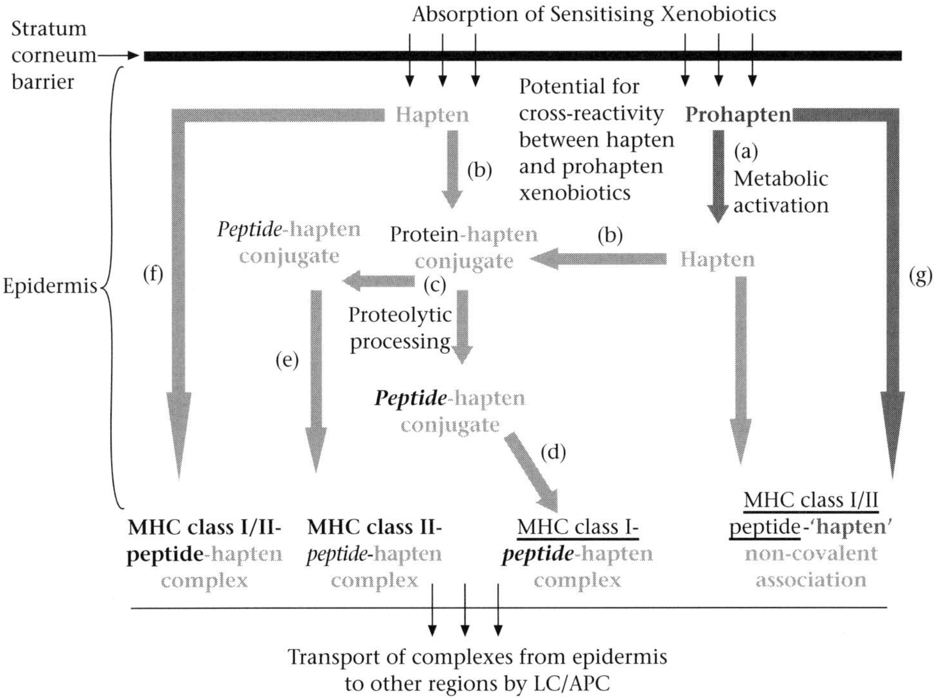

Figure 7.1: An MHC-peptide-hapten hypothesis. Sensitising xenobiotics that penetrate the stratum corneum barrier of the skin and are absorbed into the epidermis can either be haptens (protein-reactive) or prohaptens (not protein-reactive). Pathways involving haptens are shown in light grey and pathways involving prohaptens are shown in dark grey. (a) It has previously been postulated that prohaptens require cutaneous metabolic activation to haptens in order to become sensitising (Dupuis and Benezra, 1982). Once a hapten is present in the epidermis, it can potentially bind to full-length, folded skin proteins (b), thus forming a macromolecular, potentially multihaptenated, conjugate. This haptenated conjugate may then be proteolytically processed (c) into a variety of haptenated and non-haptenated peptide fragments. Different subsets of immunogenic peptide-hapten complexes may be recognised, either by MHC class I (d) or MHC class II (e) molecules. Alternatively, a hapten could covalently bind to (f) or non-covalently associate with (g) a self-peptide already residing in the MHC (class I or class II) groove. Whether non-covalent association of a xenobiotic would lead to stable immune recognition remains arguable. Once MHC-peptide-hapten complexes have been formed, they will then be presented differentially to either a $CD4^+$ T cell (by a Langerhans' cell (LC) in the case of MHC class II) or a $CD8^+$ T cell (by an antigen-presenting cell (APC) in the case of MHC class I).

(a) an individual possesses (or has the capacity to generate) specific MHC-binding 'carrier' peptides and corresponding MHC alleles, and (b) whether they possess or lack cutaneous xenobiotic-metabolising enzymes. Such data could ultimately aid the clinician in informing an individual of their potential susceptibility to a particular allergenic chemical.

APPENDIX

I

In vivo *sensitisation data and physico-chemical properties of xenobiotics*

(discussed in Chapter 5)

Chemical name	Classif.	GPMT	Human	Murine Local Lymph Node Assay Data* Vehicle	Dose	LowSI	Dose	HighSI	EC3	Physico-chemical parameters FW	BP (K)	MP (K)	Gibbs (kJ/mol)	log Po/w	MR cm^3/mol	Henry's
Aliphatic alcohols (Fig. 5.3)																
1,2-propanediol	non									76.1	428.33	229.71	−301.7	−0.81	18.97	5.15
carbowax 600	non									546	NC	NC	NC	−0.661	132.99	NC
butyl dioxitol	non									162.23	513.19	284.7	−330.34	0.85	44.22	7.21
2-butoxyethanol	non									118.18	454.32	239.93	−242.18	0.93	33.18	5.4
geraniol	non	−	−							154.25	513.06	224.70	39.84	2.46	51.18	3.73
1,4-butanediol	non									90.12	468.74	255.98	−290.84	−0.16	24.06	5.03
ethanol	weak		+							46.04	338.29	172.62	−170.86	0.1	13.01	3.64
isooctanol	weak		+							130.23	461.69	225.24	−122.78	2.809	40.49	2.9
1-decanol	weak		+							158.28	511.79	262.78	−103.5	3.75	49.74	2.65
Phenols (Fig. 5.4)																
phenylethyl alcohol	non								NC	122.17	498.03	266.66	−7.93	1.57	37.63	5.26
2-isopropyleugenol	non			AOO	12	1.8	59	2.2	NC	192.25	559.94	380.63	−21.28	3.23	57.67	5.46
3,5,6-trimethyleugenol	non								NC	206.28	583.57	444.46	−39.31	3.94	63.63	5.58
butylated hydroxytoluene	non								NC	220.36	569.66	426.33	19.63	5.64	70.13	3.33
topanol	non								NC	544.81	904.15	NC	79.89	12.22	170.39	13.01
methyleugenol	weak			AOO	11	1.9	27	4.9	16.87	178.23	520.88	307.39	12.73	3.21	53.27	2.95
4-methylol phenol	mod		+							124.14	533.75	367.11	−170.97	0.73	34.57	9.03
quinol	mod	+								110.11	502.87	394.22	−187.56	1.09	29.45	8.62
cinnamic alcohol	mod		+							134.18	521.78	272.85	80.71	1.58	43.19	5.74
eugenol	mod	+	+	AOO	10	2.4	25	5.5	12.9	164.2	537.44	373.09	−35.68	2.69	48.5	5.71
9,9,9-trimethylisoeugenol	mod									206.28	574.77	406	−15.2	3.95	63.2	5.6
2-isopropylisoeugenol	mod	+	+	AOO	3	11.1	12	11.9	NC							
4-methyl catechol	strong	+		AOO	7.6	9.8	3.8	10	NC	124.05	520.92	418.01	−188.77	1.5	34.49	8.58
2-methoxy-4-methyl phenol	strong	+	+	AOO	4.2	1.8	8.4	5	5.78	138.17	503.53	352.31	−140.36	2.02	39.26	5.82
isoeugenol	strong	+	+	AOO	2.5	2.3	5	4.1	3.47	164.2	543.78	369.77	−43.3	2.49	49.58	5.96
dihydroeugenol	strong	+		AOO	5.1	2.7	10.1	3.6	6.77	166.22	538.69	374.85	−123.52	2.94	48.46	5.58
urushiol	strong		+							320.51	703.39	575.79	−70.89	7.89	98.9	6.86
propyl gallate	strong	+		AOO	10	18.3	25	33.6	NC	212.2	636.76	605.87	−628.5	1.27	51.94	14.55
Aliphatic aldehydes (Fig. 5.5)																
formaldehyde	strong	+	+	AOO	5	3.7	10	4	NC							
octanal	strong									128.21	449.13	221.42	−83.04	2.79	39.35	1.82
furfural	strong									96.08	433.32	243.36	−99.87	0.4	25.07	3.26

Chemical name	Classif.	GPMT	Human	Murine Local Lymph Node Assay Data* Vehicle	Dose	LowSI	Dose	HighSI	EC3	Physico-chemical parameters FW	BP (K)	MP (K)	Gibbs (kJ/mol)	log Po/w	MR cm³/mol	Henry's
citral	strong	+	+	AOO	5	2.1	10	5	6.55	154.25	478.24	209.92	3.03	2.8	49.27	2.1
citronellal	strong		+							154.25	478.24	209.92	3.03	2.26	49.3	2.1
Hydroxycitronellal	mod	+	+	AOO	10	1.7	25	3.2	23	172.26	514.37	292.2	−202.62	1.42	50.28	NC
Aromatic aldehydes (Fig. 5.6)																
benzaldehyde	non		+	AOO	2.5	1.7	5	2.2	NC	106.12	454.39	236.57	20.95	1.34	32.65	2.95
anisic aldehyde	non	+								136.15	494.8	282.59	−85.26	1.47	39.11	4.49
vanillin	weak	+								152.15	547.48	394.31	−239.88	1.09	40.81	8.47
heliotropin	weak	+								150.13	530.13	348.2	−93.67	0.58	38.42	6.19
α-methyl-cinnamaldehyde	weak			AOO	2.5	1.5	5	3.4	4.47							
α-butyl-cinnamaldehyde	weak			AOO	5	1.5	10	4.4	7.59	216.32	591.91	307.69	159.98	4.35	69.5	3.96
α-amyl-cinnamaldehyde	weak	+	+	AOO	10	2.1	25	13	11.24							
α-hexyl-cinnamaldehyde	weak			AOO	10	2.5	25	6.3	11.97							
phenyl acetic aldehyde	strong			AOO	2.5	1.6	5	3.2	4.69	120.15	474.69	247.84	29.37	1.53	36.44	4.23
cyclamen aldehyde	strong	+								190.28	543.46	286.71	56.96	3.26	59.81	3.52
lillialP	strong	+								204.31	553.2	315.4	70.66	4.06	64.28	3.34
syringa aldehyde	strong	+								134.18	494.07	271.63	28.16	1.94	41.48	4.07
bourgeonal	strong	+								190.28	546.83	319.13	64.68	3.86	59.71	3.49
phenyl propionaldehyde	strong	+								134.18	482.5	244.11	35.35	1.73	41.01	4.08
cinnamic aldehyde	strong	+	+	AOO	1	2.4	2.5	4.7	1.39	132.16	499.87	254.03	118.01	2.08	42.13	4.71
Ketones and diketones (Fig 5.7a)																
Parsol DAM	non									284.31	671.27	503.05	−170.02	2.47	79.55	9.73
Parsol 1789	weak									310.39	682.43	517.05	−36.92	4.3	91.75	8.09
4-t-butylphenylacetone	weak									190.28	537.24	327.06	35.28	3.65	59.75	2.63
Cyasorb UV53	mod									326.43	717.8	575.17	−47.41	5.64	97.07	8.45
Eusolex 8020	strong									266.33	651.77	442.34	55.59	3.96	80.81	6.98
α,β-Diketones (Fig 5.7b)																
Furil	non									190.15	586.45	413.32	−207.66	0.01	46.92	6.5
Butane-2,3-dione	weak			AOO	10	2.8	25	5.2	11.25	86.09	390.88	234.2	−275.04	−0.66	21.77	NC
Glyoxal	mod	+	+							58.04	371.03	195.8	−233.08	−0.61	12.56	NC
Camphorquine	mod			AOO	25	1.7	10	3	NC	166.22	529.13	414.32	−121.15	1.7	45.49	5.07
21-Dehydro-hydrocortisone	mod									344.44	729.7	649.42	−193.19	2.01	95.34	12.28
1-Phenylpropane-1,2-dione	strong									148.16	519.2	316.97	−120.53	0.63	41.92	5.8
Carboxylic acids (Fig. 5.8)																
p-benzoic acid	non		−							138.12	571.2	466.89	−378.06	0.83	34.51	9.34
p-aminobenzoic acid	non	−	−	AOO	2.5	1.1	5	1.6	NC	137.14	580.88	450.95	−166.62	0.41	37.52	8.8

3,5,5-trimethylhexanoic acid	non									158.24	507.39	338.71	−318.61	2.97	44.65	3.91
lactic acid	non			DMSO	5	1	25	2.2	NC	90.08	477.37	329.49	−508.79	−0.97	18.84	NC
dodecanedioic acid	non									230.3	656.43	545.7	−637.66	3.17	60.35	NC
alpha-hydroxycaprylic acid	non									160.21	564.67	385.84	−466.69	1.31	41.77	NC
alpha-hydroxycaproic acid	non									132.16	532.46	363.3	−483.53	0.4	32.57	NC
cinnamic acid	non		−							148.16	560.71	372.63	−126.38	1.96	43.06	7.07
Aliphatic esters (Fig. 5.9)																
triethylcitrate	non									276.28	615.89	414.73	−1014.9	0.12	64.18	NC
methyllaurate	non									214.34	538.07	278.1	−251.79	4.96	63.45	NC
inonylacetate	non									186.29	472.02	242.98	−268.23	3.72	54.06	NC
cosmol	non									639.04	NC	NC	NC	17.48	192.6	NC
acetyltributylcitrate	non									402.29	NC	NC	NC	4.78	102.09	NC
ethyllactate	non									118.13	NC	NC	NC	0.31	28.38	NC
methylglycolate	non									90.08	NC	NC	NC	−0.53	19.11	NC
methyl stearate	weak									298.5	622.16	345.72	−201.27	7.7	91.05	NC
2-hydroxypropyl methacrylate	mod									144.17	NC	NC	NC	0.56	38.16	NC
methylglyoxalate	mod									88.06	388.16	207.4	−435.51	−0.26	18.27	NC
methacroleindiacetate	mod									256.34	574.17	300.98	−476.89	3.72	68.67	NC
ethylidene heptanoate acetate	mod									230.3	548.78	294.16	−573.02	2.93	60.14	NC
triethylaconitate	strong									258.27	591.63	332.45	−809.28	0.81	63.78	NC
2-hydroxyethylacrylate	strong			AOO	25	8.2	10	9	NC	116.12	457.25	247	−368.13	0.28	28.35	NC
Aromatic esters (Fig. 5.10)																
methyl cinnamate	non									162.19	513.08	265.63	−84.42	2.43	47.83	4.33
gardocyclene	non									220.31	556.74	331.95	−58.68	2.65	63.28	3.24
dimethyl isophthalate	non			AOO	10	1	25	0.9	NC	194.18	546.43	325.56	−484.64	1.67	49.11	5.04
parsol MDX	weak									290.4	633.71	375.54	−134.13	4.96	86.44	4.14
ethylidene benzoate acetate	weak									208.21	552.82	309.31	−469.03	2.09	52.68	5.35
anther	weak									192.25	532.15	278.25	−150.24	2.83	55.88	3.44
aspartame	weak									294.3	772.6	695.86	−472.38	−0.39	73.22	18.58
benzocaine	weak	+	+	DMF	50	2.2	10	3.2	18	165.19	553.07	355.22	−116.24	1.17	47.03	6.18
benzylbenzoate	mod	+		AOO	5	2.3	25	3.5	16.67	212.24	591.06	342.21	−18.55	3	62.2	4.82
3-carboxyphenyl heptanoate	strong									264.32	661.1	500.18	−476.08	3.9	71.58	6.53
3-acetylphenyl benzoate	strong									240.25	627.47	415.93	−148.68	2.83	67.77	6.02
BBCA	strong									286.24	746.46	699.72	−717.21	2.63	70.88	12.67
4-acetylphenyl benzoate	strong									240.25	627.47	415.93	−148.68	2.83	67.77	6.02
3-methoxyphenyl benzoate	strong									228.24	604.64	376.96	−133.18	3.02	63.83	4.51
3-trifluoromethylphenyl benzoate	strong									266.22	581.28	358.92	−609.77	4.44	63.34	2.34
3-t-butyl phenyl benzoate	strong									254.32	616.34	390.96	−0.08	4.77	76.03	4.33
3-chlorophenyl benzoate	strong									232.66	599.17	373.38	−48.53	3.51	62.17	3.41
Epoxy esters (Fig. 5.11)																
ethylphenyl glycidate	strong									192.21	544.72	322.25	−189.3	1.58	50.67	5.9
ethylmethyl phenyl glycidate	strong									206.24	552.34	357.42	−186.37	1.97	55.39	5.78

Chemical name	Murine Local Lymph Node Assay Data*									Physico-chemical parameters						
	Classif.	GPMT	Human	Vehicle	Dose	LowSI	Dose	HighSI	EC3	FW	BP (K)	MP (K)	Gibbs (kJ/mol)	log Po/w	MR cm^3/mol	Henry's
Peroxides and peroxy acids (Fig. 5.12)																
diperoxyazelaic acid	non									220.22	603.61	441.45	NC	1.47	NC	NC
diperoxydodecanedioic acid	weak									262.3	639.12	475.26	NC	2.84	NC	NC
diacetyl-diperoxy adipic acid	weak									262.21	594.58	371.28	NC	2.51	NC	NC
pernonanoic acid	weak									174.24	522.72	316.07	NC	2.96	NC	4.24
monoperoxyphthalic acid	weak									182.13	615.8	504.34	NC	0.42	NC	9.65
benzoyl peroxide	strong	+	+							242.23	619.37	384.54	NC	3.55	NC	3.84
linalyl hydroperoxide	strong	+		DMF	1	2.2	3	13.8	1.14	170.25	480.15	266.63	NC	3	51.27	2.56
Salicylates (Fig. 5.13)																
amyl salicylate	non									208.25	579.19	389.97	−304.86	2.71	57.7	6.34
methyl salicylate	non	−	−							152.15	525.36	359.89	−336.1	1.3	39.28	6.83
cis-3-hexenyl salicylate	non									220.26	604.88	411.16	−213.78	2.7	63.47	6.27
salicylic acid	non	−	−							138.12	571.2	466.89	−378.06	0.83	34.51	9.34
butyl paraben	non									194.23	573.43	393.7	−310.84	2.5	53.15	6.46
propyl paraben	non									180.21	NC	NC	NC	3.04	48.86	NC
methyl paraben	non									152	NC	NC	NC	1.99	39.58	NC
ethyl-m-hydroxybenzoate	non									166.17	542.29	371.16	−327.68	1.59	44.03	6.71
benzyl salicylate	weak									228.24	628.04	453.93	−173.17	2.61	63.89	7.92
phenylethyl salicylate	weak									242.27	639.64	465.2	−164.75	3.07	68.65	7.8
phenyl salicylate	mod									214.22	616.36	442.66	−181.59	2.5	59.06	7.26
Coumarins and Anhydrides (Fig. 5.14)																
coumarin	non									146.14	563.91	298.42	−72.17	1.76	41.55	3.55
octahydrocoumarin	non									154.21	544.51	261.86	−188.17	2.15	41.12	2.12
6-methylcoumarin	non	−	−	Acetone	25	0.8	5	1.2	NON	160.17	578.7	322.21	−73.38	2.18	46.59	3.51
1,2,4-benzene carboxylic anhydride	mod									192.13	709.52	520.15	−741.84	0.99	43.13	8.28
Phthalic anhydride	strong			AOO	10	20.9	2.5	26	NC	148.12	627.09	335.76	−396.72	1.43	36.37	3.59
Dihydrocoumarin	strong									148.16	561.9	297.66	−102.13	1.67	40.46	2.89
Aliphatic amines (Fig. 5.15)																
1,2-diaminoethane	strong									60.1	376.62	278.32	98.86	−1.26	17.87	NC
Aromatic amines (Fig. 5.16)																
musk ambrette	non									268.27	NC	NC	NC	4.21	70.75	1.06
musk xylene	non									255.18	NC	NC	NC	2.99	76.48	0.53
musk ketone	non									294.3	NC	NC	NC	3.95	78.86	2.46

aniline	weak	+	+	AOO	25	2.1	100	7.6	37.27	93.13	457.17	266.56	178.5	1.05	30.76	4.11
4-chloroaniline	mod	+	+	AOO	5	2.6	10	3.9	6.54	127.57	489.22	309	156.94	1.67	35.56	4.24
m-amino phenol	strong	+	+	AOO	2.5	2.8	5	3.5	3.21	109.13	515.01	378.28	23.88	0.66	32.45	8.09
2-nitro-1,4-phenylenediamine	strong									153.14	NC	NC	NC	0.2	36.74	2.58
N-methyl-4-aminophenol	strong									123.15	500.4	358.95	55.24	1.4	37.95	7.75
p-phenylenediamine	strong	+	+	AOO	0.1	2.2	0.25	3.5	0.19	108.14	526.75	362.34	235.32	0.24	35.46	7.56
N-rings (Fig. 5.17)																
acetylcaprolactam	non									155.19	605.74	390.5	71.07	1.05	41.03	8.47
valerolactam	non									99.13	513.6	266.86	8.05	0.04	26.86	6.11
allantoin	non									158.12	782.71	715.48	71.67	−1.96	31.92	22.73
n-benzoylpyrrolidone	non									189.08	653.49	457.77	232.94	1.43	52	9.42
Intace B350	non									191.19	682.03	507.76	160.25	1.29	49.1	12.2
ethyl lactyl PCA	weak									229.23	NC	NC	NC	−0.25	54.2	NC
octopirox	weak									236.33	613.49	415.45	87.89		84.67	1.89
pyridine 2,6-dicarboxylic acid	weak									167.12	629.98	599.83	−499.93	0.66	36.67	12.93
iso-thiazolone	weak									101.13	527.64	332.05	73.13	0.19	25.52	0
Kathon 893	mod									215.36	614.04	416.03	126.15	3.55	62.1	4.13
penicillin G	mod	+	+	DMSO	1	1.5	25	3.8	16.65	318.36	805.27	779.15	83.56	0.55	83.12	17.61
glydant	strong									188.18	684.7	533.01	−233.94	−0.65	42.2	17.55
preventol a3	strong									280.1	704.69	570.33	54.29	3.9	60.76	8.3
kathon CG	strong	+	+	DMSO	0.5	1.5	1	4.4	0.76	149.6	535.63	380.34	75.61	NC	34.55	4.25
1,2-benzisothiazolin-3-one	strong	+	+							151.19	601.85	422.35	203.83	1.57	41.05	2.84
mercaptobenzothiazole	strong	+	+	DMF	10	4.5	25	4.6	NC	167.25	574.98	434	345.93	3.42	46.75	5.83
oxazolone	strong	+	+	AOO	0.0025	3.4	0.05	8.9	NC							
Dyes (Fig. 5.18)																
blankophor	non									924.92	NC	NC	NC	7.31	229.57	NC
Red 4 CI 14 700	non									480.42	NC	NC	NC	NC	NC	NC
Ponceau 4r	weak									604.48	NC	NC	NC	NC	NC	NC
Red oil	mod									352.39	793.72	NC	NC	7.51	112.84	10.78
yellow oil	mod									306.36	NC	NC	NC	5.95	94.67	4.64
disperse black	strong									299.37	754.33	NC	NC	3.34	92.33	12.01
violet 2r cibacet	strong									238.24	721.9	678.62	221.58	0.81	70.55	13.79
brilliant blue	strong									626.55	NC	NC	NC	NC	NC	NC
HC Red 3	strong									197.19	NC	NC	NC	0.84	52.32	2.58
Yellow 5HC	strong									197.19	NC	NC	NC	0.37	52.32	1.74
Substituted 5-atom rings (Fig. 5.19)																
Bacdanol	non									208.34	571.24	332.66	45.53	2.69	67.55	3.8
Octalactone	non									142.2	521.55	239.69	−233.14	1.91	38.69	1.88
2-pentylidenecyclopentanone	weak									152.23	509.13	295.68	0.45	2.23	47.62	3.09
2-n-hexylcyclopentanone	weak									168.28	519.47	292.35	−44.3	3.08	51.23	2.06
2-pentylcyclopent-2-enone	weak									152.23	507.52	298.6	−24.68	2.23	47.62	3.09

	Murine Local Lymph Node Assay Data*									Physico-chemical parameters						
Chemical name	Classif.	GPMT	Human	Vehicle	Dose	LowSI	Dose	HighSI	EC3	FW	BP (K)	MP (K)	Gibbs (kJ/mol)	log Po/w	MR cm^3/mol	Henry's
2-pentylcyclopenta-1,3-dione	strong									168.23	550.17	349.3	−175.31	0.94	47.55	5.61
Saturated 6-atom rings (Fig. 5.20)																
Limonene extra	non									136.23	440.83	206.9	157.39	2.41	46.48	−1.19
Cyclal C	mod									138.21	473.66	249.11	−37.55	1.21	42.87	2.83
Dihydrofloriflone	strong									192.3	529.17	304.18	43.38	3.38	62.52	3.21
2,4-dimethylcyclohexene-3-carbaldehyde	strong									138.21	473.66	249.11	−37.55	1.21	42.87	2.85
Sulphonates and Sulphanilic acids (Fig. 5.21)																
sodium p-phenol sulphonate	non									196.16	NC	NC	NC	NC	NC	NC
sodium lauryl sulphate	non									288.38	NC	NC	NC	NC	NC	NC
Sulphanilic acid	non	+	–	DMF	5	1.5	25	2.2	NC	173.19	636.43	NC	NC	NC	NC	NC
1,2-dihydroxy-3,5-benzenedisulphonate	mod									270.24	715.51	NC	NC	NC	NC	NC
benzylphenol-2,4-disulphonic acid	strong									402.31	NC	NC	NC	NC	NC	NC
norbornanacetyloxy-4-benzenesulphonate	strong									310.37	643.9	428.52	−167.3	NC	NC	NC
Halogenated compounds (Fig. 5.22)																
2,4-dichloronitrobenzene	non	–	–													
Bromostyrene	mod									183.05	494.36	260.56	223.43	3.34	43.36	2.74
Dansyl chloride	strong	+								269.75	664.65	NC	NC	3.05	71.13	3.34
2,4-Dinitrochlorobenzene	strong	+	+	AOO	0.05	2.5	0.1	4.6	0.06	202.55	NC	NC	NC	2.4	46.31	0.99
Picryl chloride	strong	+	+	DMF	0.2	2.2	0.4	4.8	0.26							

This above list corresponds to the chemicals illustrated in the figures within Chapter 5.
LLNA results and EC3 values (i.e. the effective concentration that gives a threefold stimulation index) are quoted when obtainable.

Classif. = Classification from LLNA skin sensitisation data as published in Cronin & Basketter (1994)
GPMT — sensitiser (+) or non-sensitiser (−) as tested by the guinea-pig maximisation test
Human — sensitiser (+) or non-sensitiser (−) in human patch test studies
AOO — acetone:olive oil
DMSO — dimethylsulphoxide
DMF — dimethylformamide
LowSI — low stimulation index and HighSI – high stimulation index (see Kimber *et al.*, 1986)

FW = Formula weight
BP = Boiling point in K [p = 1 atm]
MP = Melting point in K [p = 1 atm]
Gibbs = Estimated Gibbs free energy in kJ/mol @ (T = 298.15K, p = 1 atm)
Log Po/w = Calculated log octanol:water partition coefficient using Broto's method: *Eur. J. Med. Chem. — Chim. Theor.* **19**, 71 (1984)
MR = Calculated Molar refractivity in cm^3/mol using Viswanadhan's fragmentation: *J. Chem. Inf. Comput. Sci.* **29**, 163 (1989)
Henry's = Estimated Henry's constant
NC — non-calculable

APPENDIX

II

Useful web addresses

http://altweb.jhsph.edu/science/pubs/ECVAM/ecvam19.htm	Alternative Methods for Skin Sensitisation Testing The Report and Recommendations of ECVAM Workshop 19[1,2].
http://www.cplscientific.co.uk/press/	Alternatives to Animal Testing II Proceedings of the Second International Scientific Conference organised by The European Cosmetic Industry Brussels, Belgium, 1999
http://worldanimal.net/cos-alternatives.html	Alternative to Cosmetic Testing on Animals
http://www.dml.georgetown.edu/depts/pharmacology/davetab.html	Cytochrome P450 substrate/inhibitor/inducers prepared by David Flockhart
http://tray.dermatology.uiowa.edu/DermImag.htm	Dermatologic Image Database more pictures of contact dematitis!
http://telemedicine.org/	Electronic Textbook of Dermatology Anatomy of the Skin by Maged N. Kamel, M.D.
http://library.dialog.com/bluesheets/html/bl0307.html	Dictionary of Substances and Their Effects (DOSE) maintained by the Royal Society of Chemistry
http://drnelson.utmem.edu/CytochromeP450.html	David Nelson's Cytochrome P450 homepage with links to other P450 sites and the human genome project
http://www.uwcm.ac.uk/uwcm/dm/contact/	Department of Dermatology University of Wales College of Medicine, Cardiff, UK
http://www.edae.gr/contact.html	Hellenic Association of Dermatology and Venereology
http://altweb.jhsph.edu/	Alternatives to animal testing

APPENDIX III

Models and Approaches for Studying Cutaneous Metabolism

In vitro models	*In vivo* models
Organ/tissue	Whole animal/man
Diffusion chambers	Skin grafts on athymic (nude) mice
Short term organ culture	Rat-human skin flap system
Isolated perfused porcine skin flap	Rat skin flap system
Tissue sections/minced skin	
Whole human hair follicles	
Human skin biopsies	
Cells	
Isolated cells	
Epidermal keratinocyte cultures	
Hair follicle keratinocyte cultures	
Reconstructed human skin	
Living skin equivalents	
Subcellular fractions	
Whole skin homogenates	
Microsomal fraction	
Cytosolic fractions	
Mitochondrial fraction	
Sub mitochondrial preparations	
Purified enzymes	
Transfected cell lines	

Approaches for studying cutaneous metabolising enzymes using the above *in vitro* models

Spectroscopic analysis — enzyme activity assays
Immunoblotting
Immunohistochemistry
Selective probe substrates
Enzyme purification and characterisation
FACS analysis
Cell depletion studies
Flow cytometry
Molecular Biology — RT-PCR, *in situ* hybridisation etc.
Molecular Studies — 3D structure analysis of enzymes by X-ray/NMR techniques
Confocal microscopy using specific antibody probes

Adapted from Hotchkiss, 1992.

References

Abe, M., Kondo, T., Xu, H. and Fairchild, R.L. (1996) Interferon-gamma inducible protein (IP-10) expression is mediated by CD8+ T cells and is regulated by CD4+ T cells during the elicitation of contact hypersensitivity. *J. Invest. Dermatol.* **107**, 360–366.

Abele, R. and Tampe, R. (1999) Function of the transport complex TAP in cellular immune recognition. *Biochim. Biophys. Acta* **1461**, 405–419.

Ademola, J.I., Wester, R.C. and Maibach, H.I. (1993) Absorption and metabolism of 2-chloro-2,6-diethyl-N-(butoxymethyl)acetanilide (Butachlor) in human skin. *Toxicol. Appl. Pharmacol.* **12**, 78–86.

Agner, T., Flyvholm, M.A. and Menne, T. (1999) Formaldehyde allergy: A follow-up study. *Am. J. Contact Dermat.* **10**, 12–17.

Agyeman, A.A. and Sultatos, L.G. (1998) The actions of the H2-blocker cimetidine on the toxicity and biotransformation of the phosphorothionate insecticide parathion. *Toxicology* **128**, 207–218.

Ahluwalia, A. (1998) Topical glucocorticoids and the skin — mechanisms of action an update. *Mediators Inflamm.* **7**, 183–193.

Ahmad, N., Agarwal, R. and Mukhtar, H. (1996) Cytochrome P450 dependent drug metabolism in skin. *Clinics in Dermatol.* **14**, 407–415.

Ahmed, S. (1997) The mechanism of a P450 enzyme-aromatase; a molecular modelling perspective for the removal of the C(19) methyl and aromatisation of the steroid A ring. *J. Enzyme Inhib.* **12**, 59–70.

Aksoy, S., Szumlanski, C.L. and Weinshilboum, R.M. (1994) Human liver nicotinamide N-methyltranferase. cDNA cloning, expression, and biochemical characterisation. *J. Biol. Chem.* **269**, 14835–14840.

Akhtar, S.A. and Barry, B.W. (1985) Absorption through human skin of ibuprofen and flurobiprofen: effect of dose variation, deposited drug films, occlusion and a penetration enhancer. *J. Pharm. Pharmacol.* **37**, 27–37.

Alam, S.M., Travers, P.J., Wung, J.L., Nasholds, W., Redpath, S., Jameson, S.C. and Gasgoigne, N.R. (1996) T cell receptor affinity and thymocyte positive selection. *Nature* **381**, 616–620.

Allen-Hoffman, B.L. and Rheinwald, J.G. (1984) Polycyclic aromatic hydrocarbon mutagenesis of human epidermal keratinocytes in culture. *Proc. Natl. Acad. Sci.* **81**, 7802–7806.

ALVARES, A.P., KAPPAS, A., LEVIN, W. and CONNEY, A.H. (1972) Inducibility of benzo(a)pyrene hydroxylase in human skin by polycyclic hydrocarbons. *Clin. Pharmacol. Ther.* **14**, 30–40.

ALVARES, A.P., LEIGH, S., KAPPAS, A., LEVIN, W. and CONNEY, A.H. (1973) Induction of aryl hydrocarbon hydroxylase in human skin. *Drug Metab. Dispos.* **1**, 386–390.

AMIN, S., JUCHATZ, A., FURUYA, K. and HECHT, S.S. (1981) Effects of fluorine substitution on the tumour initiating activity and metabolism of 5-hydroxymethylchrysene, a tumourigenic metabolite of 5-methylchrysene. *Carcinogenesis* **2**, 1027–1032.

AMKRAUT, A.A., JORDAN, W.P. and TASKOVICH, L. (1996) Effect of coadministration of corticosteroids on the development of contact sensitization. *J. Am. Acad. Dermatol.* **35**, 27–31.

ANDERS, M.W. and DEKANT, W. (1998) Glutathione-dependent bioactivation of haloalkenes. *Ann. Rev. Pharmacol. Toxicol.* **38**, 501–537.

ANDERSEN, K.E., BOMAN, A., VOLUND, A. and WAHLBERG, J.E. (1985) Induction of formaldehyde contact sensitivity: dose response relationship in the guinea pig maximization test. *Acta Derm. Venereol.* **65**, 472–478.

ANDERSON, B.D. and RAYKER, D.V. (1989) Solute structure-permeability relationships in human stratum corneum. *J. Invest. Dermatol.* **93**, 280–286.

ANDERSON, Y.B., JACKSON, J.A. and BIRNBAUM, L.S. (1993) Maturational changes in dermal absorption of 2,3,7,8-tetrachlorodibenzo-p-dioxin (TCDD) in Fischer 344 rats. *Toxicol. Appl. Pharmacol.* **119**, 214–220.

ANDERSSON, T., PATWARDHAN, A., EMILSON, A., CARLSSON, K. and SCHEYNIUS, A. (1998) HLA-DM is expressed on the cell surface and colocalizes with HLA-DR and invariant chain in human Langerhans' cells. *Arch. Dermatol. Res.* **290**, 674–680.

ANTHONSEN, H.W., BAPTISTA, A., DRABLOS, F., MARTEL, P., PETERSEN, S.B., SEBASTIAO, M. and VAZ, L. (1995) Lipases and esterases: a review of their sequences, structure and evolution. *Biotechnol. Ann. Rev.* **1**, 315–371.

ANTON, R., ABIAN, J. and VILA, L. (1995) Characterisation of arachidonic acid metabolites through the 12-lipoxygenase pathway in human epidermis by high-performance liquid chromatography and gas-chromatography mass spectrometry. *J. Mass Spec.* **SS**, S169–S182.

ARATA, J., UMEMURA, S., YAMAMOTO, Y., HAGIYAMA, M. and NOHARA, N. (1979) Prolidase deficiency. Its dermatological manifestations and some additional biochemical studies. *Arch. Dermatol.* **115**, 62–67.

ARITA, T., HORI, R., ANMO, T., WASHITAKE, M., AKATSU, M. and YAJIMA, T. (1970) Studies on percutaneous absorption of drugs 1. *Chem. Pharm. Bull.* **18**, 1045–1052.

ARTS, J.H., DROGE, S.C., SPANHAAK, S., BLOKSMA, N., PENNINKS, A.H. and KUPER, C.F. (1997) Local lymph node activation and IgE responses in brown Norway and Wistar rats after dermal application of sensitizing and non-sensitizing chemicals. *Toxicology* **117**, 229–234.

ASAHI, M., FUJII, J., TAKAO, T.T.K., HORI, M., SHIMONISHI, Y. and TANIGUCHI, N. (1997) The oxidation of selenocysteine is involved in the inactivation of glutathione peroxidase by nitric oxide donor. *J. Biol. Chem.* **272**, 19152–19157.

ASHCROFT, J.-A., OCKENDON, M. and HOTCHKISS, S.A.M. (1997) Percutaneous absorption of ethanol and detection of ethanol-metabolising cytochrome P450 enzyme 2E1 in human skin. *Human Exp. Tox.* **17**, 400.

ASHTON-RICKARDT, P.G., BANDEIRA, A., DELANEY, J.R., VAN KAER, L., PERCHER, H.P., ZINKERNAGEL, R.M. and TONEGAWA, S. (1994) Evidence for a differential avidity model of T cell selection in the thymus. *Cell* **76**, 651–663.

ASOKAN, P., DAS, M., BIK, D.P., HOWARD, P.C., MCCOY, G.D., ROSENKRANZ, H.S., BICKERS, D.R. and MUKHTAR, H. (1986) Comparative effects of topically applied nitrated arenes and their non-nitrated parent arenes on cutaneous and hepatic drug and carcinogen metabolism in neonatal rats. *Tox. Appl. Pharmacol.* **86**, 33–43.

ATHAR, M., AGARWAL, R., BICKERS, D.R. and MUKHTAR, H. (1987) Role of Reactive Oxygen Species in Skin. In: SHROOT, B. and SCHAEFER H. (eds), *Pharmacology and the Skin*, Vol. 1, Basel, Karger, 170–183.

ATKINS, P.C., ZWEIMAN, B., LITTMAN, B., PRESTI, C., VONALLMEN, C., MOSKOVITZ, A. and ESKRA, J.D. (1995) Products of arachidonic acid metabolism and the effects of cyclooxygenase inhibition on ongoing cutaneous allergic reactions. *J. Allergy & Clin. Immunol.* **95**, 742–747.

AUCAMP, J., GASPAR, A., HARA, Y. and APOSTOLIDES, Z. (1997) Inhibition of xanthine oxidase by catechins from tea (Cammelia sinensis). *Anticancer Res.* **17**, 4381–4385.

AUCLAIR, F., BESNARD, M., DUPONT, C. and WEPIERRE, J. (1991) Importance of blood flow to the local distribution of drugs after percutaneous absorption in the bipediculated dorsal flap of the hairless rat. *Skin Pharmacol.* **4**, 1–8.

AUMANN, K.D., BEDORF, N., BRIGELIUS-FLOHE, R., SCHOMBURG, D. and FLOHE, L. (1997) Glutathione peroxidase revisited — simulation of the catalytic cycle by computer assisted molecular modelling. *Biomed. Environ. Sci.* **10**, 136–155.

AUMULLER, G., EICHELER, W., RENNEBERG, W., ADERMANN, K., VILJA, P. and FORSSMANN, W.G. (1996) Immunocytochemical evidence for differential subcellular localization of 5-alpha reductase isoenzymes in human tissues. *Acta Anatomica* **156**, 241–252.

BABIUK, C., HASTINGS, K.L. and DEAN, J.H. (1987) Induction of ethylenediamine hypersensitivity in the guinea pig and the development of ELISA and lymphocyte blastogenesis techniques for its characterisation. *Fundam. Appl. Toxicol.* **9**, 623–634.

BADEN, O.M., GOLDSMITH, L.A. and BONAR, L. (1973) Conformational changes in the beta-fibrous proteins of epidermis. *J. Invest. Dermatol.* **60**, 215–218.

BAER, H., DAWSON, C.R., BYCK, J.S. and KURTZ, A.P. (1970) The immunochemistry of immune tolerance. II. The relationship of chemical structure to the induction of immune tolerance to catechols. *J. Immunol.* **104**, 178–184.

BAILLY, J., CRETTAZ, M., SCHIFFLERS, M.H. and MARTY, J.P. (1998) In vitro metabolism by human skin and fibroblasts of retinol, retinal and retinoic acid. *Exp. Dermatol.* **7**, 27–34.

BAKER, C.A., UNO, H. and JOHNSON, G.A. (1994) Minoxidil sulfation in the hair follicle. *Skin Pharmacol.* **7**, 335–339.

BALATO, N., CUSANO, F., LEMBO, G. and AYALA, F. (1984) Ethylenediamine contact dermatitis. *Contact Dermatitis* **11**, 112–114.

BAMSHAD, J. (1969) Catechol-O-methyltransferase in epidermis, dermis and whole skin. *J. Invest. Dermatol.* **52**, 351–352.

BANDO, H., MOHRI, S., YAMASHITA, F., TAKAKURA, Y. and HASHIDA, M. (1997) Effects of skin metabolism on percutaneous penetration of lipophilic drugs. *J. Pharm. Sci.* **86**, 759–761.

BANGHA, E. and ELSNER, P. (1996) Sensitisations to allergens of the European Standard Series at the department of dermatology in Zurich 1990–1994. *Dermatology* **193**, 17–21.

BANKS, Y.B., BREWSTER, D.W. and BIRUBAUM, L.S. (1990) Age-related changes in dermal absorption of 2,3,7,8-tetrachlrodibenzop-dioxin and 2,3,4,7,8-pentachlorodibenzofuran. *Fund. Appl. Toxicol.* **15**, 163–173.

BAR-NATAN, R., LOMNITSKI, L., SOFER, Y., SEGMAN, S., NEEMAN, I. and GROSSMAN, S. (1996) Interaction between beta-carotene and lipoxygenase in human skin. *Int. J. Biochem. & Cell Biol.* **28**, 935–941.

BARBAUD, A., MODIANO, P., COCCIALE, M., REICHERT, S. and SCHMUTZ, J.L. (1996) The topical application of resorcinol can provoke a systemic allergic reaction. *Br. J. Dermatol.* **135**, 1014–1015.

BARFORD, D., DAS, A.K. and EGLOFF, M.P. (1998) The structure and mechanism of protein phosphatases: insights into catalysis and regulation. *Annu. Rev. Biophys. Biomol. Struct.* **27**, 133–164.

BARKER, C.L. and CLOTHIER, R.H. (1997) Human keratinocyte cultures as models of cutaneous esterase activity. *Toxicology In Vitro* **11**, 637–640.

BARON, J., KAWABATA, T., REDICK, J.A., KNAPP, S.A., WICK, D.G., WALLACE, R.B., JAKOBY, W.B. and GUENGERICH, F.P. (1983) Localization of carcinogen-metabolizing enzymes in human and animal tissues. In: RYDSTROM, I., MONTELIUS, J. and BENGTSSON, M. (eds), *Extrahepatic drug metabolism and chemical carcinogenesis*. Amsterdam, Elsevier, 73–89.

BARON, J.M., ZWADLO-KLARWASSER, G., SIEBEN, S., RUBBEN, A., JUGERT, F.K. and MERK, H.F. (1998) Expression of cytochrome P450 isoenzymes in different compartments of the human skin. *J. Invest. Dermatol.* **110**, 681.

BARRATT, M.D. and BASKETTER, D.A. (1992) Possible origin of the sensitisation potential of isoeugenol and related compounds, I. Preliminary studies of potential reaction mechanisms. *Contact Dermatitis* **27**, 98–104.

BARRATT, M.D., BASKETTER, D.A., CHAMBERLAIN, M., ADMANS, G.D. and LANGOWSKI, J.J. (1994) An expert system rulebase for identifying contact allergens. *Toxic in Vitro* **8**, 1053–1060.

BARRATT, M.D. and LANGOWSKI, J.J. (1999) Validation and subsequent development of the DEREK skin sensitization rulebase by analysis of the BgVV list of contact allergens. *J. Chem. Inf. Comput. Sci.* **39**, 294–298.

BARRY, B.W. (1983) Drugs and the pharmaceutical sciences. In: *Dermatological Formulations*, Vol. 18. New York, Marcel Dekker.

BARRY, B.W. (1987) Penetration enhancers: mode of action in human skin. In: SHROOT, B. and SCHRAEFER, H. (eds), *Pharmacology and the Skin*, Vol. 1. Berlin, Karger, 121–137.

BARTEK, M.J., LABUDDE, J.A. and MAIBACH, H.I. (1972) Skin permeability in vivo: comparison in rat, rabbit, pig and man. *J. Invest. Dermatol.* **58**, 114–123.

BARUA, A.B. and OLSON, J.A. (1996) Percutaneous absorption, excretion and metabolism of all trans retinoyl beta-glucuronide and of all trans retinoic acid in the rat. *Skin Pharmacol.* **9**, 17–26.

BASKETTER, D.A. and GOODWIN, B.F. (1988) Investigation of the prohapten concept. Cross reactions between 1,4-substituted benzene derivatives in the guinea pig. *Contact Dermatitis* **19**, 248–253.

BASKETTER, D.A. (1992) Skin sensitisation to cinnamic alcohol: the role of skin metabolism. *Acta Derm. Venereol.* **72**, 264–265.

BASKETTER, D.A. and LIDEN, C. (1992) Further investigation of the prohapten concept: reactions to benzene derivatives in man. *Contact Dermatitis* **27**, 90–97.

BASKETTER, D.A., SCHOLES, E.W., FIELDING, I., DEARMAN, R.J., HILTON, J. and KIMBER, I. (1996) Dichloronitrobenzene: a reappraisal of its skin sensitization potential. *Contact Dermatitis* **34**, 55–58.

BASKETTER, D.A., DEARMAN, R.J., HILTON, J. and KIMBER, I. (1997) Dinitrohalobenzenes: evaluation of relative skin sensitization potential using the local lymph node assay. *Contact Dermatitis* **36**, 97–100.

BASKETTER, D.A., RODFORD, R., KIMBER, I., SMITH, I. and WAHLBERG, J.E. (1999a) Skin sensitization risk assessment: a comparative evaluation of 3 isothiazolinone biocides. *Contact Dermatitis* **40**, 150–154.

BASKETTER, D.A., LEA, L.J., COOPER, K., STOCKS, J., DICKENS, A., PATE, I., DEARMAN, R.J. and KIMBER, I. (1999b) Threshold for classification as a skin sensitiser in the local lymph node assay: a statistical evaluation. *Food Chem. Toxicol.* **37**, 1167–1174.

BAST, G.E. and KAMPFFMEYER, H.G. (1998) Dehydrogenation of 3-phenoxybenzyl alcohol in isolated perfused rabbit skin, skin homogenate and purified dehydrogenases. *Skin Pharmacol. Appl. Skin Physiol.* **11**, 250–257.

BAUMEISTER, W., WALZ, J., ZUHL, F. and SEEMULLER, E. (1998) The proteasome: paradigm of a self-compartmentalizing protease. *Cell* **92**, 367–380.

BECKLEY-KARTEY, S.A.J., HOTCHKISS, S.A.M. and CAPEL, M. (1997) Comparative in vitro Skin Absorption and Metabolism of Coumarin (1,2-Benzopyrone) in Human, Rat and Mouse. *Toxicol. & Appl. Pharmacol.* **145**, 34–42.

BEEDHAM, C. (1997) The role of non-P450 enzymes in drug oxidation. *Pharm. World Sci.* **19**, 255–263.

BEHL, C.R., FLYNN, G.L., KURIHARA, T., HARPER, N., SMITH, W., HIGUCHI, W.I., HO, N.F.H. and PIERSON, C.L. (1980a) Hydration and percutaneous absorption: influence of hydration on alkanol permeation through hairless mouse skin. *J. Invest. Dermatol.* **75**, 346–352.

BEHL, C.R., FLYNN, G.L., KURIHARA, T., SMITH, W., GATMAITAN, O., HIGUCHI, W.I. and HO, N.F.H. (1980b) Permeability of thermally damaged skin. I. Immediate influence of 60C scalding on hairless mouse skin. *J. Invest. Dermatol.* **75**, 340–345.

BENFELDT, E., SERUP, J. and MENNE, T. (1999) Effect of barrier perturbation on cutaneous salicylic acid penetration in human skin: in vivo pharmacokinetics using microdialysis and non-invasive quantification of barrier function. *Br. J. Dermatol.* **140**, 739–748.

BENINGA, J., ROCK, K. and GOLDBERG, A. (1998) Interferon-gamma can stimulate post-proteosomal trimming of the N-termini of antigenic peptides by inducing leucine aminopeptidase. *J. Biol. Chem.* **273**, 18734–18742.

BERGH, M., SHAO, L.P., HAGELTHORN, G., GAFVERT, E., NILSSON, J.L. and KARLBERG, A.T. (1998) Contact allergens from surfactants. Atmospheric oxidation of polyoxyethylene alcohols, formation of ethoxylated aldehydes, and their allergenic activity. *J. Pharm. Sci.* **87**, 276–282.

BERGH, M. and KARLBERG, A.T. (1999) Sensitizing potential of acetaldehyde and formaldehyde using a modified cumulative contact enhancement test (CCET). *Contact Dermatitis* **40**, 139–145.

BERGHARD, A., GRADIN, K. and TOFTGARD, R. (1990) Serum and extracellular calcium modulate induction of cytochrome P4501A1 in human keratinocytes. *J. Biol. Chem.* **265**, 21086–21090.

BERKOVITZ, G.D., CHEN, S., MIGEON, C.J. and LEVINE, M.A. (1992) Induction and superinduction of messenger ribonucleic acid specific for aromatase cytochrome P450 in cultured human skin fibroblasts. *J. Clin. Endocrinol. Metab.* **74**, 629–634.

BERLINER, D.L., PASQUALINI, J.R. and GALLEGOS, A.J. (1968) The formation of water soluble steroids by human skin. *J. Invest. Dermatol.* **50**, 220–224.

BERTRAND, F., BASKETTER, D.A., ROBERTS, D.W. and LEPOITTEVIN, J.-P. (1997) Skin sensitization to eugenol and isoeugenol in mice: possible metabolic pathways involving ortho-quinone and quinone methide intermediates. *Chem. Res. Toxicol.* **10**, 335–343.

BEZARD, M., KARLBERG, A.T., MONTELIUS, J. and LEPOITTEVIN, J.P. (1997) Skin sensitization to linalyl hydroperoxide: support for radical intermediates. *Chem. Res. Toxicol.* **10**, 987–993.

BHATIA, K.S. and SINGH, J. (1999) Effect of linoleic acid/ethanol or limonene/ethanol and iontophoresis on the in vitro percutaneous absorption of LHRH and ultrastructure of human epidermis. *Int. J. Pharm.* **180**, 235–250.

BIAN, Z. and WEIXIN, F. (1991) Facial contact dermatitis. *Int. J. Dermatol.* **30**, 485–486.

BICKERS, D.R., MARCELO, C.L., DUTTA-CHOUDHURY, T. and MUKHTAR, H. (1982) Studies on microsomal cytochrome P450 monooxygenases and epoxide hydrolase in cultured keratinocytes and intact epidermis from Balb/c mice. *J. Pharmacol. Exp. Ther.* **223**, 163–168.

BICKERS, D.R., MUKHTAR, H., DUTTA-CHOUDHURY, T., MARCELO, C.L. and VOORHEES, J.J. (1984) Aryl hydrocarbon hydroxylase, epoxide hydrolase and benzo(a)pyrene metabolism in human epidermis: comparative studies in normal subjects and patients with psoriasis. *J. Invest. Dermatol.* **83**, 51–56.

BICKERS, D.R., MUKHTAR, H., MEYER, L.W. and SPECK, W.T. (1985) Epidermal enzyme mediated mutagenicity of the skin carcinogen, 2-aminoanthracene. *Mutat. Res.* **147**, 37–43.

BICKERS, D.R., DAS, M. and MUKHTAR, H. (1986) Pharmacological modification of epidermal detoxification systems. *Br. J. Dermatol.* **115**, 9–16.

BICKERS, D.R. and MUKHTAR, H. (1990) Skin as a portal entry for systemic effect; xenobiotic metabolism. In: GALLI, C.L., HENSBY, C.N. and MARINOVICH, M. (eds), *Skin Pharmacology and Toxicology, Recent Advances*. New York, Plenum Press, 85–97.

BISOGNO, T., MELCK, D., DE PETROCELLIS, L., BOBROV, M.Y., GRETSKAYA, N.M., BEZUGLOV, V.V., SITACHITTA, N., GERWICK, W.H. and DI MARZO, V. (1998) Arachidonoylserotonin and other novel inhibitors of fatty acid amide hydrolase. *Biochem. Biophys. Res. Commun.* **248**, 515–522.

BJORKNER, B., BRUZE, M., DAHLQUIST, I., FREGERT, S., GRUVBERGER, B. and PERSSON, K. (1986) Contact allergy to the preservative Kathon CG. *Contact Dermatitis* **14**, 85–90.

BLACKER, K.L., OLSON, E., VASSEY, D.A. and BOYER, T.D. (1991) Characterisation of glutathione S-transferase in cultured human keratinocytes. *J. Invest. Dermatol.* **97**, 442–446.

BLANK, I.H. and SCHEUPLEIN, R.J. (1969) Transport into and within the skin. *Br. J. Dermatol.* **81**, 4–10.

BOCK, K.W., VON CLAUSBRUCH, U.C., KAUFMANN, R., LILIENBLUM, W., OESCH, F., PFEIL, H. and PLATT, K.L. (1980) Functional heterogeneity of UDP-glucuronyltransferase in rat tissues. *Biochem. Pharmacol.* **29**, 495–500.

BODDE, H.E., VERHOEF, J. and PONEC, M. (1989) Transdermal peptide delivery. *Biochem. Soc. Trans.* **17**, 943–945.

BODERKE, P., MERKLE, H.P., CULLANDER, C., PNEC, M. and BODDE, H.E. (1997) Localization of aminopeptidase activity in freshly excised human skin: direct visualization by confocal laser scanning microscopy. *J. Invest. Dermatol.* **108**, 83–86.

BOEHNLEIN, J., SAKR, A., LICHTIN, J.L. and BRONAUGH, R.L. (1994) Characterisation of esterase and alcohol dehydrogenase activity in skin. Metabolism of retinyl palmitate to retinol (vitamin A) during percutaneous absorption. *Pharm. Res.* **11**, 1155–1159.

BOLEDA, M.D., SAUBI, N., FARRES, J. and PARES, X. (1989) Physiological substrates for rat alcohol dehydrogenase classes- aldehydes of lipid peroxidation, omega-hydro fatty acids, and retinoids. *Arch. Biochem. Biophys.* **307**, 85–90.

BOLTON, J.L. and THOMPSON, J.A. (1991) Oxidation of butylated hydroxytoluene to toxic metabolites — factors influencing hydroxylation and quinone methide formation by hepatic and pulmonary microsomes. *Drug Met. Disposit.* **19**, 467–472.

BOLTON, J.L., ACAY, N.M. and VUKOMANOVIC, V. (1994) Evidence that 4-allyl-o-quinones spontaneously rearrange to their more electrophilic quinone methides: potential bioactivation mechanism for the hepatocarcinogen safrole. *Chem. Res. Toxicol.* **7**, 443–450.

BOLTON, J.L., TURNIPSEED, S.B. and THOMPSON, J.A. (1997) Influence of quinone methide reactivity on the alkylation of thiol and amino groups in proteins: studies utilising amino acid and protein models. *Chem. Biol. Interact.* **107**, 185–200.

BOMAN, A. and MAIBACH, H.I. (2000) Influence of evaporation and solvent mixtures on the absorption of toluene and n-butanol in human skin in vitro. *Ann. Occup. Hyg.* **44**, 125–135.

BORELLI, S. and NESTLE, F.O. (1998) Sensitization and development of allergic contact dermatitis caused by a single contact with an electrosurgical grounding plate containing acrylates. *Dermatology* **197**, 381–382.

BOUR, H., PEYRON, E., GAUCHERAND, M., GARRIGUE, J.-L., DESVIGNES, C., KAISERLIAN, D., REVILLARD, J.-P. and NICOLAS, J.-F. (1995) Major histocompatibility complex class I-restricted

CD8+ T cells and class II-restricted CD4+ T cells, respectively, mediate and regulate contact sensitivity to dinitrofluorobenzene. *Eur. J. Immunol.* **25**, 3006–3010.

Bouvier, M., Guo, H.C., Smith, K.J. and Wiley, D.C. (1998) Crystal structures of HLA-A*0201 complexed with antigenic peptides with either the amino- or carboxyl-terminal group substituted by a methyl group. *Proteins* **33**, 97–106.

Branden, C. and Tooze, J. (1991) *Introduction to protein structure*. New York and London, Garland Publishing, Inc.

Breton, R., Housset, D., Mazza, C. and Fontecilla-Camps, J.C. (1996) The structure of a complex of human 17-hydroxysteroid dehydrogenase with estradiol and NADP+ identifies two principal targets for the design of inhibitors. *Structure* **4**, 905–915.

Brimfield, A.A., Zweig, L.M., Novak, M.J. and Maxwell, D.M. (1998) In vitro oxidation of the hydrolysis product of sulfur mustard, 2,2′-thiobis-ethanol, by mammalian alcohol dehydrogenase. *J. Biochem. Mol. Toxicol.* **12**, 361–369.

Brodie, A.M. and Njar, V.C. (1998) Aromatase inhibitors in advanced breast cancer: mechanism of action and clinical implications. *J. Steroid Biochem. Mol. Biol.* **66**, 1–10.

Bronaugh, R.L., Stewart, R.F. and Congdon, E.R. (1983) Differences in permeability of rat skin related to sex and body site. *J. Soc. Cosmet. Chem.* **34**, 127–135.

Bronaugh, R.L. and Stewart, R.F. (1985) Methods of in vitro percutaneous absorption studies V: permeation through damaged skin. *J. Pharm. Sci.* **74**, 1062–1066.

Bronaugh, R.L., Weingarten, D.P. and Lowe, N.J. (1986) Differential rates of percutaneous absorption through the eczematous and normal skin of a monkey. *J. Invest. Dermatol.* **87**, 451–453.

Bronaugh, R.L., Collier, S.W., Macpherson, S.E. and Kraeling, M.E.K. (1994a) Influence of metabolism in skin on dosimetry after exposure. *Environ. Health Perspect.* **102**, 71–74.

Bronaugh, R.L., Roberts, C.D. and McCoy, J.L. (1994b) Dose-response relationship in skin sensitisation. *Food Chem. Toxicol.* **32**, 113–117.

Brown, M.G., Driscoll, J. and Monaco, J.J. (1991) Structural and serological similarity of MHC-linked LMP and proteasome (multicatalytic proteinase) complexes. *Nature* **353**, 355–357.

Brown, J.H., Jardetsky, T.S., Gorga, J.C., Stern, L.J., Urban, R.G., Strominger, J.L. and Wiley, D.C. (1993) Three-dimensional structure of the human class II histocompatibility antigen HLA-DR1. *Nature* **364**, 33–39.

Bruze, M. (1985) Contact sensitizers in resins based on phenol and formaldehyde. *Acta Derm. Venereol. Suppl.* **119**, 1–83.

Bruze, M. and Zimerson, E. (1997) Cross-reaction patterns in patients with contact allergy to simple methyl phenols. *Contact Dermatitis* **37**, 82–86.

BUCKS, D.A.W., MAIBACH, H.I. and GUY, R.H. (1989) Occlusion does not uniformly enhance penetration in vivo. In: BRONAUGH, R.L. and MAIBACH, H.I. (eds), *Percutaneous Absorption: Mechanisms, Methodology, Drug Delivery*. New York, Dekker, 77–93.

BUCKS, D.A.W., GUY, R.H. and MAIBACH, H.I. (1991) Effects of occlusion. In: BRONAUGH, R.L. and MAIBACH, H.I. (eds), *In vitro percutaneous absorption: principles, fundamentals and applications*. Florida, CRC Press, 85–113.

BUNDGAARD, H. (1980) The possible implication of steroid-glyoxal degradation products in allergic reactions to corticosteroids. *Arch. Pharm. Chem. Sci. Ed.* **8**, 83–90.

BURCHELL, B. and COUGHTRIE, M.W. (1997) Genetic and environmental factors associated with variation of human xenobiotic glucuronidation and sulfation. *Environ. Health Perspect.* **105**, 739–747.

BURR, M.L. (1993) *Epidemiology of Clinical Allergy*. Berlin, Karger.

BUUS, S. (1999) Description and prediction of peptide-MHC binding: the 'human MHC project'. *Current Opin. Immunol.* **11**, 209–213.

CAMPBELL, J.A., CORRIGALL, A.V., GUY, A. and KIRSCH, R.E. (1991) Immunohistologic localization of alpha, mu, and pi class glutathione S-transferases in human tissues. *Cancer* **67**, 1608–1613.

CARDULLO, A.C., RUSZKOWSKI, A.M. and DELEO, V.A. (1989) Allergic contact dermatitis resulting from sensitivity to citrus peel, geraniol, and citral. *J. Am. Acad. Dermatol.* **21**, 395–397.

CARR, M.M., BOTHAM, P.A., GAWKRODGER, D.J., MCVITTIE, E., ROSS, J.A., STEWART, I.C. and HUNTER, J.A. (1984) Early cellular reactions induced by dinitrochlorobenzene in sensitized human skin. *Br. J. Dermatol.* **110**, 637–641.

CATANZARO, J.M. and SMITH, J.G., JR. (1991) Propylene glycol dermatitis. *J. Am. Acad. Dermatol.* **24**, 90–95.

CAVANI, A., HACKETT, C.J., WILSON, K.J., ROTHBARD, J.B. and KATZ, S.I. (1995) Characterization of epitopes recognized by hapten-specific CD4+ T cells. *J. Immunol.* **154**, 1232–1238.

CHANEZ, J.F., DE-LIGNIERES, B., MARTY, J.P. and WEPIERRE, J. (1979) Influence of the size of the area of treatment on percutaneous absorption of estradiol in the rat. *Skin Pharmacol.* **2**, 15–21.

CHAPMAN, P.H., RAWLINS, M.D. and SHUSTER, S. (1979) The activity of aryl hydrocarbon hydroxylase in adult human skin. *Br. J. Clin. Pharmacol.* **7**, 499–503.

CHASE, M.W. (1982) The induction of tolerance to allergenic chemicals. *Ann. NY Acad. Sci.* **392**, 228–247.

CHEN, S. (1998) Aromatase and breast cancer. *Front Biosci.* **3**, 922–933.

CHEN, W.C., ZOUBOULIS, C.C., FRITSCH, M., BLUME PEYTAVI, U., KODELJA, V., GOERDT, S., LUU THE, V. and ORFANOS, C.E. (1998) Evidence of heterogeneity and quantitative differences of the type I 5-alpha reductase expression in cultured human skin cells — Evidence of its presence in melanocytes. *J. Invest. Dermatol.* **110**, 84–89.

CHEUNG, C., SMITH, C.K., HOOG, J.-O. and HOTCHKISS, S.A.M. (1999) Expression and Localisation of Human Alcohol and Aldehyde Dehydrogenase Enzymes in Skin. *Biophys. Biochem. Res. Comm.* **261**, 100–107.

CHEUNG, C., EDWARDS, R.J., BOOBIS, A.R. and HOTCHKISS, S.A.M. (2000a) Expression of CYP3A enzymes in mouse liver and skin. Proceedings of the Microsomal Drug Oxidation meeting, Stresa, Italy. Abstract.

CHEUNG, C., SMITH, C.K., HOOG, J.-O. and HOTCHKISS, S.A.M. (2000b) Species Comparisons in Expression and Localisation of Cutaneous and Hepatic Alcohol and Aldehyde Dehydrogenase Enzymes. Submitted to *Toxicol. Appl. Pharmacol.*

CHIU, N.M., WANG, B., KERKSIEK, K.M., KURLANDER, R., PAMER, E.G. and WANG, C.-R. (1999) The selection of M3-restricted T cells is dependent on M3 expression and presentation of N-formylated peptides in the thymus. *J. Exp. Med.* **190**, 1869–1878.

CHOI, H.K., FLYNN, G.L. and AMIDON, G.L. (1990) Transdermal delivery of bioactive peptides: the effect of n-decylmethylsulfoxide, pH, and inhibitors on enkephalin metabolism and transport. *Pharm. Res.* **7**, 1099–1106.

CHRISTOPHERS, E. and KLIGMAN, A.M. (1965) Percutaneous absorption in aged skin. In: MONTAGNA, W. (ed.), *Advances in biology of the skin*, Vol. 6, Ageing. Oxford, Pergamon Press, 163–175.

CHUNG, K. (1983) The significance of azo-reduction in the mutagenesis and carcinogenesis of azo-dyes. *Mutat. Res.* **114**, 269–281.

CHUNG, J.G., LEVY, G.N. and WEBER, W.W. (1993) Distribution of 2-aminofluorene and p-aminobenzoic acid N-acetyltransferase activity in tissues of C57BL/6J rapid and B6.A-Nat slow acetylator congenic mice. *Drug Metab. Dispos.* **21**, 1057–1063.

CIECHANOVER, A. (1994) The ubiquitin-proteasome proteolytic pathway. *Cell* **79**, 13–21.

CLARK, N.W.E., SCOTT, R.C., BLAIN, P.G. and WILLIAMS, F.M. (1993) Fate of fluazifop butyl in rat and human skin in vitro. *Arch. Toxicol.* **67**, 44–48.

CLEMMENSEN, S. (1985) Sensitizing potential of 2-hydroxyethylmethacrylate. *Contact Dermatitis* **12**, 203–208.

CLONFERO, E., ZORDAN, M., COTTICA, D., VENIER, P., POZZOLI, L., CARDIN, E.L., SARTO, F. and LEVIS, A.G. (1986) Mutagenic activity and polycyclic aromatic hydrocarbon levels in urine of humans exposed to therapeutic coal tar. *Carcinogenesis* **7**, 819–823.

COLBY, T.D., BAHNSON, B.J., CHIN, J.K., KLINMAN, J.P. and GOLDSTEIN, B.M. (1998) Active site modifications in a double mutant of liver alcohol dehydrogenase: structural studies of two enzyme-ligand complexes. *Biochemistry* **37**, 9295–9304.

COLLIER, S.W., STORM, J.E. and BRONAUGH, R.L. (1993) Reduction of azo dyes during in vitro percutaneous absorption. *Toxicol. & Appl. Pharmacol.* **118**, 73–79.

CONDE, S.L., BAZ, M., GUIMARAENS, D. and CANNAVO, A. (1995) Contact dermatitis in hairdressers: patch test results in 379 hairdressers (1980–1993). *Contact Dermatitis* **6**, 19–23.

CONDUAH BIRT, J.E.E., SHUKER, D.E.G. and FARMER, P.B. (1998) Stable acetaldehyde-protein adducts as biomarkers of alcohol exposure. *Chem. Res. Toxicol.* **11**, 136–142.

COOMBS, R.R.A. and GELL, P.G.H. (1975) Classification of allergic reactions for clinical hypersensitivity and disease. In: GELL, P.G.H., COOMBS, R.R.A. and LACHMAN, R. (eds), *Clinical Aspects of Immunology*. London, Blackwell Scientific, 761–781.

COOMES, M.W., NORLING, A.H., POHL, R.J., MULLER, D. and FOUTS, J.R. (1983) Foreign compound metabolism by isolated skin cells from the hairless mouse. *J. Pharmacol. Exp. Ther.* **225**, 770–777.

COOMES, M.W., SPARKS, R.W. and FOUTS, J.R. (1984) Oxidation of 7-ethoxycoumarin and conjugation of umbelliferone by intact, viable epidermal cells from the hairless mouse. *J. Invest. Dermatol.* **82**, 598–601.

COOPER, A.J. (1998) Mechanisms of cysteine S-conjugate beta-lyases. *Adv. Enzymol. Relat. Areas Mol. Biol.* **72**, 199–238.

COOPMAN, S., DEGREEF, H. and DOOMS-GOOSSENS, A. (1989) Identification of cross-reaction patterns in allergic contact dermatitis from topical corticosteroids. *Br. J. Dermatol.* **121**, 27–34.

CORAZZA, M., MANTOVANI, L., TRIMURTI, S. and VIRGILI, A. (1994) Occupational contact sensitization to ethylendiamine in a nurse. *Contact Dermatitis* **31**, 328–329.

CORAZZA, M., MANTOVANI, L., MARANINI, C. and VIRGILI, A. (1996) Allergic contact dermatitis from benzyl alcohol. *Contact Dermatitis* **34**, 74–75.

CORMIER, M., LEDGER, P.W., MARTY, J.P. and AMKRAUT, A. (1991) In vitro cutaneous biotransformation of propranolol. *J. Invest. Dermatol.* **97**, 447–453.

CORONEOS, E. and SIM, E. (1993) Arylamine N-acetyltransferase activity in human cultured cell lines. *Biochem. J.* **294**, 481–486.

COS, P., YING, L., CALOMME, M., HU, J.P., CIMANGA, K., VAN POEL, B., PIETERS, L., VLIETINCK, A.J. and VANDEN BERGHE, D. (1998) Structure-activity relationship and classification of flavonoids as inhibitors of xanthine oxidase and superoxide scavengers. *J. Nat. Prod.* **61**, 71–76.

COTOVIO, J., ROGUET, R., PION, F.X., ROUGIER, A. and LECLAIRE, J. (1996) Effect of imidazole derivatives on cytochrome P450 enzyme activities in a reconstructed human epidermis. *Skin Pharmacol.* **9**, 242–249.

COTOVIO, J., LECLAIRE, J. and ROGUET, R. (1997) Cytochrome P450-dependent enzyme activities in normal adult human keratinocytes and transformed human keratinocytes. *In Vitro Toxicol.* **10**, 207–216.

COUGHTRIE, M.W. (1996) Sulphation catalysed by the human cytosolic sulphotransferases — chemical defence or molecular terrorism. *Human & Exp. Toxicol.* **15**, 547–555.

COUGHTRIE, M.W., SHARP, S., MAXWELL, K. and INNES, N.P. (1998) Biology and function of the reversible sulfation pathway catalysed by human sulfotransferases and sulfatases. *Chem. Biol. Interact.* **109**, 3–27.

COURCHAY, G., BOYERA, N., BERNARD, B.A. and MAHE, Y. (1996) Messenger RNA expression of steroidogenesis enzyme subtypes in the human pilosebaceous unit. *Skin Pharmacol.* **9**, 169–176.

CRAIU, A., AKOPIAN, T., GOLDBERG, A. and ROCK, K.L. (1997) Two distinct proteolytic processes in the generation of an MHC class-I presented peptide. *Proc. Natl. Acad. Sci. USA* **94**, 10850–10855.

CRAVATT, B.F., GIANG, D.K., MAYFIELD, S.P., BOGER, D.L., LERNER, R.A. and GILULA, N.B. (1996) Molecular characterisation of an enzyme that degrades neuromodulatory fatty-acid amides. *Nature* **384**, 83–87.

CRONIN, E. and STOUGHTON, R.B. (1962) Regional variations and the effects of hydration and epidermal stripping. *Br. J. Dermatol.* **74**, 265–272.

CRONIN, M.T.D. and BASKETTER, D.A. (1994) Multivariate QSAR analysis of a skin sensitization database. *SAR & QSAR in Environmental Research* **2**, 159–179.

CROUT, D.H. and VIC, G. (1998) Glycosidases and glycosyl transferases in glycoside and oligosaccharide synthesis. *Curr. Opin. Chem. Biol.* **2**, 98–111.

CUMMINGS, E.G. (1969) Temperature and concentration effects on percutaneous penetration of N-octylamine through human skin in situ. *J. Invest. Dermatol.* **53**, 64–68.

DANNAN, G.A. and GUENGERICH, F.P. (1982) Immunochemical comparison and quantitation of microsomal flavin-containing monooxygenases in various hog, mouse, rat, rabbit, dog and human tissues. *Mol. Pharmacol.* **22**, 787–794.

DANON, A., BEN-SHIMON, S. and BEN-ZUI, Z. (1986) Effect of exercise and heat exposure on percutaneous absorption of methyl salicylate. *Eur. J. Clin. Pharmacol.* **3**, 49–52.

DAS, M., BICKERS, D.R. and MUKHTAR, H. (1986) Epidermis: The major site of cutaneous benzo(a)pyrene and benzo(a)pyrene-7,8-diol metabolism in neonatal BALB/c mice. *Drug Metab. Dispos.* **14**, 637–642.

DAVEY, C.A. and FENNA, R.E. (1996) 2.3A resolution X-ray crystal structure of the bisubstrate analogue inhibitor salicylhydroxamic acid bound to human myeloperoxidase: a model for a prereaction complex with hydrogen peroxide. *Biochemistry* **35**, 10967–10973.

DAVIS, G.J., BOSRON, W.F., STONE, C.L., OWUSU-DEKYI, K. and HURLEY, T.D. (1996) X-ray structure of human beta3beta3 alcohol dehydrogenase. The contribution of ionic interactions to coenzyme binding. *J. Biol. Chem.* **271**, 17057–17061.

DE BERSAQUES, J. (1972) Peptidases and naphthylamidases in human skin: Influence of buffers, EDTA and metals on dipeptide arylamidase III. *Enzymologia* **43**, 253–259.

DE GROOT, A.C. and WEYLAND, J.W. (1988) Kathon CG: A review. *J. Am. Acad. Dermatol.* **18**, 350–358.

DEARMAN, R.J., MOUSSAVI, A., KEMENY, D.M. and KIMBER, I. (1996) Contribution of CD4+ and CD8+ T lymphocyte subsets to the cytokine secretion patterns induced in mice during sensitization to contact and respiratory chemical allergens. *Immunology* **89**, 502–510.

DEARMAN, R.J., HILTON, J., EVANS, P., HARVEY, P., BASKETTER, D.A. and KIMBER, I. (1998) Temporal stability of local lymph node assay responses to hexyl cinnamic aldehyde. *J. Appl. Toxicol.* **18**, 281–284.

DEARMAN, R.J. and KIMBER, I. (1999) Cytokine fingerprinting: characterization of chemical allergens. *Methods* **19**, 56–63.

DEBORD, J., DANTOINE, T., BOLLINGER, J.C., ABRAHAM, M.H., VERNEUIL, B. and MERLE, L. (1998) Inhibition of arylesterase by aliphatic alcohols. *Chem. Biol. Interact.* **113**, 105–115.

DEKANT, W. and VAMVAKAS, S. (1993) Glutathione-dependent bioactivation of xenobiotics. *Xenobiotica* **23**, 873–887.

DEL TITO, B.J. JNR., MUKHTAR, H. and BICKERS, D.R. (1984) In vivo metabolism of topically applied benzo(a)pyrene-4,5-oxide in neonatal rat skin. *J. Invest. Dermatol.* **82**, 378–380.

DELAFORGE, M., JANIAUD, P., LEVI, P. and MORIZOT, J.P. (1980) Biotransformation of allylbenzene analogues in vivo and in vitro through the epoxide-diol pathway. *Xenobiotica* **10**, 737–744.

DELICONSTANTINOS, G., VILLIOTOU, V. and STAVRIDES, J.C. (1996) Alterations of nitric oxide synthase and xanthine oxidase activities of human keratinocytes by ultraviolet B radiation. Potential role for peroxynitrite in skin inflammation. *Biochem. Pharmacol.* **51**, 1727–1738.

DENNEY, R.M. (1998) Relationship between monoamine oxidase (MAO) A specific activity and proportion of human skin fibroblasts which express the enzyme in culture. *J. Neural. Transm. Suppl.* **52**, 17–27.

DENNEY, R.M., KOCH, H. and CRAIG, I.W. (1999) Association between monoamine oxidase A activity in human male skin fibroblasts and genotype of the MAOA promoter-associated variable number tandem repeat. *Hum. Genet.* **105**, 542–551.

Dery, O., Corvera, C.U., Steinhoff, M. and Bunnett, N.W. (1998) Proteinase-activated receptors: novel mechanisms of signalling by serine proteases. *Am. J. Physiol.* **274**, C1429–1452.

Dessen, A., Lawrence, C.M., Cupo, S., Zaller, D.M. and Wiley, D.C. (1997) X-ray crystal structure of HLA-DR4 (DRA*0101, DRB1*0401) complexed with a peptide from human collagen II. *Immunity* **7**, 473–481.

Dias, M., Farinha, A., Faustino, E., Hadgraft, J., Pais, J. and Toscano, C. (1999) Topical delivery of caffeine from some commercial formulations. *Int. J. Pharm.* **182**, 41–47.

Dick, I.P. and Scott, R.C. (1992) The influence of different strains and age on in vitro rat skin permeability to water and mannitol. *Pharmaceut. Res.* **9**, 884–887.

Dietrich, A., Kawakubo, Y., Rzany, B., Mockenhaupt, M., Simon, J.C. and Schopf, E. (1995) Low N-acetylating capacity in patients with Stevens-Johnson syndrome and toxic epidermal necrolysis. *Exp. Dermatol.* **4**, 313–316.

Dijkstra, A.C., Misdom, L.W., Goos, C.M., Hukkelhoven, M.W. and Vermorken, A.J. (1986) Glutathione-S-epoxide transferase in human hair follicles. *Cancer Lett.* **31**, 105–112.

Dilulio, N.A., Engeman, T., Armstrong, D., Tannenbaum, C., Hamilton, T.A. and Fairchild, R.L. (1999) Groalpha-mediated recruitment of neutrophils is required for elicitation of contact hypersensitivity. *Eur. J. Immunol.* **29**, 3485–3495.

Ditlow, C.C., Holmquist, B., Morelock, M.M. and Vallee, B.L. (1984) Physical and enzymatic properties of a class II alcohol dehydrogenase isozyme of human liver: pi-ADH. *Biochemistry* **23**(26), 6363–6368.

Dolphin, C.T., Cullingford, T.E., Shephard, E.A., Smith, R.L. and Phillips, I.R. (1996) Differential developmental and tissue-specific regulation of expression of the genes encoding three members of the flacin-containing monooxygenase family of man, FMO1, FMO3 and FMO4. *Eur. J. Biochem.* **235**, 683–689.

Dooley, T.P., Walker, C.J., Hirshey, S.J., Falany, C.N. and Diani, A.R. (1991) Localization of minoxidil sulfotransferase in rat liver and the outer root sheath of anagen pelage and vibrissa follicles. *J. Invest. Dermatol.* **96**, 65–70.

Dooms-Goossens, A., Meinardi, M.M.H.M., Bos, J.D. and Degreef, A.H. (1994) Contact allergy to corticosteroids: the results of a two-centre study. *Br. J. Dermatol.* **130**, 42–47.

Duell, E.A., Kang, S. and Voorhees, J.J. (1996a) Retinoic acid isomers applied to human skin in vivo each induce a 4-hydroxylase that inactivates only trans retinoic acid. *J. Invest. Dermatol.* **106**, 316–320.

Duell, E.A., Derguini, F., Kang, S., Elder, J.T. and Voorhees, J.J. (1996b) Extraction of human epidermis treated with retinol yields retro-retinoids in addition to free retinol and retinyl esters. *J. Invest. Dermatol.* **107**, 178–182.

DUESTER, G., FARRES, J., FELDER, M.R., HOLMES, R.S., HOOG, J.-O., PARES, X., PLAPP, B.V., YIN, S.J. and JORNVALL, H. (1999) Recommended nomenclature for the vertebrate alcohol dehydrogenase gene family. *Biochem. Pharmacol.* **58**, 389–395.

DUMONT, M., VAN, L.T., DUPONT, E., PELLETIER, G. and LABRIE, F. (1992) Characterisation, expression, and immunohistochemical localization of 3 beta-hydroxysteroid dehydrogenase/delta 5-delta 4 isomerase in human skin. *J. Invest. Dermatol.* **99**, 415–421.

DUPUIS, G. (1979) Studies on poison ivy. In vitro lymphocyte transformation by urushiol-protein conjugates. *Br. J. Dermatol.* **101**, 617–624.

DUPUIS, G. and BENEZRA, C. (1982) *Allergic Contact Dermatitis to Simple Chemicals: A Molecular Approach.* New York & Basel, Marcel Dekker Inc.

EDELSTEIN, S.B. and BREAKEFIELD, X.O. (1986) Monoamine oxidases A and B are differentially regulated by glucocorticoids and aging in human skin fibroblasts. *Cell Mol. Neurobiol.* **6**, 121–150.

EDWARDS, R.J., ADAMS, D.A., WATTS, P.S., DAVIES, D.S. and BOOBIS, A.R. (1998) Development of a comprehensive panel of antibodies against major xenobiotic metabolising forms of cytochrome P450 in humans. *Biochem. Pharmacol.* **56**, 377–387.

EGGLESTON, S.T. and LUSH, L.W. (1996) Understanding allergic reactions to local anesthetics. *Ann. Pharmacother.* **30**, 851–857.

EICHELER, W., HAPPLE, R. and HOFFMANN, R. (1998) 5-alpha reductase activity in the human follicle concentrates in the dermal papilla. *Arch. Dermatological Res.* **290**, 126–132.

EIERMANN, B., EDLUND, P.O., TJERNBERG, A., DALEN, P., DAHL, M.L. and BERTILSSON, L. (1998) 1- and 3-hydroxylations, in addition to 4-hydroxylation, of debrisoquine are catalysed by cytochrome P450 2D6 in humans. *Drug Metab. Dispos.* **26**, 1096–1101.

EINOLF, H.J., STORY, W.T., MARCUS, C.B., LARSEN, M.C., JEFCOATE, C.R., GREENLEE, W.F., YAGI, H., JERINA, D.M., AMIN, S., PARK, S., GELBOIN, H.V. and BAIRD, W.M. (1997) Role of cytochrome P450 enzyme induction in the metabolic activation of benzo(c)phenanthrene in human cell lines and mouse epidermis. *Chem. Res. Toxicol.* **10**, 609–617.

ELAHI, E., SMITH, C.K. and HOTCHKISS, S.A.M. (2000) Immunochemical detection of hapten-modified proteins in cinnamaldehyde-treated human skin. *Drug Metabolism Reviews*, **32**, Suppl 1, 104.

ELIAS, P.M. (1981) Percutaneous transport in relation to stratum corneum structure and lipid composition. *J. Invest. Dermatol.* **76**, 297–301.

ELIAS, P.M., COOPER, E.R., KORC, A. and BROWN, B.E. (1981) Percutaneous transport in relation to stratum corneum structure and lipid composition. *J. Invest. Dermatol.* **76**, 297–301.

ELIAS, P.M., FEINGOLD, K.R., MENON, G.K., GRAYSON, S., WILLIAMS, M.L. and GRUBAUER, G.

(1987) The stratum corneum two-compartment model and its functional implications. In: SHROOT, B. and SCHAEFER, H. (eds), *Pharmacology and the Skin*, Vol. 1. Berlin, Karger, 1–9.

ELIASSON, E., GARDNER, I.H.H.-S., DE WAZIERS, I., BEAUNE, P. and KENNA, J.G. (1998) Interindividual variability in P450-dependent generation of neoantigens in halothane hepatitis. *Chem. Biol. Interact.* **116**, 123–141.

EL-KATTAN, A.F., ASBILL, C.S. and MICHNIAK, B.B. (2000) The effect of terpene enhancer lipophilicity on the percutaneous permeation of hydrocortisone formulated in HPMC gel systems. *Int. J. Pharm.* **198**, 179–189.

EMERIT, I. (1992) Free radicals and aging of the skin. *EXS* **62**, 328–341.

EMMETT, E.A. (1991) Toxic responses of the skin. In: AMDUR, M.O., DOULL, J. and KLASSEN, C.D. (eds), *Casarett and Doull's Toxicology*. New York, Pergamon Press, 463–483.

ENGELAND, K. and MARET, W. (1993) Extrahepatic, differential expression of four classes of human alcohol dehydrogenase. *Biochem. Biophys. Research Comm.* **193**, 47–53.

ENGLAND, P.A., HARFORD-CROSS, C.F., STEVENSON, J.A., ROUCH, D.A. and WONG, L.L. (1998) The oxidation of naphthalene and pyrene by cytochrome P450cam. *FEBS Lett.* **424**, 271–274.

ENGLISH, J.S. and RYCROFT, R.J. (1989) Occupational sensitization to ethylenediamine in a floor polish remover. *Contact Dermatitis* **20**, 220–221.

ENK, A.H. and KATZ, S.I. (1992) Early molecular events in the induction phase of contact sensitivity. *Proc. Natl. Acad. Sci.* **89**, 1398–1402.

EPSTEIN, E. and MAIBACH, H.I. (1966) Formaldehyde allergy. Incidence and patch test problems. *Arch. Dermatol.* **94**, 186–190.

EPSTEIN, W.L., BAER, H., DAWSON, C.R. and KHURANA, R.G. (1974) Poison oak hyposensitization. Evaluation of purified urushiol. *Arch. Dermatol.* **109**, 356–360.

EPSTEIN, E.H. JR., BONIFAS, J.M., BARBER, T.C. and HAYNES, M. (1984) Cholesterol sulfotransferase of newborn mouse epidermis. *J. Invest. Dermatol.* **83**, 332–335.

EPSTEIN, E.H. JR., LANGSTON, A.W. and LEUNG, J. (1988) Sulfation reactions of the epidermis. In: MILSTONE, L.M. and EDELSON, R.L. (eds), *Endocrine, metabolic and immunologic function of keratinocytes*, New York, New York Academy of Sciences, 97–101.

ESTONIUS, M., HOOG, J.O., DANIELSSON, O. and JORNVALL, H. (1994) Residues specific for class-III alcohol dehydrogenase — site-directed mutagenesis of the human enzyme. *Biochemistry* **33**, 15080–15085.

FALANY, C.N., JOHNSON, M.R., BARNES, S. and DIASIO, R.B. (1994) Glycine and taurine conjugation of bile acids by a single enzyme. Molecular cloning and expression of human liver bile acid CoA:amino acid N-acyltransferase. *J. Biol. Chem.* **269**, 19375–19379.

FALK, K., ROTZSCHKE, O., STEVANOVIC, S., JUNG, G. and RAMMENSEE, H.-G. (1991) Allele-specific motifs revealed by sequencing of self-peptides eluted from MHC molecules. *Nature* **351**, 290–295.

FANG, J., COUTTS, R.T., MCKENNA, K.F. and BAKER, G.B. (1998) Elucidation of individual cytochrome P450 enzymes involved in the metabolism of clozapine. *Naunyn Schmiedebergs Arch. Pharmacol.* **358**, 592–599.

FAREDIN, I., TOTH, I., FAZEKAS, A.G., KOKAI, K. and JULESZ, M. (1968) Conjugation in vitro of [4-14C]-dihydroepiandrosterone to [4-14C]-dehydroepiandrosterone sulfate by normal human female skin slices. *J. Endocrinol.* **41**, 295–296.

FARM, G. (1998) Contact allergy to colophony. Clinical and experimental studies with emphasis on clinical relevance. *Acta Derm. Venereol. Suppl. (Stockh.)* **201**, 1–42.

FELDMANN, R.J. and MAIBACH, H.I. (1967) Regional variation in percutaneous penetration of [14C] cortisol in man. *J. Appl. Toxicol.* **9**, 239–244.

FELDMANN, R.J. and MAIBACH, H.I. (1969a) Absorption of some organic compounds through the skin in man. *J. Invest. Dermatol.* **54**, 399–404.

FESSENDEN, R.J. and FESSENDEN, J.S. (1990) 'Organic chemistry', 4th edition/Ed. Wadsworth Inc., Belmont CA.

FINNEN, M.J., HERDMAN, M.L. and SHUSTER, S. (1985) Distribution and sub-cellular localisation of drug metabolising enzymes in the skin. *Br. J. Dermatol.* **113**, 713–721.

FINNEN, M.J. and SHUSTER, S. (1985a) Phase I and phase 2 drug metabolism in isolated epidermal cells from adult hairless mice and in whole human hair follicles. *Biochem. Pharmacol.* **34**, 3571–3575.

FINNEN, M.J. (1987) Skin metabolism by oxidation and conjugation. In: SHROOT, B. and SCHAEFER, H. (eds), *Pharmacology and the Skin*, Vol 1. Skin Pharmacokinetics, Basel, Karger, 163–169.

FISCHER, T.I. and MAIBACH, H.I. (1985) The thin layer rapid use epicutaneous test (TRUE-test), a new patch test method with higher accuracy. *Br. J. Dermatol.* **112**, 63–68.

FISCHER, I.U., VON UNRUH, G.E. and DENGLER, H.J. (1990) The metabolism of eugenol in man. *Xenobiotica* **20**, 209–222.

FISHBEIN, I., CHORNY, M., RABINOVICH, L., BANAI, S., GATI, I. and GOLOMB, G. (2000) Nanoparticulate delivery system of a tyrphostin for the treatment of restenosis. *J. Control. Rel.* **65**, 221–229.

FLINT, M.S., DEARMAN, R.J., KIMBER, I. and HOTCHKISS, S.A.M. (1998) Production and in situ localisation of cutaneous tumour necrosis factor alpha (TNF-a) and interleukin 6 (IL-6) following skin sensitisation. *Cytokine* **10**, 213–219.

FLYNN, G.L. (1990) Physicochemical determinants of skin absorption. In: GERRITY, T.R. and HENRY, C.J. (eds), *Principles of route-to-route extrapolation for risk assessment*, New York, Elsevier, 93–127.

FRAKI, J.E. (1976) Human skin proteases. Separation and characterization of two acid proteases resembling cathepsin B1 and cathepsin D and of an inhibitor of cathepsin B1. *Arch. Dermatol. Res.* **255**, 317–330.

FRANOT, C., ROBERTS, D.W., SMITH, R.G., BASKETTER, D.A., BENEZRA, C. and LEPOITTEVIN, J.-P. (1994a) Structure-activity relationships for contact allergenic potential of gamma,gamma-dimethyl-gamma-butyrolactone derivatives. 1. Synthesis and electrophilic reactivity studies of alpha-(omega-substituted-alkyl)-gamma-gamma-dimethyl-gamma-butyrolactones and correlation of skin sensitisation potential and cross-sensitisation patterns with structure. *Chem. Res. Toxicol.* **7**, 297–306.

FRANOT, C., ROBERTS, D.W., BASKETTER, D.A., BENEZRA, C. and LEPOITTEVIN, J.-P. (1994b) Structure-activity relationships for contact allergenic potential of gamma,gamma-dimethyl-gamma-butyrolactone derivatives. 2. Quantitative structure-skin sensitization relationships for alpha-substituted-alpha-methyl-gamma,gamma-dimethyl-gamma-butyrolactones. *Chem. Res. Toxicol.* **7**, 307–312.

FREEMAN, S. (1995) Corticosteroid allergy. *Contact Dermatitis* **33**, 240–242.

FREGERT, S. (1970) Sensitization to phenylacetaldehyde. *Dermatologica* **141**, 11–14.

FREMONT, D.H., MATSUMURA, M., STURA, E.A., PETERSON, P.A. and WILSON, I.A. (1992) Crystal structures of two viral peptides in complex with murine MHC class I H-2Kb. *Science* **257**, 919–927.

FREMONT, D.H., STURA, E.A., MATSUMURA, M., PETERSON, P.A. and WILSON, I.A. (1995) Crystal structure of an H-2Kb-ovalbumin peptide complex reveals the interplay of primary and secondary anchor positions in the major histocompatibility complex binding groove. *Proc. Natl. Acad. Sci. USA* **92**, 2479–2483.

FRIEDBERG, T., GRASSOW, M.A., BARTLOMOWICZ-OESCH, B., SIEGERT, P., ARAND, M., ADESNIK, M. and OESCH, F. (1992) Sequence of a novel cytochrome CYP2B cDNA coding for a protein which is expressed in a sebaceous gland but not in the liver. *Biochem. J.* **287**, 775–783.

FRITSCH, M., SELTMANN, H. and ZOUBOULIS, C.C. (1998) Androgen metabolism in human skin cells in vitro: sebocytes produce active androgens while keratinocytes inactivate them. *J. Invest. Dermatol.* **110**, 542.

FRUH, K. and YANG, Y. (1999) Antigen presentation by MHC class I and its regulation by interferon gamma. *Curr. Opin. Immunol.* **11**, 76–81.

FUCHS, J., FREISLEBEN, H.-J. and PACKER, L. (1987) Antioxidants in the Skin. In: SHROOT, B. and SCHAEFER, H. (eds), *Pharmacology and the Skin*, Vol. 1. Basel, Karger, 249–267.

FUCHS, J., MEHLHORN, R.J. and PACKER, L. (1989) Free radical reduction mechanisms in mouse epidermis skin homogenates. *J. Invest. Dermatol.* **93**, 633–640.

FUCHS, J., GROTH, N., HERRLING, T. and ZIMMER, G. (1997) Electron paramagnetic resonance studies on nitroxide radical 2,2,5,5-tetramethyl-4-piperidin-1-oxyl (TEMPO) redox reactions in human skin. *Free Radical Biol. and Med.* **22**, 967–976.

FUJISAWA, H., KONDO, S., WANG, B., SHIVJI, G.M. and SAUDER, D.N. (1996) The role of CD4 molecules in the induction phase of contact hypersensitivity cytokine profiles in the skin and lymph nodes. *Immunology* **89**, 250–255.

FUNK, C.D., KEENEY, D.S., OLIW, E.H., BOEGLIN, W.E. and BRASH, A.R. (1996) Functional expression and cellular localisation of a mouse epidermal lipoxygenase. *J. Biol. Chem.* **271**, 23338–23344.

GAFVERT, E., SHAO, L.P., KARLBERG, A.T., NILSSON, U. and NILSSON, J.L. (1994) Contact allergy to resin acid hydroperoxides. Hapten binding via free radicals and epoxides. *Chem. Res. Toxicol.* **7**, 260–266.

GALLEGOS, A.J. and BERLINER, D.L. (1967) Transformation and conjugation of dehydropiandrosterone by human skin. *J. Clin. Endocrinol. Metab.* **27**, 1214–1218.

GARBOCZI, D.N., GHOSH, P., UTZ, U., FAN, Q.R., BIDDISON, W.E. and WILEY, D.C. (1996) Structure of the complex between human T-cell receptor, viral peptide and HLA-A2. *Nature* **384**, 134–141.

GARCIA, K.C., DEGANO, M., PEASE, L.R., HUANG, M., PETERSON, P.A., TEYTON, L. and WILSON, I.A. (1998) Structural basis of plasticity in T cell receptor recognition of a self peptide-MHC antigen. *Science* **279**, 1166–1172.

GARMANN, E.M. and GOLLNICK, H.P. (1995) Immunophenotyping of the cellular infiltrate in the early elicitation phase of contact dermatitis in the skin of presensitized atopic individuals. *Arch. Dermatol. Res.* **287**, 129–136.

GARNETT, A. (1992) Investigation of the in vitro percutaneous absorption and skin metabolism of benzyl acetate and related compounds. PhD, University of London, London.

GARNETT, A., HOTCHKISS, S.A.M. and CALDWELL, J. (1994) Percutaneous absorption of benzyl acetate through rat skin in vitro. 3. A comparison with human skin. *Fd. Chem. Toxicol.* **32**, 1061–1065.

GARRIGUE, J.L., CATROUX, P. and LECLAIRE, J. (1995) IMPT! Predictive molecular and genetic toxicology — application to the detection of sensitising potential of xenobiotics. *Clin. Rev. in Allergy & Immunol.* **13**, 189–200.

GAUDET, S.J., SLOMINSKI, A., ETMINAN, M., PRUSKI, D., PAUS, R. and NAMBOODIRI, M.A.A. (1993) Identification and characterisation of two isozymic forms of arylamine N-acetyltransferase in Syrian-hamster skin. *J. Invest. Dermatol.* **101**, 660–665.

GAUSTAD, R., JOHNSEN, H. and FONNUM, F. (1991) Carboxylesterases in guinea pig: A comparison of the different isoenzymes with regard to inhibition by organophosphorus compounds in vivo and in vitro. *Biochem. Pharmacol.* **42**, 1335–1343.

GAWKRODGER, D.J. (1997) *Dermatology: An Illustrated Colour Text,* 2nd edition/Ed. Churchill Livingstone, Edinburgh.

GERBERICK, G.F., CRUSE, L.W. and RYAN, C.A. (1999) Local lymph node assay: differentiating allergic and irritant responses using flow cytometry. *Methods* **19**, 48–55.

GERMAIN, R.N. and MARGULIES, D.H. (1993) The biochemistry and cell biology of antigen processing and presentation. *Annu. Rev. Immunol.* **11**, 403–450.

GHOSH, M.K. and MITRA, A.K. (1990) Carboxylic ester hydrolase activity in hairless and athymic nude mouse skin. *Pharmaceut. Res.* **7**, 251–255.

GHOSH, P., AMAYA, M., MELLINS, E. and WILEY, D.C. (1995) The structure of an intermediate in class II MHC maturation: CLIP bound to HLA-DR3. *Nature* **378**, 457–462.

GIANG, D.K. and CRAVATT, B.F. (1997) Molecular characterisation of human and mouse fatty acid amide hydrolases. *Proc. Natl. Acad. Sci.* **94**, 2238–2242.

GILL, D., MERLIN, K., PLUNKETT, A., JOLLEY, D. and MARKS, R. (2000) Population based surveys on the frequency of common skin diseases in adults — is there a risk of response bias? *Clin. Experim. Dermatol.* **25**, 62–66.

GIROLOMONI, G., CRUZ , P.D. JNR. and BERGSTRESSER, P.R. (1990) Internalization and acidification of surface HLA-DR molecules by epidermal Langerhans' cells: a paradigm for antigen processing. *J. Invest. Dermatol.* **94**, 753–760.

GLAUSER, T.A., KERREMANS, A.L. and WEINSHILBOUM, R.M. (1992) Human hepatic microsomal thiol methyltransferase. Assay conditions, biochemical properties, and correlation studies. *Drug Metab. Dispos.* **20**, 247–255.

GLYNNE, R., POWIS, S.H., BECK, S., KELLY, A., KERR, L.A. and TROWSDALE, J. (1991) A proteasome-related gene between the two ABC transporter loci in the class II region of the human MHC. *Nature* **353**, 357–360.

GNIADECKI, R. and CALVERLEY, M.J. (1998) Evidence for the activation of vitamin D compounds in the skin by side-chain hydroxylation. *Pharmacol. & Toxicol.* **82**, 173–176.

GODESSART, N., CAMACHO, M., LOPEZBELMONTE, J., ANTON, R., GARCIA, M., DEMORAGAS, J.M. and VILA, L. (1996) Prostaglandin H synthase-2 is the main enzyme involved in the biosynthesis of octadecanoids from linoleic-acid in human dermal fibroblasts stimulated with interleukin-1-beta. *J. Invest. Dermatol.* **107**, 726–732.

GOH, C.L. and NG, S.K. (1988) Bullous contact allergy from cinnamon. *Derm. Beruf. Umwelt.* **36**, 186–187.

GOLDRATH, A.W. and BEVAN, M.J. (1999) Selecting and maintaining a diverse T-cell repertoire. *Nature* **402**, 255–262.

GONZALEZ, F.J. and GELBOIN, H.V. (1994) Role of human cytochromes P450 in the metabolic activation of chemical carcinogens and toxins. *Drug Metab. Rev.* **26**, 165–183.

GOSSRAU, R., FREDERIKS, W.M. and VAN NOORDEN, C.J. (1990) Histochemistry of reactive oxygen-species (ROS)-generating oxidases in cutaneous and mucous epithelia of laboratory rodents with special reference to xanthine oxidase. *Histochemistry* **94**, 539–544.

GOULDEN, V. and WILKINSON, S.M. (2000) Evaluation of a contact allergy clinic. *Clin. Experim. Dermatol.* **25**, 67–70.

GRAHAM, M.J., WILLIAMS, F.M. and RAWLINS, M.D. (1991) Metabolism of aldrin to dieldrin by rat skin following topical application. *Food Chem. Toxicol.* **29**, 707–711.

GRAMMER, L.C., SHAUGHNESSY, M.A., ZEISS, C.R., GREENBERGER, P.A. and PATTERSON, R. (1997) Review of trimellitic anhydride (TMA) induced respiratory response. *Allergy Asthma Proc.* **18**, 235–237.

GRANDO, S.A., KIST, D.A., QI, M. and DAHL, M.V. (1993) Human keratinocytes synthesize, secrete and degrade acetylcholine. *J. Invest. Dermatol.* **101**, 32–36.

GREEN, M.D. and TEPHLY, T.R. (1998) Glucuronidation of amine substrates by purified and expressed UDP-glucuronosyltransferase proteins. *Drug Metab. Disposit.* **26**, 860–867.

GREENSTEIN, J.P. and WINITZ, M. (1961) *Chemistry of the Amino Acids*. New York, John Wiley & Sons.

GREGUS, Z., FEKETE, T., HALASZI, E. and KLAASSEN, C.D. (1996) Does hepatic ATP depletion impair glycine conjugation in vivo? *Drug Metab. Disposit.* **24**, 1347–1354.

GREINER, D., WEBER, J., KAUFMANN, R. and BOEHNCKE, W.-H. (1999) Benzoyl peroxide as a contact allergen in adhesive tape. *Contact Dermatitis* **41**, 233.

GRIFFIN, R.I., RUTT, D.B., HENESEY, C.M. and HARVISON, P.J. (1996) In vitro metabolism of the nephrotoxicant N-(3,5-dichlorophenyl)succinimide in the Fischer 344 rat and New Zealand white rabbit. *Xenobiotica* **26**, 369–380.

GROSHONG, R., GIBSON, D.A. and BALDESSARINI, R.J. (1977) Monoamine oxidase activity in cultured human skin fibroblasts. *Clin. Chim. Acta* **80**, 113–120.

GUENGERICH, F.P., HOSEA, N.A., PARIKH, A., BELL-PARIKH, L.C., JOHNSON, W.W., GILLAM, E.M.J. and SHIMADA, T. (1998) Twenty years of biochemistry of human P450s. Purification, expression, mechanisms, and relevance to drugs. *Drug Metab. Disposit.* **26**, 1175–1178.

GUIN, J.D., MEYER, B.N., DRAKE, R.D. and HAFFLEY, P. (1984) The effect of quenching agents on contact urticaria caused by cinnamic aldehyde. *J. Am. Acad. Dermatol.* **10**, 45–51.

GUY, G.J. and BUTTERWORTH, J. (1978) Carboxypeptidase A activity of cultured human skin fibroblasts and relationship to cystic fibrosis. *Clin. Chim. Acta* **87**, 63–69.

GUY, R.H. and HADGRAFT, J. (1988) Physicochemical aspects of percutaneous penetration and its enhancement. *Pharmaceut. Res.* **5**, 753–758.

GUY, R.H. and HADGRAFT, J. (1989) Structure-activity correlations in percutaneous absorption. In: BRONAUGH, R.L. and MAIBACH, H.I. (eds), *Percutaneous absorption: mechanisms, methodology, drug delivery*, New York, Marcel Dekker Inc., 95–109.

GUY, R.H., MAK, V.H.W., KAI, T., BOMMANNAN, D. and POTTS, R.O. (1990) Percutaneous penetration enhancers: mode of action. In: SCOTT, R.C., GUY, R.H. and HADGRAFT, J.I. (eds), *Prediction of percutaneous penetration methods measurements and modelling*. London, IBC, 213–233.

GUZEK, D.B., KENNEDY, A.H., MCNIELL, S.C., WAKSHULL, E. and POTTS, R.O. (1989) Transdermal drug transport and metabolism. 1. Comparison of in vitro and in vivo results. *Pharm. Res.* **6**, 33–39.

GYSLER, A., LANGE, K., KORTING, H.C. and SCHAFERKORTING, M. (1997) Prednicarbate biotransformation in human foreskin keratinocytes and fibroblasts. *Pharmaceut. Res.* **14**, 793–797.

HAGDRUP, H., EGSGAARD, H., CARLSEN, L. and ANDERSEN, K.E. (1994) Contact allergy to 2-hydroxy-5-tert-butyl benzylalcohol and 2,6- bis(hydroxymethyl)-4-tert-butylphenol, components of a phenolic resin used in marking pens. *Contact Dermatitis* **31**, 154–156.

HAKANSON, R. and MOLLER, H. (1963) On the metabolism of noradrenaline in the skin: activity of catechol-O-methyltransferase and monoamine oxidase. *Acta Dermatovener. (Stockh.)* **43**, 552–555.

HAMAMOTO, T. and MORI, Y. (1989) Sulfation of minoxidil in keratinocytes and hair follicles. *Res. Commun. Chem. Pathol. Pharmacol.* **66**, 33–44.

HAMMARLUND, K. and SEDIN, G. (1979) Transepidermal water loss in newborn infants III. relation to gestational age. *Acta Paediatrica Scandinavia* **68**, 795–801.

HAN, S.K., JUN, Y.H., RHO, Y.J., HONG, S.C. and KIM, Y.M. (1999) Percutaneous absorption-enhancing activity of urea derivatives. *Arch. Pharm. Res.* **14**, 12–18.

HANDSCHIN, R., MALY, I.P., CROTET, V., TORANELLI, M. and SASSE, D. (1997) Qualitative and quantitative analysis of various classes of alcohol dehydrogenase in structures of rat skin. *Acta Histochem. Cytochem.* **30**, 567–574.

HANSEN, J. and MOLLGARD, B. (1991) Biotransformation of contact allergens in the skin. In: CZERNIELEWSKI, J.M. (ed.), *Immunological and pharmacological aspects of atopic and contact eczema. Pharmacol Skin*, Vol. 4. Basel, Karger, 89093.

HARADA, N. (1992) A unique aromatase (P450AROM) mRNA formed by alternative use of tissue-specific exons 1 in human skin fibroblasts. *Biochem. Biophys. Res. Commun.* **189**, 1001–1007.

HARRISON, E.H. (1998) Lipases and carboxylesterases: possible roles in the hepatic metabolism of retinol. *Annu. Rev. Nutr.* **18**, 259–276.

HASELBECK, R.J. and DUESTER, G. (1997) Regional restriction of alcohol/retinol dehydrogenases along the mouse gastrointestinal epithelium. *Alcohol Clin. Exp. Res.* **21**, 1484–1490.

HASELBECK, R.J., ANG, H.L. and DUESTER, G. (1997) Class IV alcohol/retinol localization in epidermal basal layer: potential site of retinoic acid synthesis during skin development. *Dev. Dyn.* **208**, 447–453.

HASSON, A., GUIMARAENS, D. and CONDE-SALAZAR, L. (1990) Patch test sensitivity to the preservative Kathon CG in Spain. *Contact Dermatitis* **22**, 257–261.

HAUSEN, B.M. and BERGER, M. (1989) The sensitising capacity of coumarins. *Contact Dermatitis* **21**, 141–147.

HAUSEN, B.M. and BEYER, W. (1992) The sensitizing capacity of the antioxidants propyl, octyl, and dodecyl gallate and some related gallic acid esters. *Contact Dermatitis* **26**, 253–258.

HAUSER, C. (1990) Cultured epidermal Langerhans' cells activate effector T cells for contact sensitivity. *J. Invest. Dermatol.* **95**, 436–440.

HAUSMANN, S., BIDDISON, W.E., SMITH, K.J., DING, Y.H., GARBOCZI, D.N., UTZ, U., WILEY, D.C. and WUCHERPFENNIG, K.W. (1999) Peptide recognition by two HLA-A2/Tax11-19-specific T cell clones in relationship to their MHC/peptide/TCR crystal structures. *J. Immunol.* **162**, 5389–5397.

HAWES, E.M. (1998) N+-glucuronidation, a common pathway in human metabolism of drugs with a tertairy amine group. *Drug Metab. Disposit.* **26**, 830–837.

HECHT, S.S., RADOK, L., AMIN, S., HUIE, K., MELIKIAN, A.A., HOFFMANN, D., PATAKI, J. and HARVEY, R.G. (1985) Tumorogenicity of 5-methylchrysene dihydrodiols and dihydrodiolepoxides in newborn mice and on mouse skin. *Cancer Res.* **45**, 1449–1452.

HEIN, D.W., RUSTAN, T.D., DOLL, M.A., BUCHER, K.D., FERGUSON, R.J., FENG, Y., FURMAN, E.J. and GRAY, K. (1992) Acetyltransferases and suceptibility to chemicals. *Toxicol. Lett.* **64–65**, 123–130.

HELLERSTROM, S., THYRESSON, N., BLOHM, S.-G. and WIDMARK, G. (1955) On the nature of eczematogenic component of oxidised delta3-carotene. *J. Invest. Dermatol.* **24**, 217–224.

HENNEBOLD, J.D. and DAYNES, R.A. (1998) Inhibition of skin 11 beta-hydroxysteroid dehydrogenase activity in vivo potentiates the anti-inflammatory actions of glucocorticoids. *Arch. Dermatol. Res.* **290**, 413–419.

HENRIKUS, B.M., BREUER, W. and KAMPFFMEYER, H.G. (1991) Dermal metabolism of 4-nitrophenol and 4-nitroanisole in single-pass perfused rabbit ears. *Xenobiotica* **21**, 1229–1241.

HENRISSAT, B. (1998) Glycosidase families. *Biochem. Soc. Trans.* **26**, 153–156.

HEWITT, P.G., HOTCHKISS, S.A.M. and CALDWELL, J. (1993) Cutaneous reservoir formation and localization after topical application of 4,4′-methylene-bis-(2-chloroaniline) and 4,4′-methylenedianiline to rat and human skin in vitro. In: BRAIN, K.R., JAMES, V.J. and WALTERS, K.A. (eds), *Prediction of Percutaneous Penetration: Methods, Measurements & Modelling*, Vol. 3b. Cardiff, STS Publishing Ltd, 638–645.

HEWITT, P.G., HOTCHKISS, S.A.M. and CALDWELL, J. (1995) Decontamination procedures after in vitro topical exposure of human and rat skin to 4,4′-methylenebis[2-chloroaniline] and 4,4′-methylenedianiline. *Fundam. Appl. Toxicol.* **26**, 91–98.

HEWITT, P.G. (1995) In vitro percutaneous absorption: kinetic and metabolic studies. PhD, University of London, London.

HEWITT, P.G., HOTCHKISS, S.A.M., PERKINS, J.M. and ROWE, R.R. (1996) Transdermal metabolism of fluoroxypyr 1-methylheptyl ester during percutaneous absorption through fresh human and rat skin in vitro. In: BRAIN, K.R., JAMES, V.J. and WALTERS, K.A. (eds), *Prediction of Percutaneous Penetration*, Vol. 4b. Cardiff, STS Publishing Ltd, 303–306.

HEWITT, P.G., PERKINS, J. and HOTCHKISS, S.A. (2000a) Metabolism of fluroxypyr, fluroxypyr methyl ester, and the herbicide fluroxypyr methylheptyl ester. I: during percutaneous absorption through fresh rat and human skin in vitro. *Drug Metab. Disposit.* **28**, 748–754.

HEWITT, P.G., PERKINS, J. and HOTCHKISS, S.A. (2000b) Metabolism of fluroxypyr, fluroxypyr methyl ester, and the herbicide fluroxypyr methylheptyl ester. II: in rat skin homogenates. *Drug Metab. Disposit.* **28**, 755–759.

HICKMAN, D., RISCH, A., CAMILLERI, J.P. and SIM, E. (1992) Genotyping human polymorphic arylamine N-acetyltransferase: identification of new slow allotypic variants. *Pharmacogenetics* **2**, 217–226.

HIGO, N., SATO, S., IRIE, T. and UEKAMA, K. (1995) Percutaneous penetration and metabolism of salicylic acid derivatives across hairless mouse skin in diffusion cell in vitro. *STP Pharma. Sci.* **5**, 302–308.

HIGUCHI, W.I. and YU, C.-D. (1987) Prodrugs in transdermal delivery. In: KYDONIEUS, A.F. and BERNER, B. (eds), *Transdermal Delivery of Drugs*, Vol. 3. Florida, CRC Press, 43–83.

HIKIMA, T. and TOJO, K. (1997) Binding of prednisolone and its ester prodrugs in the skin. *Pharmaceut. Res.* **14**, 197–202.

HIRAI, A., MINAMIYAMA, Y., HAMADA, T., ISHII, M. and INOUE, M. (1997) Glutathione metabolism in mice is enhanced more with hapten-induced allergic contact dermatitis than with irritant contact dermatitis. *J. Invest. Dermatol.* **109**, 314–318.

HIROI, T., IMAOKA, S. and FUNAE, Y. (1998) Dopamine formation from tyramine by CYP2D6. *Biochem. Biophys. Res. Commun.* **249**, 838–843.

HODAM, J.R. and CREEK, K.E. (1998) Comparison of the metabolism of retinol delivered to human keratinocytes either bound to serum retinol-binding protein or added directly to the culture medium. *Experimental Cell Res.* **238**, 257–264.

HODGSON, E. and LEVI, P.E. (1992) The role of the flavin-containing monooxygenase (EC 1.14.13.8) in the metabolism and mode of action of agricultural chemicals. *Xenobiotica* **22**, 1175–1183.

HOGQUIST, K.A., JAMESON, S.C. and BEVAN, M.J. (1995) Strong agonist ligands for the T cell receptor do not mediate positive selection of functional CD8+ T cells. *Immunity* **3**, 79–86.

HOLMANN, B.P., SPIES, F. and BODDE, H.E. (1990) An optimised freeze facture replication procedure for human skin. *J. Invest. Dermatol.* **94**, 332–335.

HOMEY, B., WANG, W., SOTO, H., BUCHANAN, M.E., WIESENBORN, A., CATRON, D., MULLER, A., MCCLANAHAN, T.K., DIEU-NOSJEAN, M.C., OROZCO, R., RUZICKA, T., LEHMANN, P., OLDHAM, E. and ZLOTNIK, A. (2000) Cutting edge: the orphan chemokine receptor G-protein-coupled receptor-2 (GPR-2, CCR10) binds the skin-associated chemokine CCL27. *J. Immunol.* **164**, 3465–3467.

HOOD, H.L., KRAELING, M.E., ROBL, M.G. and BRONAUGH, R.L. (1999) The effects of an alpha hydroxy acid (glycolic acid) on hairless guinea pig skin permeability. *Fd. Chem. Toxicol.* **37**, 1105–1111.

HOPSU-HAVU, V.K. and JANSEN, C.T. (1969) Peptidases in the skin II. Demonstration and partial separation of several specific dipeptidyl naphthylamidases in the rat and human skin. *Arch. Klin. Exp. Dermatol.* **235**, 53–62.

HOPSU-HAVU, V.K., JANSEN, C.T. and JARVINEN, M. (1970a) Partial purification and characterization of an acid dipeptide naphthylamidase (carboxytripeptidase) of the rat skin. *Arch. Klin. Exp. Dermatol.* **236**, 282–296.

HOPSU-HAVU, V.K., JANSEN, C.T. and JARVINEN, M. (1970b) Partial purification and characterization of an alkaline dipeptide naphthylamidase (Arg-Arg-NAase) of the rat skin. *Arch. Klin. Exp. Dermatol.* **236**, 267–281.

HOPSU-HAVU, V.K., FRAKI, J.E. and JARVINEN, M. (1977) Proteolytic enzymes in the skin. In: BARRET, A.J. (ed.), *Proteinases in Mammalian Cells and Tissues*, Amsterdam, Elsevier, North Holland Biomedical Press, 545–581.

HORI, H., FENNA, R.E., KIMURA, S. and IKEDA-SAITO, M. (1994) Aromatic substrate molecules bind at the distal heme pocket of myeloperoxidase. *J. Biol. Chem.* **269**, 8388–8392.

HOTCHKISS, S.A.M., CHIDGEY, M.A.J., ROSE, S. and CALDWELL, J. (1990) Percutaneous absorption of benzyl acetate through rat skin in vitro. 1. Validation of an in vitro model against in vivo data. *Fd. Chem. Toxicol.* **28**, 443–447.

HOTCHKISS, S.A.M. (1992) Skin as a xenobiotic metabolising organ. In: GIBSON, G.G. (ed.), *Progress in Drug Metabolism*, Vol. 13. London, Taylor & Francis, 217–262.

HOTCHKISS, S.A.M., HEWITT, P., CALDWELL, J., CHEN, W.L. and ROWE, R.R. (1992) Percutaneous absorption of nicotinic acid, phenol, benzoic acid and triclopyr butoxyethyl ester through rat and human skin in vitro, further validation of an in vitro model by comparison with in vivo data. *Fd. Chem. Toxicol.* **30**, 891–899.

HOTCHKISS, S.A.M., MILLER, J.M. and CALDWELL, J. (1992a) Percutaneous absorption of benzyl acetate through rat skin in vitro. 2. Effect of vehicle and occlusion. *Fd. Chem. Toxicol.* **30**, 145–153.

HOTCHKISS, S.A.M., HEWITT, P. and CALDWELL, J. (1993) Percutaneous absorption of 4,4′-methylene-bis-(2-chloroaniline) and 4,4′-methylenedianiline through rat and human skin in vitro. *Toxicol. in Vitro* **7**, 141–148.

HOTCHKISS, S.A.M. (1995) Skin absorption of occupational chemicals. In: 'Handbook of Occupational Hygiene (Instalment 46)', Vol. 1. Kingston-upon-Thames, Croner, 1–38.

HOTCHKISS, S.A.M., HEWITT, P.G. and EDWARDS, R. (1996) Immunochemical detection of specific cytochrome P450 enzymes in uninduced BALB/c mouse skin. *Proceedings ISSX* **10**, 172.

HOTCHKISS, S.A.M. (1998) Dermal Metabolism. In: ROBERTS, M.S. and WALTERS, K.A. (eds), *Dermal Absorption and Toxicity Assessment. Drugs and the Pharmaceutical Sciences*, Vol. 91. New York, Marcel Dekker, 43–101.

HOTCHKISS, S.A.M. (1999) Measurement of bioavailability: measurement of absorption through skin *in vitro*. In: MAINES, M.D., COSTA, L.G., REED, D.J., SASSA, S. and SIPES, I.G. (eds), *Current Protocols in Toxicology*, Vol. 1. New York, Wiley, 5.1.1–5.1.14.

HU, Q., BAZEMORE WALKER, C.R., GIRAO, C., OPFERMAN, J.T., SUN, J., SHABANOWITZ, J., HUNT, D.F. and ASHTON-RICKARDT, P.G. (1997) Specific recognition of thymic self-peptides induces the positive selection of cytotoxic T lymphocytes. *Immunity* **7**, 221–231.

HUBER, R., HOF, P., DUARTE, R.O., MOURA, J.J., MOURA, I., LIU, M.Y., LEGALL, J., HILLE, R., ARCHER, M. and ROMAO, M.J. (1996) A structure-based catalytic mechanism for the xanthine oxidase family of molybdenum enzymes. *Proc. Natl. Acad. Sci.* **93**, 8846–8851.

HUEBER, F., WEPIERRE, J. and SCHAEFER, H. (1992) Role of transepidermal and transfollicular routes of percutaneous absorption of hydrocortisone and testosterone: in vivo study in the hairless rat. *Skin Pharmacol.* **5**, 99–107.

HUGHES, S.V., ROBINSON, E., BLAND, R., LEWIS, H.M., STEWART, P.M. and HEWISON, M. (1997) 1,25-dihydroxyvitamin D-3 regulates estrogen metabolism in cultured keratinocytes. *Endocrinology* **138**, 3711–3718.

HUNT, D.F., HENDERSON, R.A., SHABANOWITZ, J., SAKAGUCHI, K., MICHEL, H., SEVILIR, N., COX, A.L., APPELLA, E. and ENGELHARD, V.H. (1992a) Characterization of peptides bound to the class I MHC molecule HLA-A2.1 by mass spectrometry. *Science* **255**, 1261–1263.

HUNT, D.F., MICHEL, H., DICKINSON, T.A., SHABANOWITZ, J., COX, A.L., SAKAGUCHI, K., APPELLA,

E., GREY, H.M. and SETTE, A. (1992b) Peptides presented to the immune system by the murine class II major histocompatibility complex molecule I-Ad. *Science* **256**, 1817–1820.

ICHIKAWA, T., HAYASHI, S.I., NOSHIRO, N., TAKADA, K. and OKUDA, K. (1989) Purification and characterisation of cytochrome P450-induced by benzo(a)anthracene in mouse skin microsomes. *Cancer Res.* **49**, 806–809.

ILLEL, B., SCHAEFER, H., WEPIERRE, J. and DOUCET, O. (1991) Follicles play an important role in percutaneous absorption. *J. Pharm. Sci.* **80**, 424–427.

ISAKSSON, M., ZIMERSON, E. and BRUZE, M. (1999) Occupational dermatoses in composite production. *J. Occup. Environ. Med.* **41**, 261–266.

ISHIDA, T., TOYOTA, M. and ASAKAWA, Y. (1989) Terpinoid biotransformation in mammals. V. Metabolism of (+)-citronellal, (+/−)-7-hydroxycitronellal, (−)-perillaldehyde, (−)-myrtenal, cuminaldehyde, thujone and (+/−)-carvone in rabbits. *Xenobiotica* **19**, 843–855.

ITAMI, S. and TAKAYASU, S. (1982) Activity of 3 beta-hydroxysteroid dehydrogenase delta 4-5 isomerase in the human skin. *Arch. Dermatol. Res.* **274**, 289–294.

IVERSEN, L., ZIBOH, V.A., SHIMIZU, T., OHISHI, N., RADMARK, O., WETTERHOLM, A. and KRAGBALLE, K. (1994) Identification and subcellular localization of leukotriene A4-hydrolase activity in human epidermis. *J. Dermatol. Sci.* **7**, 191–201.

IVERSEN, L., DELEURAN, B., HOBERG, A.M. and KRAGBALLE, K. (1996) LTA(4) hydrolase in human skin — decreased activity, but normal concentration in lesional psoriatic skin — evidence for different LTA(4) hydrolase activity in human lymphocytes and human skin. *Arch. Dermatol. Res.* **288**, 217–224.

JARVINEN, M. and HOPSU-HAVU, V.K. (1975) alpha-N-Benzoylarginine-2-naphthylamide hydrolase (cathepsin B1?) from rat skin. II. Purification of the enzyme and demonstration of two inhibitors in skin. *Acta Chem. Scand.* **B29**, 772–780.

JEDRYCHOWSKI, R.A., STETKIEWICZ, J. and STETKIEWICZ, I. (1990) Acute toxicity of 1,4-butanediol in laboratory animals. *Pol. J. Occup. Med.* **3**, 415–420.

JETZER, W.E., HOU, S.Y.E., HUG, A.S., DURAISWAMY, N., HO, W.F.S. and FLYNN, G.L. (1988) Temperature dependency of skin permeation of waterborn organic compounds. *Pharm. Acta Helv.* **63**, 197–201.

JOHANSEN, J.D. and MENNE, T. (1995) The fragrance mix and its constituents: a 14-year material. *Contact Dermatitis* **32**, 18–23.

Johansen, J.D., Rastogi, S.C. and Menne, T. (1996) Exposure to selected fragrance materials. A case study of fragrance-mix-positive eczema patients. *Contact Dermatitis* **34**, 106–110.

JOHANSEN, J.D., SKOV, L., VOLUND, A., ANDERSEN, K. and MENNE, T. (1998) Allergens in combination have a synergistic effect on the elicitation response: a study of fragrance-sensitised individuals. *Br. J. Dermatol.* **139**, 264–270.

JOHNSON, R.A., HAER, H., KIRKPATRICK, C.H., DAWSON, C.R. and KHURANA, R.G. (1972) Comparison of the contact allergenicity of the four pentadecylcatechols derived from poison ivy urushiol in human subjects. *J. Allergy Clin. Immunol.* **49**, 27–35.

JONES, E.Y. (1997) MHC class I and class II structures. *Current Opin. Immunol.* **9**, 75–79.

JORNVALL, H., DANIELSSON, O., HJELMQVIST, L., PERSSON, B. and SHAFQAT, J. (1995) The alcohol dehydrogenase system. *Adv. Exp. Med. Biol.* **372**, 281–294.

JORNVALL, H. and HOOG, J.-O. (1995) Nomenclature of alcohol dehydrogenases. *Alcohol and Alcoholism* **30**, 153–161.

JORUNDSSON, E., PRESS, C.M., ULVUND, M. and LANDSVERK, T. (1999) Prominence of gammadelta T cells in the elicitation phase of dinitrochlorobenzene-induced contact hypersensitivity in lambs. *Vet. Pathol.* **36**, 42–50.

JUDGE, M.R., GRIFFITHS, H.A., BASKETTER, D.A., WHITE, I.R., RYCROFT, R.J. and MCFADDEN, J.P. (1996) Variation in response of human skin to irritant challenge. *Contact Dermatitis* **34**, 115–117.

JUGERT, F.K., AGARWAL, R., KUHN, A., BICKERS, D., MERK, H.F. and MUKHTAR, H. (1994) Multiple cytochrome P450 isozymes in murine skin: induction of P450 1A, 2B, 2E and 3A by dexamethasone. *J. Invest. Dermatol.* **102**, 970–975.

KALERGIS, A.M., LOPEZ, C.B., BECKER, M.I., DIAZ, M.I., SEIN, J., GARBARINO, J.A. and DEIOANNES, A.E. (1997) Modulation of fatty acid oxidation alters contact hypersensitivity to urushiols: role of aliphatic chain beta oxidation in processing and activation of urushiols. *J. Invest. Dermatol.* **108**, 57–61.

KALISH, R.S. and ASKENASE, P.W. (1999) Molecular mechanisms of CD8+ T cell-mediated delayed hypersensitivity: implications for allergies, asthma, and autoimmunity. *J. Allergy Clin. Immunol.* **103**, 192–199.

KANERVA, L., JOLANKI, R. and ESTLANDER, T. (1997a) 10 years of patch testing with the (meth)acrylate series. *Contact Dermatitis* **37**, 255–258.

KANERVA, L., HYRY, H., JOLANKI, R., HYTONEN, M. and ESTLANDER, T. (1997b) Delayed and immediate allergy caused by methylhexahydrophthalic anhydride. *Contact Dermatitis* **36**, 34–38.

KANG, S., DUELL, E.A., KIM, K.J. and VOORHEES, J.J. (1996) Liarozole inhibits human epidermal retinoic acid 4-hydroxylase activity and differentially augments human skin responses to retinoic acid and retinol in vivo. *J. Invest. Dermatol.* **107**, 183–187.

KAO, J., PATTERSON, F.K. and HALL, J. (1985) Skin penetration and metabolism of topically applied chemicals in six mammalian species, including man: an in vitro study with benzo(a)pyrene and testosterone. *Toxicol. & Appl. Pharmacol.* **81**, 502–516.

KAO, J., HALL, J. and HELMAN, G. (1988) In vitro percutaneous absorption in mouse skin: influence of skin appendages. *Toxicol. Appl. Pharmacol.* **94**, 93–103.

KAO, J. and CARVER, M.P. (1990) Cutaneous Metabolism of Xenobiotics. *Drug Metab. Rev.* **22**, 363–410.

KARLBERG, A.-T., BERGSTEDT, E., BOMAN, A., BOHLINDER, K., LIDEN, C., NILSSON, J.L.G. and WAHLBERG, J.E. (1985) Is abietic acid the allergenic component of colophony? *Contact Dermatitis* **13**, 209–215.

KARLBERG, A.-T., BOHLINDER, K., BOMAN, A., HACKSELL, U., HERMANSSON, J., JACOBSSON, S. and NILSSON, J.L.G. (1988) Identification of 15-hydroperoxyabietic acid as a contact allergen in Portuguese colophony. *J. Pharm. Pharmacol.* **40**, 42–47.

KARLBERG, A.-T. (1991) Air oxidation increases the allergenic potential of tall oil rosin. Colophony contact allergens also identified in tall oil rosin. *Am. J. Contact Dermat.* **2**, 43–49.

KARLBERG, A.-T., SHAO, L.P., NILSSON, U., GAFVERT, E. and NILSSON, J.L.G. (1994) Hydroperoxides in oxidised d-limonene identified as potent contact allergens. *Arch. Dermatol. Res.* **286**, 97–103.

KARLBERG, A.-T. and DOOMS-GOOSSENS, A. (1997) Contact allergy to oxidised d-limonene among dermatitis patients. *Contact Dermatitis* **36**, 201–206.

KARLBERG, A.-T., BASKETTER, D.A., GOOSSENS, A. and LEPOITTEVIN, J.-P. (1999) Regulatory classification of substances oxidised to skin sensitisers on exposure to air. *Contact Dermatitis* **40**, 183–188.

KATSAROU, A., ARMENAKA, M., KALOGEROMITROS, D., KOUFOU, V. and GEORGALA, S. (1999) Contact reactions to fragrances. *Ann. Allergy Asthma Immunol.* **82**, 449–455.

KATSUNO, K., MANABE, A., ITOH, K., NAKAMURA, Y., WAKAMOTO, S., HISAMITSU, H. and YOSHIDA, T. (1996) Contact dermatitis caused by 2-HEMA and GM dentin primer solutions applied to guinea-pigs and humans. *Dent. Mater. J.* **15**, 22–30.

KATZ, M. and POULSEN, B.J. (1971) In: BRODIE, B.B. and GILLETE, J.R. (eds), *Handbook of Experimental Pharmacology*, Vol. 28. New York, Springer-Verlag, 103.

KAWAKUBO, Y., MANABE, S., YAMAZOE, Y., NISHIKAWA, T. and KATO, R. (1988) Properties of cutaneous acetyltransferase catalyzing N- and O-acetylation of carcinogenic arylamines and N-hydroxylamine. *Biochem. Pharmacol.* **37**, 265–270.

KAWAKUBO, Y., YAMAZOE, Y., KATO, R. and NISHIKAWA, T. (1990) High capacity of human skin for N-acetylation of arylamines. *Skin Pharmacol.* **3**, 180–185.

KAWAKUBO, Y., NAKAMORI, M., SCHOPF, E. and OHKIDO, M. (1997) Acetylator phenotype in patients with p-phenylenediamine allergy. *Dermatology* **195**, 43–45.

KAWAKUBO, Y., BLOEKE, B. and MERK, H. (1998) p-Phenylenediamine (PPD) N-acetylation in human skin cytosol. *J. Invest. Dermatol.* **110**, Int Invest Dermatol meeting abstract.

KEENEY, D.S., SKINNER, C., WEI, S.Z., FRIEDBERG, T. and WATERMAN, M.R. (1998) A keratinocyte specific epoxygenase, CYP2B12, metabolizes arachidonic acid with unusual selectivity, producing a single major epoxyeicosatrienoic acid. *J. Biol. Chem.* **273**, 9279–9284.

KEHREN, J., DESVIGNES, C., KRASTEVA, D.M.-T.O.A., HORAND, F., HAHNE, M., KAGI, D., KAISERLIAN, D. and NICOLAS, J.-F. (1999) Cytotoxicity is mandatory for CD8+ T cell-mediated contact hypersensitivity. *J. Exp. Med.* **189**, 779–786.

KEIL, J.E. and SHMUNES, E. (1983) The epidemiology of work-related skin disease in South Carolina. *Arch. Dermatol.* **119**, 650–654.

KELLEY, M. and VESSEY, D.A. (1994) Characterisation of the acyl-CoA:amino acid N-acyltransferase from primate liver mitochondria. *J. Biochem. Toxicol.* **9**, 153–158.

KENNEY, G.E., SAKR, A., LICHTIN, J.L., CHOU, H. and BRONAUGH, R.L. (1995) In vitro skin absorption and metabolism of padimate-O and a nitrosamine formed in padimate-O-containing cosmetic products. *J. Soc. Cosmetic Chem.* **46**, 117–127.

KENOUCH, S., LOMBES, M., DELAHAYE, F., EUGENE, E., BONVALET, J.P. and FARMAN, N. (1994) Human skin as target for aldosterone: coexpression of mineralocorticoid receptors and 11 beta-hydroxysteroid dehydrogenase. *J. Clin. Endocrinol. Metab.* **79**, 1334–1341.

KEOGH, B.P., ALLEN, R.G., PIGNOLO, R., HORTON, J., TRESINI, M. and CRISTOFALO, V.J. (1996) Expression of hydrogen peroxide and glutathione metabolising enzymes in human skin fibroblasts derived from donors of different ages. *J. Cell Physiol.* **167**, 512–522.

KHAN, W.A., DAS, M., STICK, S., JAVED, S., BICKERS, D.R. and MUKHTAR, H. (1987) Induction of epidermal NAD(P)H:quinone reductase by chemical carcinogens: a possible mechanism for the detoxification. *Biochem. Biophys. Res. Commun.* **146**, 126–133.

KHAN, W.A., PARK, S.S., GELBOIN, H.V., BICKERS, D.R. and MUKHTAR, H. (1989a) Epidermal cytochrome P450: immunochemical characterization of isoform induced by topical application of 3-methylcholanthrene to neonatal rat. *J. Pharmacol. Exper. Therapeut.* **249**, 921–927.

KHAN, W.A., PARK, S.S., GELBOIN, H.V., BICKERS, D.R. and MUKHTAR, H. (1989b) Monoclonal antibodies directed characterization of epidermal and hepatic cytochrome P450 isoenzymes induced by skin application of therapeutic crude coal tar. *J. Invest. Dermatol.* **93**, 40–45.

KHAN, I.U., BICKERS, D.R., HAQQI, T.M. and MUKHTAR, H. (1992) Induction of CYP1A1 mRNA in rat epidermis and cultured human epidermal keratinocytes by benz(a)anthracene and beta-naphthoflavone. *Drug Metab. Disposit.* **20**, 620–624.

KIKONYOGO, A. and PIETRUSZKO, R. (1997) Cimetidine and other H2-receptor antagonists as inhibitors of human E3 aldehyde dehydrogenase. *Mol. Pharmacol.* **52**, 267–271.

KIKUCHI, M., FUKUYAMA, K. and EPSTEIN, W.L. (1988) Soluble dipeptidyl peptidase IV from terminal differentiated rat epidermal cells: purification and its activity on synthetic and natural peptides. *Arch. Biochem. Biophys.* **266**, 369–376.

KIM, H.P., MANI, I., IVERSEN, L. and ZIBOH, V.A. (1998) Effects of naturally occurring flavonoids and biflavonoids on epidermal cyclooxygenase and lipoxygenase from guinea-pigs. *Prostaglandins Leukotrienes & Essential Fatty Acids* **58**, 17–24.

KIM, N., EL-KHALILI, M., HENARY, M.M., STREKOWSKI, L. and MICHNIAK, B.B. (1999) Percutaneous penetration enhancement activity of aromatic S, S-dimethyliminosulfuranes. *Int. J. Pharm.* **187**, 219–229.

KIMBER, I., MITCHELL, J.A. and GRIFFIN, A.C. (1986) Development of a murine local lymph node assay for the determination of sensitising potential. *Food Chem. Toxicol.* **24**, 585–586.

KIMBER, I. and WEISENBERGER, C. (1989) A murine local lymph node assay for the identification of contact allergens. Assay development and results of an initial validation study. *Arch. Toxicol.* **63**, 274–282.

KIMBER, I., HOLLIDAY, M.R. and DEARMAN, R.J. (1995) Cytokine regulation and chemical sensitization. *Toxicol. Lett.* **82–83**, 491–496.

KIMBER, I., DEARMAN, R.J., CUMBERBATCH, M. and HUBY, R.J. (1998a) Langerhans' cells and chemical allergy. *Curr. Opin. Immunol.* **10**, 614–619.

KIMBER, I., HILTON, J., DEARMAN, R.J., GERBERICK, G.F., RYAN, C.A., BASKETTER, D.A., LEA, L., HOUSE, R.V., LADICS, G.S., LOVELESS, S.E. and HASTINGS, K.L. (1998b) Assessment of the skin sensitization potential of topical medicaments using the local lymph node assay: an interlaboratory validation. *J. Toxicol. Environ. Health* **53**, 563–579.

KIMBER, I., CUMBERBATCH, M., DEARMAN, R.J., BHUSHAN, M. and GRIFFITHS, C.E. (2000) Cytokines and chemokines in the initiation and regulation of epidermal Langerhans' cell mobilisation. *Br. J. Dermatol.* **142**, 401–412.

KLEIJMEER, M.J., OORSCHOT, V.M.J. and GEUZE, H.J. (1994) Human resident Langerhans' cells display a lysosomal compartment enriched in MHC class II. *J. Invest. Dermatol.* **103**, 516–523.

KLENIEWSKA, D. and MAIBACH, H.I. (1980) Allergenicity of aminobenzene compounds: structure-function relationships. *Dermatosen.* **28**, 11–13.

KLIGMAN, A.M. (1983a) Skin permeability: dermatological aspects of transdermal delivery. *Am. Heart J.* **108**, 200–206.

KNUDSEN, B.B. and MENNE, T. (1990) Kathon CG — a new contact sensitizing preservative. *Ugeskr. Laeger* **152**, 656–657.

KOBAYASHI, K., YAMAMOTO, T., CHIBA, K., TANI, M., SHIMADA, N., ISHIZAKI, T. and KUROIWA, Y. (1998) Human buprenorphine N-dealkylation is catalysed by cytochrome P450 3A4. *Drug Metab. Dispos.* **26**, 818–821.

KOBAYASHI, I., HOSAKA, K., MARUO, H., SAEKI, Y., KAMIYAMA, M., KONNO, C. and GEMBA, M. (1999) Skin toxicity of propranolol in guinea pigs. *J. Toxicol. Sci.* **24**, 103–112.

KODA, A., NAKATOMI, I., NAKAMURA, K., INOUE, H. and KAMIMURA, T. (1985) Inhibition of delayed hypersensitivity reactions by a new agent, cis-1- methyl-4-isohexylcyclohexane carboxylic acid (IG-10). *Int. J. Immunopharmacol.* **7**, 41–49.

KOIVUSALO, M., BAUMANN, M. and UOTILA, L. (1989) Evidence for the identity of glutathione-dependent formaldehyde dehydrogenase and class III alcohol dehydrogenase. *FEBS Lett.* **257**, 105–109.

KONDO, S. and SAUDER, D.N. (1995) Epidermal cytokines in allergic contact dermatitis. *J. Am. Acad. Dermatol.* **33**, 786–800.

KRAELING, M.E.K., LIPICKY, R.J. and BRONAUGH, R.L. (1996) Metabolism of benzocaine during percutaneous absorption in the hairless guinea-pig: acetylbenzocaine formation and activity. *Skin Pharmacol.* **9**, 221–230.

KRECISZ, B. and KIEC-SWIERCZYNSKA, M. (1998) The role of formaldehyde in the occurrence of contact allergy. *Med. Pr. (Polish journal)* **49**, 609–614.

KROEMER, H.K. and KLOTZ, U. (1992) Glucuronidation of drugs. A re-evaluation of the pharmacological significance of the conjugates and modulating factors. *Clin. Pharmacokinet.* **23**, 292–310.

KROL, E.S. and BOLTON, J.L. (1997) Oxidation of 4-alkylphenols and catechols by tyrosinase: ortho-substituents alter the mechanism of quinoid formation. *Chem. Biol. Interact.* **104**, 11–27.

KUHN, U., BRAND, P., WILLEMSEN, J., JONULEIT, H., ENK, A.H., VAN BRANDWIJK-PETERSHANS, R., SALOGA, J., KNOP, J. and BECKER, D. (1998) Induction of tyrosine phosphorylation in human MHC class II-positive antigen-presenting cells by stimulation with contact sensitizers. *J. Immunol.* **160**, 667–673.

KUROKI, T., CHIDA, K., HOSOMI, J. and KONDO, S. (1989) Use of human epidermal cells in the study of carcinogenesis. *J. Invest. Dermatol.* **92**, 271S–274S.

LAMB, K.A., DENYER, S.P., SANDERSON, F.D. and SHAW, P.N. (1994) The metabolism of a series of ester pro-drugs by NCTC-2544 cells, skin homogenate and LDE testskin. *J. Pharm. & Pharmacol.* **46**, 965–973.

LANDSTEINER, K. and JACOBS, J. (1936) Studies on the sensitization of animals with simple chemical compounds. *J. Exp. Med.* **64**, 625–639.

LANKAT-BUTTGEREIT, B. and TAMPE, R. (1999) The transporter associated with antigen processing TAP: structure and function. *FEBS Lett.* **464**, 108–112.

LAUERMA, A.I., TARVAINEN, K., FORSTROM, L. and REITAMO, S. (1993) Contact hypersensitivity to hydrocortisone-free-alcohol in patients with allergic patch test reactions to tixocortol pivalate. *Contact Dermatitis* **28**, 10–14.

LAWRENCE, C.M., FINNEN, M.J. and SHUSTER, S. (1984) Effect of coal tar on cutaneous aryl hydrocarbon hydroxylase induction and anthralin irritancy. *Br. J. Dermatol.* **110**, 671–675.

LAWTON, M.P., CASHMAN, J.R., CRESTEIL, T., DOLPHIN, C.T., ELFARRA, A.A., HINES, R.N., HODGSON, E., KIMURA, T., OZOLS, J., PHILLIPS, I.R. and ET AL (1994) A nomenclaturem for the mammalian flavin-containing monooxygenase gene family based on amino acid sequence identities. *Arch. Biochem. Biophys.* **308**, 254–257.

LE POOLE, I.C., RMJGJ, V., SMIT, N.P.M., OOSTING, J., WESTERHOF, W. and PAVEL, S. (1994) Catechol-O-methyltransferase in vitiligo. *Arch. Dermatol. Res.* **286**, 81–86.

LECHLER, R. (1994) The roles of class I and II molecules of the major histocompatibility complex in T-cell immunity. In: LECHLER, R. (ed.), *HLA & Disease*, London, Academic Press Limited, 49–72.

LEE, H.K., ALARIE, Y. and KAROL, M.H. (1984) Induction of formaldehyde sensitivity in guinea pigs. *Toxicol. Appl. Pharmacol.* **75**, 147–155.

LEE, A.R.C. and TOJO, K. (1996) Metabolism of vitamin E during skin permeation. *J. Soc. Cosmetic Chem.* **47**, 85–95.

LEONG, J., HUGHESFULFORD, M., RAKHLIN, N., HABIB, A., MACLOUF, J. and GOLDYNE, M.E. (1996) Cyclooxygenases in human and mouse skin and cultured human keratinocytes — association of COX-2 expression with human keratinocyte differentiation. *Experimental Cell Res.* **224**, 79–87.

LEPOITTEVIN, J.P. and BENEZRA, C. (1986) Saturated analogues of poison ivy allergens. Synthesis of trans,trans- and cis,trans-3-alkyl-1,2-cyclohexanediols and sensitizing properties in allergic contact dermatitis. *J. Med. Chem.* **29**, 287–291.

LEPOITTEVIN, J.-P. and KARLBERG, A.-T. (1994) Interactions of allergenic hydroperoxides with proteins: a radical mechanism. *Chem. Res. Toxicol.* **7**, 130–133.

LEPOITTEVIN, J.-P., DRIEGHE, J. and DOOMS-GOOSENS, A. (1995) Studies in patients with corticosteroid contact allergy: understanding cross-reactivity among different steroids. *Arch. Dermatol.* **131**, 31–37.

LEPOITTEVIN, J.-P. and LEBLOND, I. (1997) Hapten-peptide-T cell receptor interactions: molecular basis for the recognition of haptens by T lymphocytes. *Eur. J. Dermatol.* **7**, 151–154.

LEPOITTEVIN, J.-P. and GOOSENS, A. (1998) Molecular basis for the recognition of haptens by T lymphocytes. In: LEPOITTEVIN, J.-P., BASKETTER, D.A., GOOSENS, A. and KARLBERG, A.-T. (eds), *Allergic Contact Dermatitis: the Molecular Basis*, Berlin, Springer-Verlag, 112–128.

LESSARD, E., FORTIN, A., BELANGER, P.M., BEAUNE, P., HAMELIN, B.A. and TURGEON, J. (1997) Role of CYP2D6 in the N-hydroxylation of procainamide. *Pharmacogenetics* **7**, 381–390.

LEVANG, A.K., ZHAO, K. and SINGH, J. (1999) Effect of ethanol/propylene glycol on the in vitro percutaneous absorption of aspirin, biophysical changes and macroscopic barrier properties of the skin. *Int. J. Pharm.* **181**, 255–263.

LEVIN, W., CONNEY, A.H., ALVARES, A.P., MERKATZ, I. and KAPPAS, A. (1972) Induction of benzo(a)pyrene hydroxylase in human skin. *Science* **176**, 419–420.

LI, T.-K. and BOSRON, W.F. (1981) Distribution and properties of human alcohol dehydrogenase isozymes. In: 'Annals New York Acad Sci, Part I. Alcohol and acetaldehyde metabolism', 1–10.

LI, H., HALLOWS, W.H., PUNZI, J.S., PANKIEWICZ, K.W., WATANABE, K.A. and GOLDSTEIN, B.M. (1994a) Crystallographic studies of isosteric NAD analogues bound to alcohol dehydrogenase: specificity and substrate binding in two ternary complexes. *Biochemistry* **33**, 11734–11744.

LI, X.-Y., DUELL, E.A., QIN, L., WATKINS, P.B. and VOORHEES, J.J. (1994b) Cytochrome P450 3A5 is the major 3A subfamily member expressed in normal human skin in vivo. *J. Invest. Dermatol.* **102**, 624.

LI, X.-Y., ASTROM, A., DUELL, E.A., QIN, L., GRIFFITHS, C.E.M. and VOORHEES, J.J. (1995) Retinoic acid antagonizes basal as well as coal tar and glucocorticoid induced cytochrome P450 1A1 expression in human skin. *Carcinogenesis* **16**, 519–624.

LI, Q., INAGAKI, H. and MINAMI, M. (1996) Evaluation of cross-sensitization among dye-intermediate agents using modified lymphocyte transformation test. *Arch. Toxicol.* **70**, 414–419.

LIEBER, C.S. (1988) Biochemical and molecular basis of alcohol-induced injury to liver and other tissues. *N. Engl. J. Med.* **319**, 1639–1650.

LIEBER, C.S. (1999) Microsomal ethanol-oxidising system (MEOS): The first 30 years (1968–1998) — A review. *Alcoholism: Clin. and Exp. Res.* **23**, 991–1007.

LILIENBLUM, W., IRMSCHER, G., FUSENIG, N.E. and BOCK, K.W. (1986) Induction of UDP-glucuronosyltransferase and arylhydrocarbon hydroxylase activity in mouse skin and in normal and transformed skin cells in culture. *Biochem. Pharmacol.* **35**, 1517–1520.

LIN, S.X., ZHU, D.W., AZZI, A., CAMPBELL, R.L., BRETON, R., LABRIE, F., GHOSH, D., PLETNEV, V., DUAX, W.L. and PANGBORN, W. (1996) Studies on the three-dimensional structures of estrogenic 17 beta-hydroxysteroid dehydrogenase. *J. Endocrinol.* **150**, S13–20.

LINDEMAYR, H. and DROBIL, M. (1981) Contact sensitisation to benzoyl peroxide. *Contact Dermatitis* **7**, 137–140.

LISI, P. and HANSEL, K. (1998) Is benzoquinone the prohapten in cross-sensitivity among aminobenzene compounds. *Contact Dermatitis* **39**, 304–306.

LIU, Z., SUN, Y.-J., ROSE, J., CHUNG, Y.-J., HSIAO, C.-D., CHANG, W.-R., KUO, I., PEROZICH, J., LINDAHL, R., HEMPEL, J. and WANG, B.-C. (1997) The first structure of an aldehyde dehydrogenase reveals novel interactions between NAD and the Rossmann fold. *Nat. Struct. Biol.* **4**, 317–323.

LODEN, M. (1985) The in vitro hydrolysis of diisopropyl fluorophosphate during penetration through human full-thickness skin and isolated epidermis. *J. Invest. Dermatol.* **85**, 335–339.

LODI, A., MANCINI, L.L., AMBONATI, M., COASSINI, A., RAVANELLI, G. and CROSTI, C. (2000) Epidemiology of occupational contact dermatitis in a North Italian population. *Eur. J. Dermatol.* **10**, 128–132.

LOMNITSKI, L., SKLAN, D. and GROSSMAN, S. (1995) Lipoxygenase activity in rat dermis and epidermis — partial purification and characterisation. *Biochim. et Biophys. Acta — Lipids and Lipid Metab.* **1255**, 351–359.

LOMNITSKI, L., GROSSMAN, S., BERGMAN, M., SOFER, Y. and SKLAN, D. (1997) In vitro and in vivo effects of beta-carotene on rat epidermal lipoxygenase. *Int. J. Vitamin & Nutrit. Res.* **67**, 407–414.

LOPEZ-SOLACHE, I., LUU-THE, V., SERALINI, G.E. and LABRIE, F. (1996) Heterogeneity of rat type 1 5-alpha-reductase cDNA: cloning, expression and regulation by pituitary implants and dihydrotestosterone. *Biochem. Biophys. Acta* **1305**, 139–144.

LOTTE, C., WESTER, R.C., ROUGIER, A. and MAIBACH, H.I. (1993) Racial differences in the in vivo percutaneous absorption of some organic compounds: a comparison between black, caucasian & asian subjects. *Arch. Dermatol. Res.* **284**, 456–459.

LOVELESS, S.E., LADICS, G.S., GERBERICK, G.F., RYAN, C.A., BASKETTER, D.A., SCHOLES, E.W., HOUSE, R.V., HILTON, J., DEARMAN, R.J. and KIMBER, I. (1996) Further evaluation of the local lymph node assay in the final phase of an international collaborative trial. *Toxicology* **108**, 141–152.

LU, C.Y., LEE, H.C., FAHN, H.J. and WEI, Y.H. (1999) Oxidative damage elicited by imbalance of free radical scavenging enzymes is associated with large-scale mtDNA deletions in aging human skin. *Mutat. Res.* **423**, 11–21.

LUSHNIAK, B.D. (1995) The epidemiology of occupational contact dermatitis. *Dermatol. Clin.* **12**, 671–680.

LUTZ, M.E. and EL-AZHARY, R.A. (1997) Allergic contact dermatitis due to topical application of corticosteroids: review and clinical implications. *Mayo Clin. Proc.* **72**, 1141–1144.

LYNCH, D.H., ROBERTS, L.K. and DAYNES, R.A. (1987) Skin immunology: the achilles heel to transdermal drug delivery? *J. Control. Rel.* **6**, 39–50.

MCAULIFFE, D.J. and BLANK, I.H. (1991) Effects of UVA (320–400nm) in the barrier characteristics of the skin. *J. Invest. Dermatol.* **96**, 758–762.

MCCORMACK, J.J., BOISITS, E.K. and FISCHER, L.B. (1982) An in vitro comparison of the permeability of adult versus neonatal skin. In: MAIBACH, H.I. and BOISITS, E.K. (eds), *Neonatal skin. Structure and functions*. New York, Marcel Dekker, 149–164.

McCormick, K. and Abdel-Rahman, A. (1991) The role of testosterone in trichloroethylene penetration in vitro. *Environ. Res.* **54**, 82–92.

McCracken, N.W., Blain, P.G. and Williams, F.M. (1993) Nature and role of xenobiotic metabolizing esterases in rat liver, lung, skin and blood. *J. Biochem. Pharmacol.* **45**, 31–36.

McFarland, B.J., Beeson, C. and Sant, A.J. (1999) Cutting edge: a single, essential hydrogen bond controls the stability of peptide-MHC class II complexes. *J. Immunol.* **163**, 3567–3571.

McKenzie, A.W. and Stoughton, R.B. (1962) Method of comparing percutaneous absorption of steroids. *Arch. Dermatol.* **86**, 608–614.

Macpherson, S.E., Scott, R.C. and Williams, F.M. (1991) Fate of carbaryl in rat skin in vitro. *Arch. Toxicol.* **65**, 594–598.

Magnusson, B. and Kligman, A.M. (1969) The identification of contact allergens by animal assay. The guinea pig maximisation test. *J. Invest. Dermatol.* **52**, 268–276.

Mahgoub, A., Idle, J.R., Dring, L.G., Lancaster, R. and Smith, R.L. (1977) Polymorphic hydroxylation of debrisoquine in man. *Lancet* **ii**, 584–586.

Maibach, H.I. and Menne, T. (1989) 'Nickel and the Skin'. Florida, CRC Press.

Majeti, V.A. and Suskind, R.R. (1977) Mechanism of cinnamaldehyde sensitization. *Contact Dermatitis* **3**, 16–18.

Malanin, K. (1993) Active sensitization to camphorquinone and double active sensitization to acrylics with long-lasting patch test reactions. *Contact Dermatitis* **29**, 284–285.

Manome, H., Aiba, S. and Tagami, H. (1999) Simple chemicals can induce maturation and apoptosis of dendritic cells. *Immunology* **98**, 481–490.

Mardh, G., Dingley, A.L., Auld, D.S. and Vallee, B.L. (1986) Human class II (pi) alcohol dehydrogenase has a redox-specific function in norepinephrine metabolism. *Proc. Natl. Acad. Sci. USA* **83**(23), 8908–8912.

Marks, J.G. and DeLeo, V.A. (1997) *Contact and occupational dermatology*, 2nd ed/Ed. Mosby–Year Book, 400 pp.

Marks, J.G., Belsito, D.V., DeLeo, V.A., Fowler, J.F., Fransway, A.F., Maibach, H.I., Mathias, C.G.T., Nethercott, J.R., Rietschel, R.L., Sherertz, E.F., Storrs, F.J. and Taylor, J.S. (1998) North American Contact Dermatitis Group patch test results for the detection of delayed-type hypersensitivity to topical allergens. *J. Am. Acad. Dermatol.* **38**, 911–918.

Martin, G.P., Ladenheim, D., Marriott, C., Hollingsbee, D.A. and Brown, M.B. (2000) The influence of hydrocolloid patch composition on the bioavailability of triamcinolone acetonide in humans. *Drug Dev. Ind. Pharm.* **26**, 35–43.

MARTIN, S., ORTMANN, B., PFLUGFELDER, U., BIRSNER, U. and WELTZEIN, H.U. (1992) Role of hapten-anchoring peptides in defining hapten-epitopes for MHC-restricted cytotoxic T cells. Cross-reactive TNP-determinants on different peptides. *J. Immunol.* **149**, 2569.

MARTIN, S. and WELTZIEN, H.U. (1994) T cell recognition of haptens, a molecular view. *Int. Arch. Allergy Immunol.* **104**, 10–16.

MARTINEZ, C.K. and MONACO, J.J. (1991) Homology of proteasome subunits to a major histocompatibility complex-linked LMP gene. *Nature* **353**, 664–667.

MARZULLI, F.N. and TREGEAR, K.T. (1961) Identification of a barrier layer in the skin. *J. Physiol.* **52**, 1957.

MARZULLI, F.N. (1962) Barriers to skin penetration. *J. Invest. Dermatol.* **39**, 387–393.

MARZULLI, F.N. and MAIBACH, H.I. (1987) *Dermatotoxicology*, 3rd ed/Ed. Hemisphere Publishing Corporation, New York.

MASON, R.P., PETERSON, F.J. and HOLTZMAN, J.L. (1977) The formation of an azo anion free radical metabolite during the microsomal azo reduction of sulfonazo III. *Biochem. Biophys. Res. Commun.* **75**, 532–540.

MATHEWS, J.M., GARNER, C.E., BLACK, S.L. and MATTHEWS, H.B. (1997) Diethanolamine absorption, metabolism and disposition in rat and mouse following oral, intravenous and dermal administration. *Xenobiotica* **27**, 733–746.

MATHEWS, J.M., GARNER, C.E. and MATTHEWS, H.B. (1995) Metabolism, bioaccumulation, and incorporation of diethanolamine into phospholipids. *Chem. Res. Toxicol.* **8**, 625–633.

MATHIAS, C.G. (1985) The Cost of Occupational Skin Disease. *Arch. Dermatol.* **121**, 332–334.

MATHIAS, C.G.T. and MORRISON, J.H. (1988) Occupational skin diseases, United States. *Arch. Dermatol.* **124**, 1519–1524.

MATHIAS, C.G.T. (1989) Contact dermatitis and workers' compensation: criteria for establishing occupational causation and aggravation. *J. Am. Acad. Dermatol.* **20**, 842–848.

MATSUNAGA, T., KATAYAMA, I., YOKOZEKI, H. and NISHIOKA, K. (1998) Epidermal cytokine mRNA expression induced by hapten differs from that induced by primary irritant in human skin organ culture system. *J. Dermatol.* **25**, 421–428.

MATSUZAWA, T., WADA, Y., SHIMOYAMA, M., NAKAJIMA, K., SEKI, T., SUGIBAYASHI, K. and MORIMOTO, Y. (1994) The effect of different routes of administration on the metabolism of morphine: the disposition of morphine and its metabolites after topical application. *Biopharm. Drug Dispos.* **15**, 665–678.

MATTHIEU, L., WEYLER, J., DECKERS, I., VAN SPUNDEL, M., VAN ANDEL, A. and DOCKX, P. (1993)

Occupational contact sensitization to ethylenediamine in a wire-drawing factory. *Contact Dermatitis* **29**, 39.

Mayer, R.L. (1954) Group sensitisation to compounds of quinone structure and its biochemical base. *Progr. Allergy* **4**, 79–82.

Meding, B. (1993) Skin symptoms among workers in a spice factory. *Contact Dermatitis* **29**, 202–205.

Menczel, E. and Maibach, H.I. (1972) Chemical binding to human dermis in vitro testosterone and benzyl alcohol. *Acta Dermatol. Venereol.* **52**, 38–42.

Menne, T., Frosch, P., Veien, N.K. et al. (1991) Contact sensitization to 5-chloro-2-methyl-4-isothiazolinon-3-one and 2-methyl-4-isothiazolin-3-one (MCI/MI). A European multicentre study. *Contact Dermatitis* **24**, 334–341.

Mercurio, M.G., Bickers, D.R. and Sassa, S. (1995) Demonstration of messensger RNAs for 3 major forms of cytochrome P450 in normal human skin. *J. Invest. Dermatol.* **104**, 676.

Merk, H., Rumpf, M., Bolsen, K., Wirth, G. and Goerz, G. (1984) Inducibility of arylhydrocarbon hydroxylase activity in human hair follicles by topical application of liquor carbonis detergens (coal tar). *Br. J. Dermatol.* **111**, 279–284.

Merk, H. and Jugert, F. (1991) Cutaneous NAD(P)H:quinone reductase: a xenobiotic metabolizing enzyme with potential cancer and oxidative stress protecting properties. *Skin Pharmacol.* **4**, 95–100.

Merk, H., Jugert, F., Bonnekoh, B. and Mahrle, G. (1991) Induction and inhibition of NAD(P)H: quinone reductase in murine and human skin. *Skin Pharmacol.* **4**, 183–190.

Meyer, W. and Neurand, K. (1976) The distribution of enzymes in the skin of the domestic pig. *Lab. Anim.* **10**, 237–247.

Meyer, W., Neurand, K., Godynicki, S., Kojda, G. and Mayer, B. (1996) Demonstration of NADPH diaphorase (NO-synthase) in sebaceous glands of the mammalian integument, with remarks on the glandular capillary net. *Cellul. & Molec. Biol.* **42**, 241–248.

Mier, P.D. and van den Hurk, J.J.M.A. (1975) Lysosomal hydrolases of the epidermis. *Br. J. Dermatol.* **93**, 509–517.

Mint, A., Hotchkiss, S.A.M. and Caldwell, J. (1994) Percutaneous absorption of diethyl phthalate through rat and human skin in vitro. *Toxicol. In Vitro* **8**, 251–256.

Mint, A. (1995) Investigation into the topical disposition of the phthalic acid esters, dimethyl phthalate, diethyl phthalate and dibutyl phthalate in rat and human skin. PhD, University of London, London.

Moloney, S.J., Fromson, J.M. and Bridges, J.W. (1982) The metabolism of 7-ethoxycoumarin and 7-hydroxycoumarin by rat and hairless mouse skin strips. *Biochem. Pharmacol.* **31**, 4005–4009.

MOMMAAS, A.M., MULDER, A.A., JORDENS, R., OUT, C., TAN, M.C., CRESSWELL, P., KLUIN, P.M. and KONING, F. (1999) Human epidermal Langerhans' cells lack functional mannose receptors and a fully developed endosomal/lysosomal compartment for loading of HLA class II molecules. *Eur. J. Immunol.* **29**, 571–580.

MONKS, T.J. and LAU, S.S. (1992) Toxicology of quinone-thioethers. *Crit. Rev. Toxicol.* **22**, 243–270.

MONKS, T.J. and LAU, S.S. (1994) Glutathione conjugation as a mechanism for the transport of reactive metabolites. *Adv. Pharmacol.* **27**, 183–210.

MOODY, R.P., NADEAU, B. and CHU, I. (1995) In-vivo and in-vitro dermal absorption of benzo[a]pyrene in rat, guinea-pig, human and tissue-cultured skin. *J. Dermatol. Sci.* **9**, 48–58.

MOON, K.C., WESTER, R.C. and MAIBACH, H.I. (1990) Diseased skin models in the hairless guinea pig: in vivo percutaneous absorption. *Dermatological* **180**, 8–12.

MORALES, J., HOMEY, B., VICARI, A.P., HUDAK, S., OLDHAM, E., HEDRICK, J., OROZCO, R., COPELAND, N.G., JENKINS, N.A., MCEVOY, L.M. and ZLOTNIK, A. (1999) CTACK, a skin associated chemokine that preferentially attracts skin homing memory T lymphocytes. *Proc. Natl. Acad. Sci. USA* **96**, 14470–14475.

MORELLI, J.G., NORRIS, D.A., BRADLEY LYONS, M. and MURPHY, R. (1990) Metabolism of exogenous leukotrienes by cultured human keratinocytes. *J. Invest. Dermatol.* **94**, 681–684.

MORENO, A. and PARES, X. (1991) Purification and characterization of a new alcohol dehydrogenase from human stomach. *J. Biol. Chem.* **266**(2), 1128–1133.

MORIMOTO, K., IWAKURA, Y., NAKATANI, E., MIYAZAKI, M. and TOJIMA, H. (1992) Effects of proteolytic enzyme inhibitors as absorption enhancers on the transdermal iontophoretic delivery of calcitonin in rats. *J. Pharm. Pharmacol.* **44**, 216–218.

MORIMOTO, K., IWAKURA, Y., MIYAZAKI, M. and NAKATANI, E. (1992a) Effects of proteolytic enzyme inhibitors of enhancement of transdermal iontophoretic delivery of vasopressin and an analogue in rats. *Int. J. Pharm.* **81**, 119–125.

MORIWAKI, Y., YAMAMOTO, T., YAMAGUCHI, K., TAKAHASHI, S. and HIGASHINO, K. (1996) Immunohistochemical localisation of aldehyde and xanthine oxidase in rat tissues using polyclonal antibodies. *Histochem. Cell Biol.* **105**, 71–79.

MORONI, P., NAVA, C., ZERBONI, R., PIERINI, F., ARBOSTI, G.G.B.V., BRAMBILLA, G., MARCHISIO, M., VENERONI, C. and BERTUCCI, R. (1985) Le dermopatie allergiche professionali: cinque anni di esperienza. *Med. Lav.* **76**, 294–303.

MOSLEMI, S. and SERALINI, G.E. (1997) Inhibition and inactivation of equine aromatase by steroidal and non-steroidal compounds. A comparison with human aromatase inhibition. *J. Enzyme Inhib.* **12**, 214–254.

MUKHTAR, H. and BRESNICK, E. (1976) Glutathione-S-epoxide transferase in mouse skin and human foreskin. *J. Invest. Dermatol.* **66**, 161–164.

MUKHTAR, H. and BICKERS, D.R. (1981) Drug metabolism in skin: comparative activity of the mixed function oxidases, epoxide hydrolase and glutathione S-transferase in liver and skin of the neonatal rat. *Drug Metab. Dispos.* **9**, 311–314.

MUKHTAR, H. and BICKERS, D.R. (1982) Evidence that coal tar is a mixed inducer of microsomal metabolising enzymes. *Toxicol. Lett.* **11**, 221–227.

MUKHTAR, H. and BICKERS, D.R. (1983) Age related changes in benzo(a)pyrene metabolism and epoxide metabolizing enzyme activities in rat skin. *Drug Metab. Disposit.* **11**, 562–567.

MUKHTAR, H., DAS, M. and BICKERS, D.R. (1986) Skin tumor initiating activity of therapuetic crude coal tar as compared to other polycyclic aromatic hydrocarbons in Sencar mice. *Cancer Lett.* **31**, 147–151.

MUKHTAR, H., BIK, D.P., RUZICKA, T., MERK, H.F. and BICKERS, D.R. (1989) Cytochrome P450-dependent omega-oxidation of leukotriene B4 in rodent and human epidermis. *J. Invest. Dermatol.* **93**, 231–235.

MUKHTAR, H. and KHAN, W.A. (1989) Cutaneous cytochrome P450. *Drug Metab. Rev.* **20**, 657–673.

MULLER, K. and GAWLIK, I. (1996) Inactivation of mouse epidermal 12-lipoxygenase by anthralin-implications for the role of oxygen radicals. *Biochem. Pharmacol.* **51**, 1173–1179.

MULLER, G., KNOP, J. and ENK, A.H. (1996) Is cytokine expression responsible for differences between allergens and irritants? *Am. J. Contact Dermat.* **7**, 177–184.

MULLER-GOYMANN, C.C. and ALBERG, U. (1999) Modified water containing hydrophilic ointment with suspended hydrocortisone-21-acetate — the influence of the microstructure of the cream on the in vitro drug release and in vitro percutaneous penetration. *Eur. J. Pharm. Biopharm.* **47**, 139–143.

MURTHY, V.L. and STERN, L.J. (1997) The class II MHC protein HLA-DR1 in complex with an endogenous peptide: implications for the structural basis of the specificity of peptide binding. *Structure* **5**, 1385–1396.

NACHT, S., YEUNG, D., BEASLEY, J.N. JNR., ANJO, M.D. and MAIBACH, H.I. (1981) Benzoyl peroxide: percutaneous penetration and metabolic disposition. *J. Am. Acad. Dermatol.* **4**, 31–37.

NAJBAUER, J., JOHNSON, B.A. and ASWAD, D.W. (1992) Analysis of stable protein methylation in cultured cells. *Arch. Biochem. Biophys.* **293**, 85–92.

NAKAGAWA, S. and TANIOKU, K. (1972) The induction of delayed sensitivity to 2,4-dinitrophenyl conjugates in guinea pigs sensitized with DNCB. *Dermatologica* **144**, 19–26.

NAKAGAWA, M., KAWAI, K. and KAWAI, K. (1996) Multiple azo disperse dye sensitization mainly due to group sensitizations to azo dyes. *Contact Dermatitis* **34**, 6–11.

NAKAJIMA, T., WANG, R.S., ELOVAARA, E., GONZALEZ, F.J., GELBOIN, H.V., RAUNIO, H., PELKONEN, O., VAINIO, H. and AOYAMA, T. (1997) Toluene metabolism by cDNA-expressed human hepatic cytochrome P450. *Biochem. Pharmacol.* **53**, 271–277.

NAKAMURA, K., YOKOI, T., KODAMA, T., INOUE, K., NAGASHIMA, K., SHIMADA, N., SHIMIZU, T. and KAMATAKI, T. (1998) Oxidation of histamine H1 receptor antagonist mequitazine is catalysed by cytochrome P450 2D6 in human liver microsomes. *J. Pharmacol. Exp. Ther.* **284**, 437–442.

NAKATOMI, I., NAKAMURA, K., FURUKAWA, K. and KODA, A. (1987) Inhibition of delayed hypersensitivity reactions by a new agent, cis-1- methyl-4-isohexylcyclohexane carboxylic acid (IG-10)–II. The mechanism regarding the action on lymphokines. *Int. J. Immunopharmacol.* **9**, 243–253.

NAKAYAMA, T., KIMURA, T., KODAMA, M. and NAGATA, C. (1983) Generation of hydrogen peroxide and superoxide anion from active metabolites of naphthylamines and aminoazo dyes: its possible role in carcinogenesis. *Carcinogenesis* **4**, 765–769.

NASSERI-SINA, P., HOTCHKISS, S.A.M. and CALDWELL, J. (1997) Cutaneous xenobiotic metabolism: glycine conjugation in human and rat keratinocytes. *Food Chem. Toxicol.* **35**, 409–416.

NATHAN, D., SAKR, A., LICHTIN, J.L. and BRONAUGH, R.L. (1990) In vitro skin absorption and metabolism of benzoic acid, p-aminobenzoic acid and benzocaine in the hairless guinea-pig. *Pharm. Res.* **7**, 1147–1151.

NEBERT, D.W. (1997) Polymorphisms in drug-metabolising enzymes: what is their clinical relevance and why do they exist. *Am. J. Hum. Genet.* **60**, 265–271.

NELSON, D.R., KOYMANS, L., KAMATAKI, T., STEGEMAN, J.J., FEYEREISEN, R., WAXMAN, D.J., WATERMAN, M.R., GOTOH, O., COON, M.J., ESTABROOK, R.W., GUNSALUS, I.C. and NEBERT, D.W. (1996) P450 superfamily: update on new sequences, gene mapping, accession numbers and nomenclature. *Pharmacogenetics* **6**, 1–42.

NICHOLLS, R., DE JERSEY, J., WORRALL, S. and WILCE, P. (1992) Modification of proteins and other biological molecules by acetaldehyde: adduct structure and functional significance. *Int. J. Biochem.* **24**, 1899–1906.

NICOLAU, G. and YACOBI, A. (1990) Transdermal absorption and skin metabolism of viprostol, a synthetic prostaglandin E2 analogue. *Drug Metab. Rev.* **21**, 401–425.

NIELSEN, G.D., NIELSEN, J.B., ANDERSEN, K.E. and GRANDJEAN, P. (2000) Effects of industrial detergents on the barrier function of human skin. *Int. J. Occup. Environ. Health* **6**, 138–142.

NILSSON, U., BERGH, M., SHAO, L.P. and KARLBERG, A.-T. (1996) Analysis of contact allergenic compounds in oxidised d-limonene. *Chromatographia* **42**.

NISHIOKA, K., AOKI, T. and TASHIRO, M. (1971) Studies on carrier substances of DNCB contact allergy. *Dermatologica* **142**, 232–240.

NORDEN, G. (1953) The role of appearance, metabolism and disappearance of 3,5-benzopyrene in the epithelium of mouse skin. *Acta Pathol. Microbiol. Scand.* **96**, 1–87.

NORRED, W.P. and AKIN, F.J. (1976) Induction of aryl hydrocarbon hydroxylase and carbon monoxide-binding hemoproteins in mouse epidermis by tobacco carcinogens. *Biochem. Pharmacol.* **25**, 732–734.

OBATA, Y., SESUMI, T., TAKAYAMA, K., ISOWA, K., GROSH, S., WICK, S., SITZ, R. and NAGAI, T. (2000) Evaluation of skin damage caused by percutaneous absorption enhancers using fractal analysis. *J. Pharm. Sci.* **89**, 556–561.

OESCH, F., TEGTMEYER, F., KOHL, F.V., RUDIGER, H. and GLATT, H.R. (1980) Interindividual comparison of epoxide hydratase and glutathione S-transferase activities in cultured human fibroblasts. *Carcinogenesis* **1**, 305–309.

OKUDA, H., NOJIMA, H., WATANABE, N., MIWA, K. and WATABE, T. (1988) Activation of the carcinogne, 5-hydroxymethylchrysene, to the mutagenic sulphate ester by mouse skin sulphotransferase. *Biochem. Pharmacol.* **37**, 970–973.

OLIVER, C.J. and SHENOLIKAR, S. (1998) Physiologic importance of protein phosphatase inhibitors. *Front Biosci.* **3**, D961–972.

OLSON, J.A., MOON, R.C., ANDERS, M.W., FENSELAU, C. and SHANE, B. (1992) Enhancement of biological activity by conjugation reactions. *J. Nutr.* **122**, 615–624.

OMIECINSKI, C.J., REDLICH, C.A. and COSTA, P. (1990) Induction and development expression of cytochrome P4501A1 messenger RNA in rat and human tissue, detection by the polymerase chain reaction. *Cancer Res.* **50**, 4315.

OMURA, T. and SATO, R. (1964) The carbon monoxide-binding pigment of liver microsomes. I. Evidence for its hemoprotein nature. *J. Biol. Chem.* **239**, 2370–2378.

OPHASWONGSE, S. and MAIBACH, H.I. (1994) Alcohol dermatitis: allergic contact dermatitis and contact urticaria syndrome. *Contact Dermatitis* **30**, 1–6.

ORTIZ DE MONTELLANO, P.R. (1989) Cytochrome P450 catalysis: radical intermediates and dehydrogenase reactions. *TIPS Rev.* **10**, 354–359.

OTTERNESS, D.M., KEITH, R.A., KERREMANS, A.L. and WEINSHILBOUM, R.M. (1986) Mouse liver thiol methyltransferase. Assay conditions, biochemical properties, and strain variation. *Drug Metab. Dispos.* **14**, 680–688.

PANNATIER, A., JENNER, P., TESTA, B. and ETTER, J.C. (1978) The skin as a drug metabolizing organ. *Drug Metab. Rev.* **8**, 319–343.

PARK, B.K., KITTERINGHAM, N.R., PIRMOHAMED, M. and TUCKER, G.T. (1996) Relevance of induction of human drug-metabolising enzymes: pharmacological and toxicological implications. *Br. J. Clin. Pharmacol.* **41**, 477–491.

PARK, K.K., SOHN, Y., LIEM, A., KIM, H.J., STEWART, B.C. and MILLER, J.A. (1997) The electrophilic, mutagenic and tumorigenic activities of phenyl and 4-nitrophenyl vinyl ethers and their epoxide metabolites. *Carcinogenesis* **18**, 431–437.

PASCHOUD, J.M., KELLER, W. and SCHMIDLI, B. (1956) Untersuchungen uber Peptidasen in der gesunden und der befallenen Haut von Psoriasiskranken. *Arch. Klin. Exp. Dermatol.* **203**, 203–216.

PATLEWICZ, G., BASKETTER, D.A., SMITH, C.K., HOTCHKISS, S.A.M. and ROBERTS, D.W. (2001) Skin Sensitisation Structure Activity Relationships for Aldehydes. Accepted by *Contact Dermatitis.*

PATRICK, E. and MAIBACH, H.I. (1989) Dermatotoxicology. In: HAYES, A.W. (ed.), *Principles and Methods of Toxicology*, New York, Raven Press, 383–406.

PAYNE, P.A. (1991) Measurement of properties and function of skin. *Clinical, Physical and Physiological Measurements* **12**, 105–129.

PAYTON, M.A. and SIM, E. (1998) Genotyping human arylamine N-acetyltransferase type 1 (NAT1): the identification of two novel allelic variants. *Biochem. Pharmacol.* **55**, 361–366.

PENDLINGTON, R.U., WILLIAMS, D.L., NAIK, J.T. and SHARMA, R.K. (1994) Distribution of xenobiotic metabolizing enzymes in skin. *Toxicology in Vitro* **8**, 525–527.

PENNING, T.M. (1997) Hydroxysteroid dehydrogenases. New drug targets of the aldo-keto reductase superfamily. *Adv. Exp. Med. Biol.* **414**, 475–490.

PENNING, T.M., BENNETT, M.J., SMITH-HOOG, S., SCHLEGEL, B.P., JEZ, J.M. and LEWIS, M. (1997) Structure and function of 3 alpha-hydroxysteroid dehydrogenase. *Steroids* **62**, 101–111.

PERRENOUD, D., BIRCHER, A., HUNZIKER, T., SUTER, H., BRUCKNER-TUDERMAN, L., STAGER, J., THURLIMANN, W., SCHMID, P., SUARD, A. and HUNZIKER, N. (1994) Frequency of sensitization to 13 common preservatives in Switzerland. Swiss Contact Dermatitis Research Group. *Contact Dermatitis* **30**, 276–279.

PETERS, W.H.M., ALLEBES, W.A., JANSEN, P.L.M., POELS, L.G. and CAPEL, P.J.A. (1987) Characterization and tissue specificity of a monoclonal antibody against human uridine 5′-diphosphate-glucuronyltransferase. *Gastroenterology* **93**, 162–169.

PHAM, M.A., MAGDALOU, J., TOTIS, M., FOURNEL-GIGLEUX, S., SIEST, G. and HAMMOCK, B.D. (1989) Characterization of distinct forms of cytochromes-P450, epoxide metabolizing enzymes and UDP-glucuronyltransferases in rat skin. *Biochem. Pharmacol.* **38**, 2187–2194.

PHAM, M.A., MAGDALOU, J., SIEST, G., LENOIR, M.C., BERNARD, B.A., JAMOULLE, J.C. and SHROOT, B. (1990) Reconstituted epidermis: a novel model for the study of long metabolism in human epidermis. *J. Invest. Dermatol.* **94**, 749–752.

PICARD-AMI, L.A., MACKAY, A. and KERRIGAN, C.L. (1992) Effect of allopurinol on the survival of experimental pig flaps. *Plast. Reconstr. Surg.* **89**, 1098–1103.

PICARDO, M., CANNISTRACI, C., CRISTAUDO, A., DE LUCA, C. and SANTUCCI, B. (1990) Study on cross-reactivity to the para group. *Dermatologica* **181**, 104–108.

PICARDO, M., ZOMPETTA, C., MARCHESE, C., DE LUCA, C., FAGGIONI, A., SCHMIDT, R.J. and SANTUCCI, B. (1992) Paraphenylenediamine, a contact allergen, induces oxidative stress and ICAM-1 expression in human keratinocytes. *Br. J. Dermatol.* **126**, 450–455.

PICARDO, M., ZOMPETTA, C., GRANDINETTI, M., AMEGLIO, F., SANTUCCI, B., FAGGIONI, A. and PASSI, S. (1996) Paraphenylenediamine, a contact allergen, induces oxidative stress in normal human keratinocytes in culture. *Br. J. Dermatol.* **134**, 681–685.

PIGATTO, P., BIGARDI, A., LEGORI, A., VALSECCHI, R. and PICARDO, M. (1996) Cross-reactions in patch testing and photopatch testing with ketoprofen, thiaprophenic acid, and cinnamic aldehyde. *Am. J. Contact Dermat.* **7**, 220–223.

PIROG, E.C. and COLLINS, D.C. (1994) 3-alpha-hydroxysteroid dehydrogenase activity in rat liver and skin. *Steroids* **59**, 259–264.

PODDA, M., ZOLLNER, T., GRUNDMANN-KOLLMANN, M., KAUFMANN, R. and BOEHNCKE, W.H. (1999) Allergic contact dermatitis from benzyl alcohol during topical antimycotic treatment. *Contact Dermatitis* **41**, 302–303.

POHL, R.J., PHILPOT, R.M. and FOUTS, J.R. (1976) Cytochrome P-450 content and mixed function oxidase activity in microsomes isolated from mouse skin. *Drug Metab. Dispos.* **4**, 442–450.

POLAK, L. and MACHER, E. (1974) In vitro sensitisation to dinitrochlorobenzene in guinea-pigs. *Nature* **252**, 748–749.

POTTS, R.O. and FRANCOEUR, M.L. (1991) The influence of stratum corneum morphology on water permeability. *J. Invest. Dermatol.* **96**, 495–499.

POTTS, R.O., BOMMANNAN, B. and GUY, R.H. (1992) Percutaneous absorption. In: MUKHTAR, H. (ed.), *Pharmacology of the skin*. CRC Press, 13–27.

POTTS, R.O. and GUY, R. (1992) Predicting skin permeability. *Pharm. Res.* **9**, 663–669.

POULOS, T.L. (1995) Cytochrome P450. *Curr. Opin. Struct. Biol.* **5**, 767–774.

PRUE, C., MARTINSON, M.E., MCANALLY, P.M. and STAGNER, W.C. (1998) Postmarketing survey results of T.R.U.E. test, a new allergen patch test. *Am. J. Contact Dermat.* **9**, 6–10.

RAFFALI, F., ROUGIER, A. and ROGUET, R. (1994) Measurement and modulation of cytochrome P450 dependent enzyme activity in cultured human keratinocytes. *Skin Pharmacol.* **7**, 345–354.

RAFFERTY, T.S., MCKENZIE, R.C., HUNTER, J.A., HOWIE, A.F., ARTHUR, J.R., NICOL, F. and BECKETT, G.J. (1998) Differential expression of selenoproteins by human skin cells and protection by selenium from UVB-radiation-induced cell death. *Biochem. J.* **332**, 231–236.

RAFII, F. and CERNIGLIA, C.E. (1995) Reduction of azo dyes and nitroaromatic compounds by bacterial enzymes from the human intestinal tract. *Environ. Health Perspect.* **103**, 17–19.

RAMASWAMY, S., EKLUND, H. and PLAPP, B.V. (1994) Structures of horse liver alcohol dehydrogenase complexed with NAD+ and substituted benzyl alcohols. *Biochemistry* **33**, 5230–5237.

RAMBUKKANA, A., BOS, J.D., IRIK, D., MENKO, W.J., KAPSENBERG, M.L. and DAS, P.K. (1995) In situ behaviour of human Langerhans' cells in skin organ culture. *Lab. Invest.* **73**, 521–529.

RAMCHAND, C.N., CLARK, A.E., RAMCHAND, R. and HEMMINGS, G.P. (1995) Cultured human keratinocytes as a model for studying the dopamine metabolism in schizophrenia. *Medical Hypotheses* **44**, 53–57.

RAMMENSEE, H., BACHMANN, J., EMMERICH, N.P., BACHOR, O.A. and STEVANOVIC, S. (1999) SYFPEITHI: database for MHC ligands and peptide motifs. *Immunogenetics* **50**, 213–219.

RANDOLPH, R.K. and SIMON, M. (1997) Metabolism of all-trans retinoic acid by cultured human epidermal keratinocytes. *J. Lipid Res.* **38**, 1374–1383.

RAZA, H., AWASTHI, Y.C., ZAIM, M.T., ECKERT, R.L. and MUKHTAR, H. (1991) Glutathione S-transferases in human and rodent skin:multiple forms and species specific expression. *J. Invest. Dermatol.* **96**, 463–467.

RAZA, H., AGARWAL, R., BICKERS, D.R. and MUKHTAR, H. (1992) Purification and molecular characterisation of B-naphthoflavone-inducible cytochrome P450 from rat epidermis. *J. Invest. Dermatol.* **98**, 233–240.

REES, R., SMITH, D., LI, T.D., CASHMER, B., GARNER, W., PUNCH, J. and SMITH, D.J. JNR. (1994) The role of xanthine oxidase and xanthine dehydrogenase in skin ischemia. *J. Surg. Res.* **56**, 162–167.

REILLY, T.P., LASH, L.H., DOLL, M.A., HEIN, D.W., WOSTER, P.M. and SVENSSON, C.K. (2000) A role for bioactivation and covalent-binding within epidermal keratinocytes in sulfonamide-induced cutaneous drug reactions. *J. Invest. Dermatol.* **114**, 1164–1173.

REINERS, J.J., CANTU, A.R. and PAVONE, A. (1990) Modulation of constitutive cytochrome P450 expression in vivo and in vitro in murine keratinocytes as a function of differentiation and extracellular Ca2+ concentration. *Proc. Natl. Acad. Sci.* **87**, 1825–1829.

REINERS, J.J.J., THAI, G., RUPP, T. and CANTU, A.R. (1991) Assessment of the antioxidant/prooxidant status of murine skin following topical treatment with 12-O-tetradecanoylphorbol-13-acetate and throughout the ontogeny of skin cancer. Part 1: quantitation of superoxide dismutase, catalase, glutathione peroxidase and xanthine oxidase. *Carcinogenesis* **12**, 2337–2343.

REINERS, J.J., JONES, C.L., HONG, N. and MYRAND, S.P. (1998) Differential induction of CYP1A1, CYP1B1, AHD4 and NMO1 in murine skin tumours and adjacent normal epidermis by ligands of the aryl hydrocarbon receptor. *Molecular Carcinogenesis* **21**, 135–146.

REINHERZ, E.L., TAN, K., TANG, L., KERN, P., LIU, J., XIONG, Y., HUSSEY, R.E., SMOLYAR, A., HARE, B., ZHANG, R., JOACHIMIAK, A., CHANG, H.C., WAGNER, G. and WANG, J. (1999) The crystal structure of a T cell receptor in complex with peptide and MHC class II. *Science* **286**, 1913–1921.

REN, B., HUANG, W., AKESSON, B. and LADENSTEIN, R. (1997) The crystal structure of seleno-glutathione peroxidase from human plasma at 2.9A resolution. *J. Mol. Biol.* **268**, 869–885.

RENDIC, S. and DI CARLO, F.J. (1997) Human cytochrome P450 enzymes: a status report summarizing their reactions, substrates, inducers, and inhibitors. *Drug Metab. Rev.* **29**, 413–580.

RETTIE, A.E., WILLIAMS, F.M., RAWLINS, M.D., MAYER, R.T. and BURKE, D.M. (1986) Major differences between lung, skin and liver in the microsomal metabolism of homologous series of resorufin and coumarin ethers. *Biochem. Pharmacol.* **35**, 3495–3500.

RICCI, C., VACCARI, S., CAVALLI, M. and VINCENZI, C. (1997) Contact sensitization to sunscreens. *Am. J. Contact Dermat.* **8**, 165–166.

RITSCHEL, W.A., SABOUNI, A. and HUSSAIN, A.S. (1989) Percutaneous absorption of coumarin griseofulvin and propranolol hydrochloride across human scalp and abdominal skin. *Methods & Findings in Experimental & Clinical Pharmacol.* **11**, 643–646.

ROBERTS, D.W. and WILLIAMS, D.L. (1982) The derivation of quantitative correlation between skin sensitization and physico-chemical parameters for alkylating agents and their application to experimental data for sultone. *J. Theor. Biol.* **99**, 807–825.

ROBERTS, D.W. and BASKETTER, D.A. (1990) A quantitative structure activity/dose response relationship for contact allergic potential of alkyl group transfer agents. *Contact Dermatitis* **23**, 331–335.

ROBERTS, D.W., FRAGINALS, R., LEPOITTEVIN, J.-P. and BENEZRA, C. (1991) Refinement of the relative alkylation index (RAI) model for skin sensitization and application to mouse and guinea-pig test data for alkylsulfonates. *Arch. Dermatol. Res.* **283**, 387–394.

ROBERTS, D.W. and BENEZRA, C. (1993) Quantitative structure-activity relationships for skin sensitization potential of urushiol analogues. *Contact Dermatitis* **29**, 78–83.

ROBERTS, D.W. (1995) Linear free energy relationships for reactions of electrophilic halo- and pseudohalobenzenes, and their application in prediction of skin sensitization potential for SNAr electrophiles. *Chem. Res. Toxicol.* **8**, 545–551.

ROBERTS, D.W. and LEPOITTEVIN, J.-P. (1998) Hapten-Protein Interactions. In: LEPOITTEVIN,

J.-P., BASKETTER, D.A., GOOSSENS, A. and KARLBERG, A.-T. (eds), *Allergic Contact Dermatitis: the Molecular Basis*. Berlin, Springer-Verlag, 81–111.

ROBERTS, M.S. and WALTERS, K.A. (eds) (1998), *Dermal Absorption and Toxicity Assessment*. New York, Marcel Dekker.

ROBERTS, D.W., YORK, M. and BASKETTER, D.A. (1999) Structure-activity relationships in the murine local lymph node assay for skin sensitization: alpha,beta-diketones. *Contact Dermatitis* **41**, 14–17.

ROBERTS, M.S., ANDERSON, R.A., SWARBRICK, J. and MOORE, D.E. (1978) The percutaneous absorption of phenolic compounds: the mechanisms of diffusion across the stratum corneum. *J. Pharm. Pharmacol.* **30**, 486–492.

ROBINSON, M.K., FLETCHER, E.R., JOHNSON, G.R., WYDER, W.E. and MAURER, J.K. (1990) Value of the cutaneous basophil hypersensitivity (CBH) response for distinguishing weak contact sensitization from irritation reactions in the guinea pig. *J. Invest. Dermatol.* **94**, 636–643.

ROBINSON, M.K. (1999) Population differences in skin structure and physiology and the susceptibility to irritant and allergic contact dermatitis: implications for skin safety testing and risk assessment. *Contact Dermatitis* **41**, 65–79.

ROCK, K.L. and GOLDBERG, A.L. (1999) Degradation of cell proteins and the generation of MHC class I-presented peptides. *Annu. Rev. Immunol.* **17**, 739–779.

RONGONE, E.L. (1987) Skin structure function and biochemistry. In: MARZULLI, F.N. and MAIBACH, H.J. (eds), *Dermatotoxicology*. New York, Hemisphere, 1–70.

ROPER, C.S., HOWES, D., BLAIN, P.G. and WILLIAMS, F.M. (1995) Prediction of the percutaneous penetration and metabolism of dodecyl decathoxylate in rats using in vitro models. *Archives of Toxicol.* **69**, 649–654.

ROPER, C.S., HOWES, D., BLAIN, P.G. and WILLIAMS, F.M. (1998) Percutaneous penetration of 2-phenoxyethanol through rat and human skin. *Food & Chem. Toxicol.* **35**, 1009–1016.

ROSKOS, K.V. and MAIBACH, H.I. (1992) Percutaneous absorption and age. *Drugs and Aging* **2**, 432–449.

ROSS, R., ROSS, X.-L., GHADIALLY, H., LAHR, T., SCHWING, J., KNOP, J. and RESKE-KUNZ, A.B. (1999) Mouse Langerhans' cells differentially express an activated T cell-attracting CC chemokine. *J. Invest. Dermatol.* **113**, 991–998.

ROUGIER, A., DUPUIS, D., LOTTE, C., ROGUET, R. and SCHAEFER, H. (1983) In vivo correlation between stratum corneum reservoir function and percutaneous absorption. *J. Invest. Dermatol.* **81**, 275–278.

ROUGIER, A., DUPUIS, D., LOTTE, C. and ROGUET, R. (1985) The measurement of the stratum corneum reservoir. A predictive method for in vivo percutaneous absorption studies. *J. Invest. Dermatol.* **84**, 66–68.

ROY, S.D. and FLYNN, G.L. (1990) Transdermal delivery of narcotic analgesics: pH anatomical and subject influences on cutaneous permeability of fentamyl and sufentamyl. *Pharm. Res.* **7**, 842–847.

ROZELL, B., HANSSON, H.A., LUTHMAN, M. and HOLMGREN, A. (1985) Immunohistochemical localization of thioredoxin and thioredoxin reductase in adult rats. *Eur. J. Cell Biol.* **38**, 79.

RUGSTAD, H.E. and DYBING, E. (1975) Glucuronidation in cultures of human skin epithelial cells. *Eur. J. Clin. Invest.* **5**, 133–137.

RUSSO, J., CHUNG, S., CONTRERAS, K., LIAN, B., LORENZ, J., STEVENS, D. and TROUSDELL, W. (1995) Identification of 4-(N,N-dimethylamino)benzaldehyde as a potent, reversible inhibitor of mouse and human class I aldehyde dehydrogenase. *Biochem. Pharmacol.* **50**, 399–406.

RUSTEMEYER, T., DEGROOT, J., VONBLOMBERG, B.M.E., FROSCH, P.J. and SCHEPER, R.J. (1998) Cross-reactivity patterns of contact sensitizing methacrylates. *Toxicol. & Appl. Pharmacol.* **148**, 83–90.

SADEK, C.M. and ALLEN-HOFFMANN, B.L. (1994) Cytochrome P4501A1 is rapidaly induced in normal human keratinocytes in the absence of xenobiotics. *J. Biol. Chem.* **269**, 16067–16074.

SAFFORD, R.J., BASKETTER, D.A., ALLENBY, C.F. and GOODWIN, B.F.J. (1990) Immediate contact reactions to chemicals in the fragrance mix and a study of the quenching action of eugenol. *Br. J. Dermatol.* **123**, 595–606.

SAMPOL, E., MIRRIONE, A., VILLARD, P.H., PICCERELLE, P., SCOMA, H., BARBIS, P., BARRA, Y., DURAND, A. and LACARELLE, B. (1997) Evidence for a tissue specific induction of cutaneous CYP2E1 by dexamethasone. *Biochem. Biophys. Res. Comm.* **235**, 557–561.

SANDERINK, G.J., ARTUR, Y. and SIEST, G. (1988) Human aminopeptidases: A review of the literature. *J. Clin. Chem. Clin. Biochem.* **26**, 795–807.

SANT, A.J., BEESON, C., MCFARLAND, B., CAO, J., CEMAN, S., BRYANT, P.W. and WU, S. (1999) Individual hydrogen bonds play a critical role in MHC class II: peptide interactions: implications for the dynamic aspects of class II trafficking and DM-mediated peptide exchange. *Immunol. Rev.* **172**, 239–253.

SANTAMBROGIO, L., SATO, A.K., CARVEN, G.J., BELYANSKAYA, S.L., STROMINGER, J.L. and STERN, L.J. (1999) Extracellular antigen processing and presentation by immature dendritic cells. *Proc. Natl. Acad. Sci. USA* **96**, 15056–15061.

SANTELLA, L., KYOZUKA, K., DE RISO, L. and CARAFOLI, E. (1998) Calcium, protease action and the regulation of the cell cycle. *Cell Calcium* **23**, 123–130.

SANTUS, G.C., WATARI, N., HINZ, R.S., BENET, L.Z. and GUY, R. (1987) Cutaneous metabolism of transdermally delivered nitroglycerin in vitro. In: SHROOT, B. and SCHAEFER, H. (eds), *Pharmacology and the Skin*, Vol. 1. Basel, Karger, 240–244.

SARNESTO, A., LINDER, N. and RAIVIO, K.O. (1996) Organ distribution and molecular forms of human xanthine dehydrogenase/xanthine oxidase protein. *Lab. Invest.* **74**, 48–56.

SATO, Y. (1985) Modified guinea pig maximisation test. *Curr. Probl. Derm.* **14**, 193–200.

SATO, A.K., ZARUTSKIE, J.A., RUSHE, M.M., LOMAKIN, A., NATARAJAN, S.K., SADEGH-NASSERI, S., BENEDEK, G.B. and STERN, L.J. (2000) Determinants of the peptide-induced conformational change in the human class II major histocompatibility complex protein HLA-DR1. *J. Biol. Chem.* **275**, 2165–2173.

SAWAYA, M.E. and PENNEYS, N.S. (1992) Immunohistochemical distribution of aromatase and 3B-hydroxysteroid dehydrogenase in human hair follicle and sebaceous gland. *J. Cutan. Pathol.* **19**, 309–314.

SCHAEFER, H. and REDELMEIER, T.E. (1996) *Skin Barrier: Principles of Percutaneous Absorption.* Basel, Karger.

SCHALLREUTER, K.U. and WOOD, J.M. (1986) The role of thioredoxin reductase in the reduction of free radicals at the surface of the epidermis. *Biochem. Biophys. Res. Commun.* **136**, 630–637.

SCHALLREUTER, K.U., PITTELKOW, M.R. and WOOD, J.M. (1986) Free radical reduction by thioredoxin reductase at the surface of normal and vitiliginous human keratinocytes. *J. Invest. Dermatol.* **87**, 728–732.

SCHALLREUTER, K.U., HORDINSKY, M.K. and WOOD, J.M. (1987) Thioredoxin reductase. Role in free radical reduction in different hypopigmentation disorders. *Arch. Dermatol.* **123**, 615–619.

SCHALLREUTER, K.U., WOOD, J.M., PITTELKOW, M.R., BUTTNER, G., SWANSON, N., KORNER, C. and EHRKE, C. (1996) Increased monoamine oxidase A activity in the epidermis of patients with vitiligo. *Arch. Dermatol. Res.* **288**, 14–18.

SCHAUENSTEIN, E., ESTERBAUER, H., ZOLLNER, H. and GOVE, P.H. (1977) *Aldehydes in Biological Systems. Their Natural Occurrence and Biological Activities.* London, Pion.

SCHEUPLEIN, R.J. and BLANK, I.H. (1971) Permeability of the skin. *Physiological Rev.* **51**, 702–747.

SCHEUPLEIN, R.J. and ROSS, L.W. (1974) Mechanisms of percutaneous absorption V. Percutaneous absorption of solvent deposited solids. *J. Invest. Dermatol.* **62**, 353–363.

SCHEUPLEIN, R.J. and BRONAUGH, R.L. (1983) Percutaneous Absorption. In: GOLDSMITH, L.A. (ed.), *Biochemistry and Physiology of the Skin.* Oxford, OUP, 1255–1295.

SCHMIDT, R.J., KHAN, L. and CHUNG, L.Y. (1990) Are free radicals and not quinones the haptenic species derived from urushiols and other contact allergenic mono- and dihydric alkylbenzenes? The significance of NADH, glutathione and redox cycling in the skin. *Arch. Dermatol. Res.* **282**, 56–64.

SCHMIDT, R.J. and CHUNG, L.Y. (1990) Oxidative stress occurs in skin in the preimmunologic phase of the cell-mediated immune response to allergenic 2,4-dinitrohalobenzenes. *Free Rad. Biol. Med.* **9**, 147.

SCHMIDT, R.J. and CHUNG, L.Y. (1992) Biochemical responses of skin to allergenic and non-allergenic nitrohalobenzenes. *Arch. Dermatol. Res.* **284**, 400–408.

SCHNUCH, A., UTER, W., GEIER, J., FROSCH, P.J. and RUSTEMEYER, T. (1998a) Contact allergies in healthcare workers. Results from the IVDK. *Acta Derm. Venereol.* **78**, 358–363.

SCHNUCH, A., WESTPHAL, G.A., MULLER, M.M., SCHULZ, T.G., GEIER, J., BRASCH, J., MERK, H.F., KAWAKUBO, Y., RICHTER, G., KOCK, P., FUCHS, T., GUTGESELL, T., REICH, K., GEBHARDT, M., BECKER, D., GRABBE, J., SZLISKA, C., ABERER, W. and HALLIER, E. (1998b) Genotype and phenotype of N-acetyltransferase 2 (NAT2) polymorphism in patients with contact allergy. *Contact Dermatitis* **38**, 209–211.

SCHOKET, B., HEWER, A., GROVER, P.L. and PHILLIPS, D.H. (1988) Covalent binding of components of crude coal tar, creosote, and bitumen to the DNA of the skin and lungs of mice following topical application. *Carcinogenesis* **9**, 1253–1258.

SCHOLES, E.W., PENDLINGTON, R.U., SHARMA, R.K. and BASKETTER, D.A. (1994) Skin metabolism of contact allergens. *Toxic in vitro* **8**, 551–553.

SCOTT, C.A., PETERSON, P.A., TEYTON, L. and WILSON, I.A. (1998) Crystal structures of two I-Ad-peptide complexes reveal that high affinity can be achieved without large anchor residues. *Immunity* **8**, 319–329.

SCOTT, R.C., THOMPSON, M.A., WARD, R.J., RAMSEY, J. and RHODES, C. (1986) In vitro absorption of 1-chloro, 2, 4-dinitrobenzene (DNCB) through human, hooded rat and mouse epidermis. *Br. J. Dermatol.* **115**, 47–48.

SEBZDA, E., WALLACE, V.A., MAYER, J., YEUNG, R.S., MAK, T.W. and OHASHI, P.S. (1994) Positive and negative thymocyte selection induced by different concentrations of a single peptide. *Science* **263**, 1615–1618.

SEIDEGARD, J. and EKSTROM, G. (1997) The role of human glutathione transferases and epoxide hydrolases in the metabolism of xenobiotics. *Environ. Health Perspect.* **105**, 791–799.

SEIDENARI, S., MANTOVANI, L., MANZINI, B.M. and PIGNATTI, M. (1997) Cross-sensitizations between azo dyes and para-amino compound. A study of 236 azo-dye sensitive subjects. *Contact Dermatitis* **36**, 91–96.

SENMA, M., FUJIWARA, N., SASAKI, S., TOYAMA, M., SAKAGUCHI, K. and TAKAOKA, I. (1978) Studies on the cutaneous sensitization reaction of guinea pigs to purified aromatic chemicals. *Acta Derm. Venereol.* **58**, 121–124.

SERTOLI, A., FRANCALANCI, S., ACCIAI, M.C. and GOLA, M. (1999) Epidemiological survey of contact dermatitis in Italy (1984–1993) by GIRDCA (Gruppo Italiano Ricerca Dermatiti da Contatto e Ambientali). *Am. J. Contact Dermat.* **10**, 18–30.

SHAH, P.K. and BORCHARDT, R.T. (1990) Liquid chromatographic analysis of leucine-enkephalin and its metabolites in homogenates of cultured human keratinocytes. *J. Pharm. Biomed. Anal.* **8**, 457–461.

SHAH, P.K. and BORCHARDT, R.T. (1991) A comparison of peptidase activities and peptide metabolism in cultured mouse keratinocytes and neonatal mouse epidermis. *Pharm. Res.* **8**, 70–75.

SHAH, P.V., FISCHER, H.L., SUMIER, M.R., MONROE, R.J., CHERNOFF, N. and HALL, L.L. (1987) Comparison of the penetration of 14 pesticides through the skin of young and adult rats. *J. Toxicol. Envir. Health* **21**, 353–366.

SHARMA, V.K. and CHAKRABARTI, A. (1998) Common contact sensitisers in Chandigarh, India. *Contact Dermatitis* **38**, 127–131.

SHEIKH, S., NI, L., HURLEY, T.D. and WEINER, H. (1997) The potential roles of the conserved amino acids in human liver mitochondrial aldehyde dehydrogenase. *J. Biol. Chem.* **272**, 18817–18822.

SHERMAN, M.A., RUNNELS, H.A., MOORE, J.C., STERN, L.J. and JENSEN, P.E. (1994) Membrane interactions influence the peptide binding behaviour of DR1. *J. Exp. Med.* **179**, 229–234.

SHEU, S.Y., LAI, C.H. and CHIANG, H.C. (1998) Inhibition of xanthine oxidase by purpurogallin and silymarin group. *Anticancer Res.* **18**, 263–267.

SHINDO, Y., WITT, E., HAN, D., EPSTEIN, W. and PACKER, L. (1994) Enzymic and non-enzymic antioxidants in epidermis and dermis of human skin. *J. Invest. Dermatol.* **102**, 122–124.

SINCLAIR, J. and SIM, E. (1997) A fragment consisting of the first 204 amino-terminal amino acids of human arylamine N-acetyltransferase one (NAT1) and the first transacetylation step of catalysis. *Biochem. Pharmacol.* **53**, 11–16.

SINGH, S. and SINGH, J. (1993) Transdermal drug delivery by passive diffusion and iontophoresis: a review. In: 'Medicinal Research Reviews', Vol. 13. John Wiley & Sons, 569–621.

SINGHAL, S.S., SAXENA, M., AWASTHI, S., AHMAD, H., SHARMA, R. and AWASTHI, Y.C. (1992) Glutathione S-transferase of mouse liver: sex-related differences in the expression of various isozymes. *Biochim. Biophys. Acta* **1171**, 19–26.

SINGHAL, S.S., SAXENA, M., AWASTHI, S., MUKHTAR, H., ZAIDI, S.I.A., AHMAD, H. and AWASTHI, Y.C. (1993) Glutathione S-transferases of human skin — qualitative and quantitative differences in men and women. *Biochim. et Biophys. Acta* **1163**, 266–272.

SLADEK, N.E., MANTHEY, C.L., MAKI, P.A., ZHANG, Z. and LANDKAMER, G.J. (1989) Xenobiotic oxidation catalyzed by aldehyde dehydrogenases. *Drug Metab. Rev.* **20**, 697–720.

SLIVKA, S.R. (1992) Testosterone metabolism in an in vitro skin model. *Cell Biol. & Toxicol.* **8**, 267–276.

SLOB, A. (1973) Tulip allergens in Alstroemeria and some other Liliflora. *Phytochemistry* **12**, 811–815.

SLOMINSKI, A., BAKER, J., ROSANO, T.G., GUISTI, L.W., ERMAK, G., GRANDE, M. and GAUDET, S.J. (1996) Metabolism of serotonin to N-acetylserotonin, melatonin and 5-methoxytryptamine in hamster skin culture. *J. Biol. Chem.* **271**, 12281–12286.

SMITH, B.J., CURTIS, J.F. and ELING, T.E. (1991) Bioactivation of xenobiotics by prostaglandin H synthase. *Chem. Biol. Interact.* **79**, 245–264.

SMITH, C.K., SMART, A.T.S. and HOTCHKISS, S.A.M. (1999) Effects of an alcohol dehydrogenase inhibitor on cinnamaldehyde absorption and biotransformation in human skin. *The Toxicologist* **48**, 73.

SMITH, C.K., MOORE, C.A., ELAHI, E., SMART, A.T.S. and HOTCHKISS, S.A.M. (2000a) Human Skin Absorption and Metabolism of the Contact Allergens, Cinnamic Aldehyde and Cinnamic Alcohol. *Toxicol. Appl. Pharm.* **168**, 189–199.

SMITH, C.K., ELAHI, E. and HOTCHKISS, S.A.M. (2000b) Immuno-detection of protein-cinnamaldehyde adducts in cinnamic allergen-treated human skin. Proceedings of the Microsomal Drug Oxidation Meeting, Stresa, Italy.

SOLARY, E., EYMIN, B., DROIN, N. and HAUGG, M. (1998) Proteases, proteolysis, and apoptosis. *Cell Biol. Toxicol.* **14**, 121–132.

SOLOMAN, A.E. and LOWE, N.J. (1979) Percutaneous absorption in experimental epidermal diseases. *Br. J. Dermatol.* **100**, 717–721.

SPAHN-LANGGUTH, H. and BENET, L.Z. (1992) Acyl glucuronides revisited: is the glucuronidation process a toxification as well as a detoxification mechanism. *Drug Metab. Disposit.* **24**, 5–47.

SPEIR, J.A., ABDEL-MOTAL, U.M., JONDAL, M. and WILSON, I.A. (1999) Crystal structure of an MHC class I presented glycopeptide that generates carbohydrate-specific CTL. *Immunity* **10**, 51–61.

SPRACKLIN, D.K., HANKINS, D.C., FISHER, J.M., THUMMEL, K.E. and KHARASCH, E.D. (1997) Cytochrome P450 2E1 is the principal catalyst of human oxidative halothane metabolism in vitro. *J. Pharmacol. Exp. Ther.* **281**, 400–411.

STANLEY, L.A., CORONEOS, E., CUFF, R., HICKMAN, D., WARD, A. and SIM, E. (1996) Immunochemical detection of arylamine N-acetyltransferase in normal and neoplastic bladder. *J. Histochem. Cytochem.* **44**, 1059–1067.

STANLEY, L.A., MILLS, I.G. and SIM, E. (1997) Localisation of polymorphic N-acetyltransferase (NAT2) in tissues of inbred mice. *Pharmacogenetics* **7**, 121–130.

STEINBRINK, K., PIOR, J., VOGL, T., SORG, C. and MACHER, E. (1999) Contact tolerance. *Pathobiology* **67**, 311–313.

STEINMETZ, C.G., XIE, P., WEINER, H. and HURLEY, T.D. (1997) Structure of mitochondrial aldehyde dehydrogenase: the genetic component of ethanol aversion. *Structure* **5**, 701–711.

STEINSTRASSER, I. and MERKLE, H.P. (1995) Dermal metabolism of topically applied drugs: pathways and models reconsidered. *Pharm. Acta Helv.* **70**, 3–24.

STEINSTRASSER, I., KOOPMANN, K. and MERKLE, H.P. (1997) Epidermal aminopeptidase activity and metabolism as observed in an organised HaCaT cell sheet model. *J. Pharm. Sci.* **86**, 378–383.

STELTENKAMP, R.J., BOOMAN, K.A., DORSKY, J., KING, T.O., ROTHENSTEIN, A.S., SCHWOEPPE, E.A., SEDLAK, R.I., SMITH, T.H. and THOMPSON, G.R. (1980) Citral: A survey of consumer patch-test sensitization. *Food Cosmet. Toxicol.* **18**, 413–417.

STERN, L.J. and WILEY, D.C. (1994) Antigenic peptide binding by class I and class II histocompatibility proteins. *Structure* **2**, 245–251.

STILLMAN, S.C., EVANS, B.A. and HUGHES, I.A. (1991) Androgen dependent stimulation of aromatase activity in genital skin fibroblasts from normals and patients with androgen insensitivity. *Clin. Endocrinol.* **35**, 533–538.

STORM, J.E., COLLIER, S.W., STEWART, R.F. and BRONAUGH, R.L. (1990) Metabolism of xenobiotics during percutaneous absorption: role of absorption rate and cutaneous enzyme activity. *Fund. Appl. Toxicol.* **15**, 132–141.

STOTTS, J. and ELY, W.J. (1977) Induction of human skin sensitization to ethanol. *J. Invest. Dermatol.* **69**, 219–222.

STOUGHTON, R.B. (1969) Some bioassays for measuring percutaneous absorption. In: MONTAGNA, W. VAN-SCOTT, E.J. and STOUGHTON, R.B. (eds), *Advances in biology of the skin*, Vol. 12. New York, Hemisphere, 537.

SUGIBAYASHI, K., HAYSHI, T., HATANAKA, T., OGIHARA, M. and MORIMOTO, Y. (1996) Analysis of simultaneous transport and metabolism of ethyl nicotinate in hairless rat skin. *Pharmaceut. Res.* **13**, 855–860.

SUGIMOTO, K., SENDA, T., AOSHIMA, H., MASAI, E., FUKUDA, M. and MITSUI, Y. (1999) Crystal structure of an aromatic ring opening dioxygenase LigAB, a protocatechuate 4,5-dioxygenase, under aerobic conditions. *Structure* **7**, 953–965.

SUIT, P.F. and ESTES, M.L. (1990) Methanol intoxication: clinical features and differential diagnosis. *Cleve. Clin. J. Med.* **57**, 464–471.

SUMMER, K.H. and GOGGELMANN, W. (1980) 1-chloro-2,4-dinitrobenzene depletes glutathione in rat skin and is mutagenic in Salmonella Typhimurium. *Mutat. Res.* **77**, 91–93.

SUTTER, T.R., TANG, Y.M., HAYES, C.L., WO, Y.Y., JABS, E.W. LI, X., YIN, H., CODY, C.W. and GREENLEE, W.F. (1994) Complete cDNA sequence of a human dioxin-inducible mRNA identifies a new gene subfamily of cytochrome P450 that maps to chromosome 2. *J. Biol. Chem.* **269**, 13092–13099.

SVENSSON, S., LUNDSJO, A., CRONHOLM, T. and HOOG, J.-O. (1996) Aldehyde dismutase activity of human liver alcohol dehydrogenase. *FEBS Letts.* **394**, 217–220.

SWAIN, C.G. and SCOTT, C.B. (1953) Quantitative correlation of reaction rates. Comparison of hydroxide ion with other nucleophilic reagents towards alkyl halides, esters, epoxides and acyl halides. *J. Am. Chem. Soc.* **75**, 141–147.

TAKAHARA, H., ZAIDI, S.I., MUKHTAR, H., HANDA, M., EPSTEIN, W.L. and FUKUYAMA, K. (1993) Purification and characterisation of NADPH-cytochrome P450 reductase from rat epidermis. *J. Cell Biochem.* **53**, 206–212.

TAMMI, R., AGREN, U.M., TUHKANEN, A.L. and TAMMI, M. (1994) Hyaluronan metabolism in skin — Introduction. *Progress in Histochem. & Cytochem.* **29**, 1–81.

TAMURA, M., SUEISHI, T., SUGIBAYASHI, K., MORIMOTO, Y., JUNI, K., HASEGAWA, T. and KAWAGUCHI, T. (1996) Metabolism of testosterone and its ester derivatives in organotypic coculture of human dermal fibroblasts with differentiatied epidermis. *Int. J. Pharmaceut.* **131**, 263–271.

TANG, H.L. and CYSTER, J.G. (1999) Chemokine up-regulation and activated T cell attraction by maturing dendritic cells. *Science* **284**, 819–822.

TARVAINEN, K., JOLANKI, R. and ESTLANDER, T. (1993) Occupational contact allergy to unsaturated polyester resin cements. *Contact Dermatitis* **28**, 220–224.

TAUBER, U. and ROST, K.L. (1987) Esterase activity of the skin including species variations. In: SHROOT, B. and SCHAEFER, H. (eds), *Pharmacology and the Skin,* Vol. 1. Basel, Karger, 170–183.

THIBOUTOT, D., HARRIS, G., ILES, V., CIMIS, G., GILLILAND, K. and HAGARI, S. (1995) Activity of the type 1,5-alpha reductase exhibits regional differences in isolated sebaceous glands and whole skin. *J. Invest. Dermatol.* **105**, 209–214.

THIBOUTOT, D., MARTIN, P., VOLIKOS, L. and GILLILAND, K. (1998) Oxidative activity of the type 2 isozyme of 17beta-hydroxysteroid dehydrogenase (17beta-HSD) predominates in human sebaceous glands. *J. Invest. Dermatol.* **111**, 390–395.

THOMPSON, D.C., CONSTANTIN-TEODOSIU, D. and MOLDEUS, P. (1991) Metabolism and cytotoxicity of eugenol in isolated rat hepatocytes. *Chem. Biol. Interact.* **77**, 137.

TIKKANEN, R., ROUVINEN, J., TORRONEN, A., KALKKINEN, N. and PELTONEN, L. (1996a) Large-scale purification and preliminary x-ray diffraction studies of human aspartylglucosaminidase. *Proteins* **24**, 253–258.

TIKKANEN, R., RIIKONEN, A., OINONEN, C., ROUVINEN, R. and PELTONEN, L. (1996b) Functional analyses of active site residues of human lysosomal aspartylglucosaminidase: implications for catalytic mechanism and autocatalytic activation. *EMBO J.* **15**, 2954–2960.

TIMBRELL, J.A. (1991) 'Principles of biochemical toxicology', 2nd edition/Ed. Taylor & Francis, London.

TOFTGARD, R., HAAPARANTA, T., ENG, L. and HALPERT, J. (1986) Rat lung and liver microsomal cytochrome P450 isozymes involved in the hydroxylation of n-hexane. *Biochem. Pharmacol.* **35**, 3733–3738.

TONGE, R.P. (1995) The cutaneous deposition of the sensitising chemicals hydroxycitronellal and dinitrochlorobenzene. PhD, University of London, London.

TOREN, K., BRISMAN, J. and MEDING, B. (1997) Sensitization and exposure to methylisothiazolinones (Kathon) in the pulp and paper industry — a report of two cases. *Am. J. Ind. Med.* **31**, 551–553.

TOTH, I., SZECSI, M., JULESZ, J. and FAREDIN, I. (1997) Activity and inhibition of 3-beta-hydroxysteroid dehydrogenase delta 5,4-isomerase in human skin. *Skin Pharmacol.* **10**, 160–168.

TREFFEL, P., MURET, P., MURET-D'ANIELLO, P., COUMES-MARQUET, S. and AGACHE, P. (1992) Effect of occlusion on in vitro percutaneous absorption of two different compounds with different physicochemical properties. *Skin Pharmacol.* **5**, 108–113.

TUMA, D.J., NEWMAN, M.R., DONOHUE, T.M. and SORRELL, M.F. (1987) Covalent binding of acetaldehyde to proteins: participation of lysine residues. *Clin. Exp. Res.* **11**, 579–584.

TUR, E., MAIBACH, H.I. and GUY, R.H. (1991) Percutaneous penetration of methyl nicotinate at three anatomical sites: evidence for an appendageal contribution to transport? *Skin Pharmacol.* **4**, 230–234.

UNDERWOOD, P.M., ZHOU, Q., JAEGER, M., REILMAN, R., PINNEY, S., WARSHAWSKY, D. and TALASKA, G. (1997) Chronic, topical administration of 4-aminobiphenyl induces tissue-specific DNA adducts in mice. *Toxicol. & Appl. Pharmacol.* **144**, 325–331.

VALOTI, M., FROSINI, M., PALMI, M., DE MATTEIS, F. and SGARAGLI, G. (1998) N-dealkylation of chlorimipramine and chlorpromazine by rat liver microsomal cytochrome P450 isoenzymes. *J. Pharm. Pharmacol.* **50**, 1005–1011.

VAN BLADEREN, P.J., BREIMER, D.D., ROTTEVEEL-SMIJS, G.M.T., JONG, R.A.W., BUIJS, W., GEN, A. and MOHN, G.R. (1980) The role of glutathione conjugation in the mutagenicity of 1,2-dibromoethane. *Biochem. Pharmacol.* **29**, 2975–2982.

VAN DEN STEEN, P., RUDD, P.M., DWEK, R.A., VAN DAMME, J. and OPDENAKKER, G. (1998) Cytokine and protease glycosylation as a regulatory mechanism in inflammation and autoimmunity. *Adv. Exp. Med. Biol.* **435**, 133–143.

VAN HOOIDONK, C., CEULEN, B.I., KIENHUIS, H. and BOCK, J. (1980) Rate of skin penetration of organophosphates measured in diffusion cells. In: HOLMSTEDT, B., LAUWERYS, R., MERCIER, M. and ROBERFROID, M. (eds), *Mechanisms of Toxicity and Hazard Evaluation.* Amsterdam, Elsevier, 643–646.

VAN PELT, F.N.A.M. (1990) Cultured human keratinocytes in toxicological research. PhD, University of Utrecht.

VAN ROOIJ, J.G., DEROOS, J.H., BODELIER-BADE, M.M. and JONGENEELEN, F.J. (1993) Absorption of polycyclic aromatic hydrocarbons through human skin: differences between anatomical sites and individuals. *J. Toxicol. Environ. Health* **38**, 355–368.

VANDEN BOSSCHE, H., WILLEMSENS, G. and JANSSEN, P.A.J. (1988) Cytochrome P450-dependent metabolism of retinoic acid in rat skin microsomes: inhibition by ketoconozole. *Skin Pharmacol.* **1**, 176–185.

VANE, J.R., BAKHLE, Y.S. and BOTTING, R.M. (1998) Cyclooxygenases 1 and 2. *Annu. Rev. Pharmacol. Toxicol.* **38**, 970.

VATSIS, K.P., WEBER, W.W., BELL, D.A., DUPRET, J.-M., PRICE-EVANS, D.A., GRANT, D.M., HEIN, D.W., LIN, H.J., MEYER, U.A., RELLING, M.V., SIM, E., SUZUKI, T. and YAMAZOE, Y. (1995) Nomenclature for N-acetyltransferases. *Pharmacogenetics* **5**, 1–17.

VECCHINI, F. and MICHEL, S. (1994) Importance of cytochrome P450 for the development of new drug concepts in the skin. *Eur. J. Dermatol.* **4**, 583–588.

VECCHINI, F., MACE, K., MAGDALOU, J., MAHE, Y., BERNARD, B.A. and SHROOT, B. (1995) Constitutive and inducible expression of drug metabolising enzymes in cultured human keratinocytes. *Br. J. Dermatol.* **132**, 14–21.

VENKATESH, K., LEVI, P.E. and INMAN, A.O. (1992) Enzymatic and immunohistochemical studies on the role of cytochrome P450 and the flavin containing monooxygenase of mouse skin in metabolism of pesticides and other xenobiotics. *Pest Biochem. Physiol.* **43**, 53–66.

VERECKEN, P., BIRRINGER, C., KNITELIUS, A.C., HERBAUT, D. and GERMAUX, M.A. (1998) Sensitization to benzyl alcohol: a possible cause of 'corticosteroid allergy'. *Contact Dermatitis* **38**, 106.

VERRIER, A.C., SCHMITT, D. and STAQUET, M.J. (1999) Fragrance and contact allergens in vitro modulate the HLA-DR and E-cadherin expression on human epidermal Langerhans', cells. *Int. Arch. Allergy Immunol.* **120**, 56–62.

VICKERS, C.F.H. (1963) Existence of reservoir in the stratum corneum. *Archives of Dermatology* **88**, 20–23.

VIDMAR, D.A. and IWANE, M.K. (1999) Assessment of the ability of the topical skin protectant (TSP) to protect against contact dermatitis to urushiol (Rhus) antigen. *Am. J. Contact Dermat.* **10**, 190–197.

VOLDEN, G., VAN DEN HURK, J.J.M.A. and MIER, P.D. (1976) First demonstration of cathepsin A in epidermis. *Br. J. Dermatol.* **95**, 675–676.

von Greyerz, S., Zanni, M., Schnyder, B. and Pichler, W.J. (1998) Presentation of non-peptide antigens, in particular drugs, to specific T cells. *Clin. Exp. Allergy* **28**, 7–11.

Wallace, K.B.E. (1997) 'Free Radical Toxicology'. Taylor & Francis, London.

Walter, K. and Kurz, H. (1988) Binding of drugs to human skin: influencing factors and the role of tissue lipids. *J. Pharm. Pharmacol.* **40**, 689–693.

Wang, M., Roberts, D.L., Paschke, R., Shea, T.M., Masters, B.S.S. and Kim, J.-J.P. (1997) Three-dimensional structure of NADPH-cytochrome P450 reductase: prototype for FMN and FAD containing enzymes. *Proc. Natl. Acad. Sci.* **94**, 8411–8416.

Wang, B., Amerio, P. and Sauder, D.N. (1999) Role of cytokines in epidermal Langerhans' cell migration. *J. Leukoc. Biol.* **66**, 33–39.

Wani, G. and D'Ambrosio, S.M. (1995) Differential expression of the O6=alkylguanine-DNA alkyltransferase gene in normal human breast and skin tissue: in situ mapping of cell type-specific expression. *Mol. Carcinog.* **12**, 177–184.

Warbrick, E.V., Dearman, R.J., Lea, L.J., Basketter, D.A. and Kimber, I. (1999) Local lymph node assay responses to paraphenylenediamine: intra- and inter-laboratory evaluations. *J. Appl. Toxicol.* **19**, 255–260.

Weibel, H. and Hansen, J. (1989a) Penetration of the fragrance compounds, cinnamaldehyde and cinnamyl alcohol, through human skin *in vitro*. *Contact Dermatitis* **20**, 167–172.

Weibel, H. and Hansen, J. (1989b) Interaction of cinnamaldehyde (a sensitiser in fragrance) with protein. *Contact Dermatitis* **20**, 161–166.

Weibel, H., Hansen, J. and Andersen, K.E. (1989) Cross-sensitisation patterns in guinea-pigs between cinnamaldehyde, cinnamyl alcohol and cinnamic acid. *Acta Derm. Venereol.* **69**, 302–307.

Weigand, D.A., Haygood, C., Gaylor, J.R. and Anglin, J.J.H. (1980) Racial variation in the cutaneous barrier. In: Drill, V.A. and Lazar, P. (eds), *Current concepts in cutaneous toxicity*. New York, Academic Press, 221.

Weigmann, H., Lademann, J., Meffert, H., Schaefer, H. and Sterry, W. (1999) Determination of the horny layer profile by tape stripping in combination with optical spectroscopy in the visible range as a prerequisite to quantify percutaneous absorption. *Skin Pharmacol. Appl. Skin Physiol.* **12**, 34–45.

Weiner, H. and Flynn, T.G. (1989) Nomenclature of mammalian aldehyde dehydrogenases. In: 'Enzymology and molecular biology of carbonyl metabolism', Alan Liss, New York, xix–xxi.

Weinshilboum, R. (1988) Pharmacogenetics of methylation: relationship to drug metabolism. *Clin. Biochem.* **21**, 201–210.

WEINSHILBOUM, R. (1989) Methyltransferase pharmacogenetics. *Pharmacol. Ther.* **43**, 77–90.

WEINSHILBOUM, R.M. (1992) Methylation pharmacogenetics: thiopurine methyltransferase as a model system. *Xenobiotica* **22**, 1055–1071.

WEINSHILBOUM, R. and AKSOY, I. (1994) Sulfation pharmacogenetics in humans. *Chem. Biol. Interact.* **92**, 233–246.

WEINSHILBOUM, R.M., OTTERNESS, D.M., AKSOY, I.A., WOOD, T.C., HER, C. and RAFTOGIANIS, R.B. (1997) Sulfation and solfotransferases 1: sulfotransferase molecular biology: cDNAs and genes. *FASEB J.* **11**, 3–14.

WEINSTEIN, G.D., FROST, P. and HSIA, S.L. (1968) In vitro interconversion of estrone and 17-beta estradiol in human skin and vaginal mucosa. *J. Invest. Dermatol.* **51**, 4–10.

WEPIERRE, J. and MARTY, J.P. (1979) Percutaneous absorption of drugs. *Trends in Pharmacological Sciences*. Inaugural Issue, 23–26.

WERTZ, P.W., SWARTZENDRUBER, D.C., MADISON, K.C. and DOWNING, D.T. (1987) Composition and morphology of epidermal cyst lipids. *J. Invest. Dermatol.* **89**, 419–425.

WESTER, R.C. and NOONAN, P.K. (1980) Relevance of animal models for percutaneous absorption. *Int. J. Pharmacy* **7**, 99–110.

WESTER, R.C., MAIBACH, H.I., BUCKS, D.A.W. and AUFRERE, M.B. (1984) In vivo percutaneous absorption of paraquat from hand, leg, and forearm of humans. *J. Toxicol. Envir. Health* **14**, 759–762.

WESTER, R.C. and MAIBACH, H.I. (1985) In vivo percutaneous absorption and decontamination of pesticides in humans. *J. Toxicol. Environ. Health* **16**, 25–37.

WHELAND, G.W. and PAULING, L. (1935) A quantum mechanical discussion of orientation of substituents in aromatic molecules. *J. Am. Chem. Soc.* **57**, 2086–2095.

WIEBEL, F.J., LEUTZ, B.S. and GELBOIN, H.V. (1975) Aryl hydrocarbon (benzo(a)pyrene) hydroxylase: a mixed function oxidase in mouse skin. *J. Invest. Dermatol.* **64**, 184–189.

WILKES, G.L., BROWN, I.A. and WILDNAUER, R.H. (1973) The biomechanical properties of skin. *CRC Critical Reviews in Bioengineering* **1**, 453–495.

WILKIN, J.K. and STEWART, J.H. (1987) Substrate specificity of human cutaneous alcohol dehydrogenase and erythema provoked by lower aliphatic alcohols. *J. Invest. Dermatology* **88**, 452–454.

WILLIAMS, D. and WOODHOUSE, K. (1995) The relationship between age and cutaneous aryl hydrocarbon hydroxylase (AHH) activity. *Age Ageing* **24**, 213–216.

WILSON, D.R. and MAIBACH, H.I. (1982) An in vivo comparison of barrier function. In: MAIBACH, H.I. and BOISITS, E.K. (eds), *Neonatal skin. Structure and functions*. New York, Marcel Dekker, 101–110.

WOLKENSTEIN, P., TAN, C., LECOEUR, S., WECHSLER, J., GARCIA-MARTIN, N., CHARUE, D., BAGOT, M. and BEAUNE, P. (1998) Covalent binding of carbamazepine reactive metabolites to P450 isoforms present in the skin. *Chem. Biol. Interact.* **113**, 39–50.

WONG, C.Y., GUU, Y.B., WANG, M.T. and WANG, D.P. (1999) Percutaneous transport of diclofenac sodium from mixtures of fatty alcohol (or fatty acid) and propylene glycol through the rabbit abdominal skin. *Drug Dev. Ind. Pharm.* **25**, 1209–1213.

WONG, K.O., TAN, A.Y., LIM, B.G. and WONG, K.P. (1993) Sulphate conjugation of minoxidil in rat skin. *Biochem. Pharmacol.* **45**, 1180–1182.

WOUTERS, J. and BAUDOUX, G. (1998) First partial three-dimensional model of human monoamine oxidase A. *Proteins* **32**, 97–110.

WOUTERS, J. (1998) Structural aspects of monoamine oxidase and its reversible inhibition. *Curr. Med. Chem.* **5**, 137–162.

XIE, P., PARSONS, S.H., SPECKHARD, D.C., BOSRON, W.F. and HURLEY, T.D. (1997) X-ray structure of human class IV $\sigma\sigma$ alcohol dehydrogenase. *J. Biol. Chem.* **272**, 18558–18563.

XU, H., BANERJEE, A., DILULIO, N.A. and FAIRCHILD, R.L. (1997) Development of effector CD8+ T cells in contact hypersensitivity occurs independently of CD4+ T cells. *J. Immunol.* **158**, 4721–4728.

YAMADA, H., SHIIYAMA, S., SOEJIMA-OHKUMA, T., HONDA, S., KUMAGAI, Y., CHO, A.K., OGURI, K. and YOSHIMURA, H. (1997) Deamination of amphetamines by cytochromes P450: studies on substrate specificity and regioselectivity with microsomes and purified CYP2C subfamily isozymes. *J. Toxicol. Sci.* **22**, 65–73.

YAMADA, K. and TOJO, K. (1997) Bioconversion of estradiol esters in the skin of various animal models in vitro. *Eur. J. Pharm. Biopharmaceut.* **43**, 253–258.

YANG, Z.-N., BOSRON, W.F. and HURLEY, T.D. (1997) Structure of human $\chi\chi$ alcohol dehydrogenase: a glutathione dependent formaldehyde dehydrogenase. *J. Mol. Biol.* **265**, 330–343.

YANG, T.J., SHOU, M., KORZEKWA, K.R., GONZALEZ, F.J., GELBOIN, H.V. and YANG, S.K. (1998) Role of cDNA-expressed human cytochromes P450 in the metabolism of diazepam. *Biochem. Pharmacol.* **55**, 889–896.

YANG, M., KOGA, M., KATOH, T. and KAWAMOTO, T. (1999a) A study for the proper application of urinary naphthols, new biomarkers for airborne polycyclic aromatic hydrocarbons. *Arch. Environ. Contam. Toxicol.* **36**, 99–108.

YANG, Z., BIRKENHAUER, P., JULMY, F., CHICKERING, D., RANIERI, J.P., MERKLE, H.P., LUSCHER, T.F. and GANDER, B. (1999b) Sustained release of heparin from polymeric particles for inhibition of human vascular smooth muscle cell proliferation. *J. Control. Rel.* **60**, 269–277.

YAWALKER, N., EGLI, F., BRAND, C.U., PICHLER, W.J. and BRAATHEN, L.R. (2000) Antigen-presenting cells and keratinocytes express interleukin-12 in allergic contact dermatitis. *Contact Dermatitis* **42**, 18–22.

YOKOYAMA, H., MORIYA, S., SUZUKI, H., NAGATA, S. and ISHII, H. (1996) Establishment of a specific antibody (Ab) against human class IV (σ) alcohol dehydrogenase (ADH) and its distribution in the human gastric mucosa. *Gastroenterology* **110**, A1366.

YOKOZEKI, H., KATAYAMA, I. and NISHIOKA, K. (1995) Experimental study for the development of an in vitro test for contact allergens. 1. Primary activation of hapten-specific T cells by hapten conjugated epidermal cells. *Int. Arch. Allergy Immunol.* **106**, 394–400.

YOSHIDA, A., RZHETSKY, A., HSU, L.C. and CHANG, C. (1998) Human aldehyde dehydrogenase gene family. *Eur. J. Biochem.* **251**, 549–557.

YOURICK, J.J. and BRONAUGH, R.L. (1997) Percutaneous absorption and metabolism of coumarin in human and rat skin. *J. Appl. Toxicol.* **17**, 153–158.

YOURICK, J.J. and BRONAUGH, R.L. (2000) Percutaneous penetration and metabolism of 2-nitro-p-phenylenediamine in human and fuzzy rat skin. *Toxicol. Appl. Pharmacol.* **166**, 13–23.

ZANNI, M.P., VON GREYERZ, S., SCHNYDER, B., BRANDER, K.A., FRUTIG, K., HARI, Y., VALITUTTI, S. and PICHLER, W.J. (1998) HLA-restricted, processing- and metabolism-independent pathway of drug recognition by human alphabeta T lymphocytes. *J. Clin. Invest.* **102**, 1591–1598.

ZARUTSKIE, J.A., SATO, A.K., RUSHE, M.M., CHAN, I.C., LOMAKIN, A., BENEDEK, G.B. and STERN, L.J. (1999) A conformational change in the human major histocompatibility complex protein HLA-DR1 induced by peptide binding. *Biochemistry* **38**, 5878–5887.

ZATZ, J. (1984) Skin structure. In: BALL, S.V.F. and BALL, L.A. (eds), *Controlled Drug Bioavailability*, Vol. 3. New York, Wiley, 190–193.

ZBAIDA, S. (1995) The mechanism of microsomal azoreduction: predictions based on electronic aspects of structure-activity relationships. *Drug Metab. Rev.* **27**, 497–516.

ZGOMBIC-KNIGHT, M., FOGLIO, M.H. and DUESTER, G. (1995) Genomic structure and expression of the ADH7 gene encoding human class IV alcohol dehydrogenase, the form most efficient for retinol metabolism in vitro. *J. Biol. Chem.* **270**, 4305–4311.

ZHANG, Z.Y. (1998) Protein-tyrosine phosphatases: biological functions, structural characteristics, and mechanisms of catalysis. *Crit. Rev. Biochem. Mol. Biol.* **33**, 1–52.

ZHAO, K. and SINGH, J. (1999) In vitro percutaneous absorption enhancement of propranolol hydrochloride through porcine epidermis by terpenes/ethanol. *J. Control. Rel.* **62**, 359–366.

ZHAO, K. and SINGH, J. (2000) Mechanism(s) of in vitro percutaneous absorption enhancement of tamoxifen by enhancers. *J. Pharm. Sci.* **89**, 771–780.

ZHOU, X.H. and LI WAN PO, A. (1990) Comparison of enzymic activities of tissues lining portals of drug absorption, using the rat as a model. *Int. J. Pharm.* **62**, 259–267.

ZIEGLER, D.M. (1990) Flavin-containing monooxygenases: enzymes adapted for multisubstrate specificity. *Trends Pharmacol. Sci.* **11**(8), 321–324.

Index